999

LITTLE-KNOWN
Natural Healing
Foods
and

Proven Home
Remedies

By the Editors of FC&A

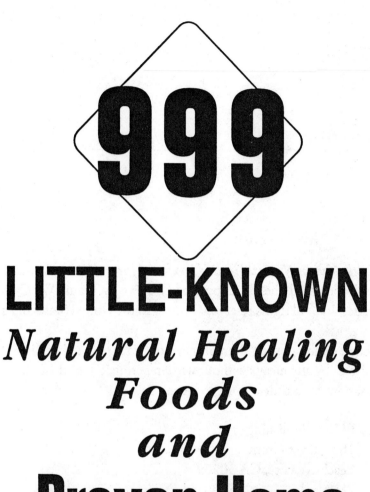

999

LITTLE-KNOWN
Natural Healing
Foods
and
Proven Home
Remedies

By the Editors of FC&A

FC&A Publishing
103 Clover Green
Peachtree City, GA 30269

Publisher: FC&A Publishing
Editors: Editorial Staff of FC&A
Production: Carol Parrott
Cover design: Diane Dunn
Printed and bound by Banta Company

First printing March 1994

ISBN 0-915099-59-4

Table of Contents

Do not be anxious about anything, but in everything, by prayer and petition, with thanksgiving, present your requests to God. And the peace of God, which transcends all understanding, will guard your hearts and your minds in Christ Jesus.

Philippians 4:6–7

But I will restore you to health and heal your wounds, declares the Lord.

Jeremiah 30:17a

Notice:

This book is for information only. It does not constitute medical advice and should not be construed as such. We cannot guarantee the safety or effectiveness of any drug, treatment or advice mentioned. Some of these tips may not be effective for everyone.

A good physician is the best judge of what medical treatment may be needed for certain conditions and diseases. We recommend in all cases that you contact your personal physician or health care provider before taking or discontinuing any medications, or before treating yourself in any way.

INTRODUCTION

Who is the most important person in your life when it comes to your health? It's not your doctor. It's you.

As the editors of *999 Little-Known Natural Healing Foods and Proven Home Remedies*, we know that you're the one in control of your body.

A healthy body is an awesome responsibility. And it's not made any easier by the fact that new medical studies are spouting out of scientific laboratories by the thousands. Medical knowledge, even concerning which foods work best to keep you healthy, is growing by leaps and bounds and changing every day.

That's where we come in. In *999 Little-Known Natural Healing Foods and Proven Home Remedies*, you'll learn all about healthy, disease-fighting foods, plus how to stay fit and trim, how the world around you affects your health, what to do when your children are sick, and how your mind can play tricks on your body. You'll even learn how to talk to your doctor about health problems and prescribed medications.

To get the latest health information to you, we searched through the top medical journals for the most significant news you can use to prevent diseases and to treat common ailments at home.

We give you recent nutrition breakthroughs and solid home remedies in a no-frills format that won't burden you with useless details.

Our book will help you make the choices and decisions that determine both how long you will live and the quality of your days. Will you suffer with allergies every day of your life? Will heart disease take you before your time?

Your health is more in your control than you think. Did you know that scientists believe that 80 percent of all cancers can be prevented by making changes in your lifestyle: quitting smoking, limiting your exposure to the sun, and, perhaps most important, eating a healthy, low-fat diet rich in vegetables, fruits and whole grains?

Since your health, and your family's, is in your hands, it's only appropriate that our book, one of the most intelligent choices you can make for your health, is in your hands as well.

Keeping your body healthy

Nutrition
Weight control
Exercise and fitness
Health risks

NUTRITION

Nutrition guidelines

The Four Basic Food Groups — It's a concept most Americans have heard since elementary school. And many health-conscious mothers and fathers try diligently to provide daily servings from those four famous food groups to keep their families healthy.

But did you know these groups have changed?

The four equal food groups have been rearranged to form the new Food Guide Pyramid. These new food guidelines emphasize a low-fat diet that includes a variety of foods.

Following the Pyramid's guidelines will help you maintain a healthy weight and reduce your risk of high blood pressure, heart disease, diabetes and osteoporosis.

Recently, interest in Americans' eating habits shifted from a focus on dietary deficiencies, such as not getting enough vitamins and minerals, to a growing concern about how much fat, sugar and salt we're eating.

To help people make more healthy food choices, the United States Department of Agriculture and the Department of Health and Human Services developed the Food Guide Pyramid. It shows you how to create healthy meals from the ground up.

Use the grains group (bread, cereal, rice and pasta) as a base; build up with fruits and vegetables, then add meat and vegetables; top it all off with fat, oils and sweets (used sparingly, of course).

Instead of the Four Basic Food Groups, the new Pyramid divides food into six different groups, listed below. We'll start at the top of the Pyramid and work our way down.

The new food pyramid

☐ Fats, oils and sweets. This group includes salad dressings, oils, cream, butter, margarine, sugars, soft drinks, candies and sweet desserts. The foods in this group provide lots of calories and/or fat, but have little nutritional value. Use foods in this category sparingly.

☐ Milk, yogurt and cheese group. Eat two to three servings from this group each day. Teens, young adults up to age 24 and women who are pregnant or breast-feeding need three servings.

☐ Meat, poultry, fish, dry beans, eggs and nuts. Eat only two to three servings from this group daily. Total servings should equal five to seven ounces. These foods are especially important for providing dietary protein, calcium, iron and zinc.

☐ Vegetables. Eat three to five servings each day.

☐ Fruits. Eat two to four servings of fruit every day. Most people need to eat more fruits and vegetables than they do now. An apple a day will no longer do the trick. It appears that you'll need at least five (three vegetables and two fruits) a day to keep the doctor away.

☐ Bread, cereal, rice and pasta. Eat six to 11 servings daily.

No one food group is more important than another. You need food from all the different groups for maximum health. You should eat at least the minimum number of servings from each group.

The actual number of servings you need from each group depends on how many calories you use each day.

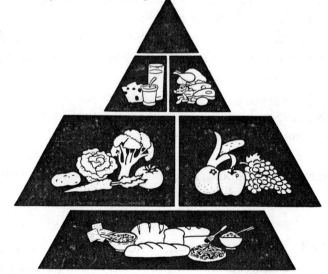

Counting calories

How many calories you need every day depends on your age, sex, size and level of physical activity.

Obviously, larger, more active men need more food than smaller, less active women.

The National Academy of Sciences created the following guidelines to help you determine your daily caloric needs:

Adults and Teens:

— 1,600 calories per day is the average number necessary for most inactive women and older adults.

— 2,200 calories per day is what most children, teenage girls, active women and inactive men need from their diets. Women who are pregnant or breast-feeding probably need more.

— 2,800 calories per day is about the right number for teen-age boys, active men and very active women.

Young Children

Young children need fewer calories per day than older children do, but they still need the same variety of foods.

Most preschool children need fewer than 1,600 calories per day, which means smaller servings, not fewer food groups. All children need at least two cups of milk every day.

If you're having trouble deciding what activity level you fit into, here are some general guidelines: An inactive person rarely or never exercises; a moderately active person exercises at least 20 minutes two or three times a week; an active person exercises four to five times a week; an extremely active person exercises six to seven times a week.

After establishing a calorie range, it is important to determine how many servings of food from each food group will provide the approximate number of calories you need each day.

The following chart of daily calorie needs and numbers of servings per day will help you figure it out:

Number of servings for	1,600 calories	2,200 calories	2,800 calories
Bread group servings	6	9	11
Vegetable servings	3	4	5
Fruit servings	2	3	4
Milk group servings	2-3	2-3	2-3
Meat group servings	2, for a total of 5 ounces	2, for a total of 6 ounces	3, for a total of 7 ounces

Many people who try to follow the Pyramid guidelines think that eating the recommended number of servings per day would mean tons of extra food. However, "serving sizes" are smaller than most people think.

Listed below are some examples of typical "serving sizes" in each of the different food groups.

- ☐ Bread, cereal, rice and pasta group: one serving equals one slice of bread, one ounce of ready-to-eat cereal or one-half cup of cooked rice, cereal or pasta.

- ☐ Fruit group: one serving equals one medium apple or banana, one-half cup of chopped, cooked or canned fruit or three-fourths cup of fruit juice.

- ☐ Vegetable group: one serving equals one cup of raw leafy vegetables, one-half cup of other types of raw or cooked vegetables or three-fourths cup of vegetable juice.

- ☐ Milk, yogurt and cheese group: one serving equals one cup of milk or yogurt, 1 1/2 ounces of natural cheese or two ounces of processed cheese.

- ☐ Meat, poultry, fish, dry beans, eggs and nuts group: one serving equals two to three ounces of cooked lean meat, poultry or fish,

1 1/2 cups of cooked dry beans, 3 eggs or six tablespoons of peanut butter.

The number of recommended servings you should eat from each food group may seem overwhelming, especially the six to 11 servings of bread, cereal, rice or pasta.

However, servings add up quicker than you might think. Consider your meals and snacks for a typical day. For breakfast, you have a small bowl of cereal and one slice of toast. That's two servings already.

For lunch, you have a sandwich. You've quickly moved up to four servings. Your afternoon snack of three or four small crackers quickly ups your daily grains total to five.

A half cup of rice or pasta at dinner brings your total up to the recommended six servings.

Although serving sizes are based on actual measurements of food amounts, you don't need to measure food at every meal. Serving sizes simply provide guidelines to help you estimate how much food you should eat without gaining or losing weight.

However, if you are interested in losing weight, exercise regularly and cut back on fats and sugars. Continue to eat the recommended number of servings from each food group.

Otherwise, you may not get all the nutrients you need to keep your body strong and healthy.

Medical Sources ————————————————

The Food Guide Pyramid, United States Department of Agriculture
Controlling Your Fat Tooth, Workman Publishing Co. Inc., New York, 1991

Fighting fat

Losing weight also means cutting excess fat from the diet. The American Heart Association recommends that people limit fat in their diets to 30 percent of the calories.

This amounts to about 53 grams of fat in a 1,600-calorie diet, 73 grams of fat in a 2,200-calorie diet, and 93 grams of fat in a 2,800-calorie diet.

To determine how much fat will make up 30 percent of your diet, simply multiply your total day's calories by .30, then divide that number by 9 (each gram of fat has 9 calories).

Your final figure is the number of grams of fat you can include in your diet each day.

For example: 1,600 calories x .30 = 480 (calories from fat)
Then, 480 / 9 = 53 grams of fat per day.

Here are some guidelines on how to determine how much fat you eat:

Step 1)   Jot down everything you ate yesterday for meals and snacks.
Step 2)   Write down the number of grams of fat in each food you list. Use nutrition labels on packaged foods or the chart below to find out how many grams of fat each food contained.
Step 3)   Add up your grams of fat. Did you have more fat than you should?

If your diet contains more than 30 percent of the calories from fat, you need to cut back on your fat intake to lower your risk of heart disease and other chronic diseases.

Food groups   Grams of fat

Bread, cereal, rice and pasta group

Bread, one slice	1
Hamburger roll, bagel or English muffin	2
Tortilla (one)	3
Rice, pasta, cooked (1/2 cup)	trace
Plain crackers, small (three to four)	3
Pancakes, 4" diameter (two)	3
Croissant, one large (2 ounces)	12
Doughnut, one medium (2 ounces)	11
Danish, one medium (2 ounces)	13
Cake, frosted (1/16, average)	13
Cookies, two medium	4
Fruit pie with top crust (1/6 of 8" pie)	19

Food groups	Grams of fat
Vegetable group	
Vegetables, cooked (1/2 cup)	trace
Vegetables, leafy, raw (1 cup)	trace
Vegetables, nonleafy, raw (1/2 cup)	trace
Potatoes, scalloped (1/2 cup)	4
Potato salad (1/2 cup)	8
French fries (approximately 10)	8
Fruit group	
Whole fruit (medium apple, banana)	trace
Fruit, raw or canned (1/2 cup)	trace
Fruit juice, unsweetened (3/4 cup)	trace
Avocado (1/4 whole)	9
Milk, yogurt and cheese group	
Skim milk (1 cup)	trace
Nonfat yogurt, plain (8 ounces)	trace
Low-fat milk, 2 percent (1 cup)	5
Whole milk (1 cup)	8
Chocolate milk, 2 percent (1 cup)	5
Low-fat yogurt, plain (8 ounces)	4
Low-fat yogurt, fruit (8 ounces)	3
Natural cheddar cheese (1-1/2 ounces)	14
Processed cheese (2 ounces)	18
Mozzarella, part skim (1-1/2 ounces)	7
Ricotta, part skim (1/2 cup)	10
Cottage cheese, 4 percent fat (1/2 cup)	5
Ice cream (1/2 cup)	7
Ice milk (1/2 cup)	3
Frozen yogurt (1/2 cup)	2
Meat, poultry, fish, dry beans, eggs and nuts group	
Lean meat, poultry, fish, cooked	6
Ground beef, lean, cooked	16
Chicken, with skin, fried	13

Food groups	Grams of fat
Meat, poultry, fish, dry beans, eggs and nuts group	
Bologna (two slices)	16
Egg (one)	5
Dry beans and peas, cooked (1/2 cup)	trace
Peanut butter (2 tablespoons)	16
Nuts (1/3 cup)	22
Fats, oils and sweets group	
Butter, margarine (1 teaspoon)	4
Mayonnaise (1 tablespoon)	11
Salad dressing (1 tablespoon)	7
Sour cream (2 tablespoons)	6
Cream cheese (1 ounce)	10
Sugar, jam, jelly (1 tablespoon)	0
Cola (12 fluid ounces)	0
Fruit drink (12 fluid ounces)	0
Chocolate bar (1 ounce)	9
Sherbet (1/2 cup)	2
Fruit sorbet (1/2 cup)	0
Gelatin dessert (1/2 cup)	0

Medical Source ————————————————————
The Food Guide Pyramid, United States Department of Agriculture

Good fat, bad fat

By now we've all heard the warnings that eating too much fat can be hazardous to your health. Just sitting down to eat a bowl of ice cream can make us feel so guilty that we can't even enjoy it.

The truth is, your body actually needs a certain amount of fat for energy and also for cell growth and repair.

You can include a reasonable amount of fat in your diet. You just need to choose your fats carefully and limit your percentage of calories that come from fat.

In general, Americans eat too much fat. Our fat consumption is one reason we have a higher rate of cardiovascular disease and some forms of cancer than other countries where people eat less fat.

You know that fats should make up 30 percent or less of your diet. But the kind of fat you eat is equally important. Fats are made up of a combination of fatty acids; saturated, polyunsaturated and monounsaturated fats (including olive and canola oils).

Polyunsaturated and monounsaturated fats lower levels of LDL (the bad cholesterol), and monounsaturated fats like olive oil even raise HDL cholesterol levels (the good kind).

A diet that contains a balance of polyunsaturated and monounsaturated fats and limits the amount of calories to less than 30 percent of your total daily caloric intake appears to be the best way to reduce your risk of fat-related diseases.

Medical Source ———————————————
The American Journal of Clinical Nutrition (56,1:77)

Artificial sweeteners: A bitter disappointment or a safe alternative?

Many sugar substitutes are being developed in laboratories these days and used in products such as foods, soft drinks, mouthwashes and pill coatings. They give you the sweet taste without the calories.

Aspartame and saccharin by any other name would taste as sweet ... but would they be as safe as good old sugar or honey?

Known by their brand names of Sweet 'n Low, NutraSweet and Equal, saccharin and aspartame now sweeten over 4,500 products used by more than 200 million people around the world. Yet some still question their safety.

Some doubters have a "sour" taste in their mouths concerning artificial sweeteners — believing that they can cause unpleasant side effects like headaches, memory loss, dizziness and even seizures.

While most people don't experience any adverse side effects, you should still try to use artificial sweeteners in moderation, advises dietician Nancy Clark, director of Nutrition Services at SportsMedicine Brookline in Boston.

She explains, "As with any food, moderation is always best. Artificial sweeteners will never be proved 100 percent safe, but then neither will any food or ingredient."

Saccharin is the granddaddy of the artificial sweeteners — it's 300 times as sweet as sugar. According to Clark, you'd have to consume more Sweet 'n Low every day than the amount contained in 850 cans of diet soda to be in danger from saccharin.

The newest generation of artificial sweeteners is aspartame (NutraSweet or Equal), and it's about 200 times as sweet as sugar. Aspartame appears to be safe unless you consume more than the amount contained in 20 cans of diet soda on a daily basis, according to the report.

However, the following people probably need to stay away from aspartame and saccharin:

- ❐ People who develop allergic reactions to these products (or to strawberries and peanuts).
- ❐ People, especially children, who are born with an inherited condition known as phenylketonuria (PKU), which is when the body fails to oxidize the amino acid phenylalanine because of a defective enzyme).

Now, what about using artificial sweeteners to help you lose weight? The bitter truth is, people gain weight because they eat too much fat, not because they eat too much sugar.

To slim down, you probably need to exercise more and eat fewer fatty foods. That means a diet drink won't help if you're eating burgers and fries with it.

Filling up on diet drinks when you're feeling hungry won't help either, says Clark. Surprisingly, most people who use artificial sweeteners don't actually reduce their calorie intake. It could be that the tongue is satisfied with the sweeteners, but the body still craves sweets and fats. When you're hungry, only foods that contain calories will raise your blood sugar back to normal.

Athletes should drink fruit juice or a sugar-sweetened drink instead of a diet soft drink after exercise. The carbohydrates will help refuel those tired muscles.

The best news about artificial sweeteners is that they don't cause tooth decay. In some cases, they even help prevent it.

Medical Source ────────────────────────
The Physician and Sportsmedicine (21,2:45)

Sweet news for sugar lovers

Do you love sweets? It's only natural. Humans are born preferring sweet over sour or bitter tastes.

Despite their popularity, sweeteners, especially table sugar, receive their share of bad publicity. Sugar has been accused of causing numerous health problems, including heart disease, diabetes, anxiety, fatigue, depression, hyperactivity and even criminal behavior.

The truth is that sugar, eaten in moderate amounts in addition to a varied diet, cannot be linked to any health problems, other than tooth decay.

In fact, even obesity can't be blamed on sugar. Thin people tend to eat more sugar than overweight people. The problem with sugar is that it's usually connected with fat. It's usually the fat in "sweets" that we are attracted to, and fat causes all kinds of health problems.

Sugar also has no nutritional value, only calories. If eating sugary foods keeps you from eating nutritious foods, you aren't getting a healthy diet.

An average "healthy" amount of sugar in a diet should be limited to six teaspoons per day on a 1,600-calorie diet, 12 teaspoons per day on a 2,200-calorie diet and 18 teaspoons of sugar per day on a 2,800-calorie diet.

These numbers represent sugars added to foods during processing or at the table, not the sugars found naturally in fruits and milk. It's the added sugars that provide calories with few vitamins and minerals.

Most of the added sugars in the typical American diet come from foods in the Pyramid tip — soft drinks, candy, jams, jellies, syrups and table sugar we add to foods like coffee or cereal.

Added sugars in the food groups come from foods such as ice cream, sweetened yogurt, chocolate milk, canned or frozen fruit with heavy syrup, and sweetened bakery products like cakes and cookies.

The following chart shows you the amounts of added sugars in some popular foods. You may be surprised!

Food groups	Amount of added sugar (teaspoons)
Bread, cereal, rice and pasta group	
Bread, one slice	0
Muffin, one medium	1
Cookies, two medium	1
Danish pastry, one medium	1
Doughnut, one medium	2
Pound cake, no-fat, 1 ounce	2
Angel food cake, 1/12 tube cake	5
Cake, frosted, 1/16 average	6
Fruit pie with two crusts, 1/6 pie	6
Fruit group	
Fruit, canned in juice, 1/2 cup	0
Fruit, canned in light syrup, 1/2 cup	2
Fruit, canned in heavy syrup, 1/2 cup	4
Milk, yogurt and cheese group	
Chocolate milk, 2 percent, 1 cup	3
Low-fat yogurt, flavored, 8 ounces	5
Low-fat yogurt, fruit, 8 ounces	7
Ice cream or frozen yogurt, 1/2 cup	3
Chocolate shake, 10 fluid ounces	9
Other	
Sugar, jam or jelly, 1 teaspoon	1
Syrup or honey, 1 tablespoon	3
Chocolate bar, 1 ounce	3
Gelatin dessert, 1/2 cup	4
Sherbet, 1/2 cup	5
Cola, 12 fluid ounces	9
Fruit drink, 12 fluid ounces	12

Medical Sources ——————————————————

FDA Report of Sugars Task Force
The Food Guide Pyramid, United States Department of Agriculture

Salting away heart disease

If you're salt sensitive, eating foods high in salt could cause you to have high blood pressure, and, as a result, heart disease.

Researchers have recently discovered that older people and people who are pear-shaped benefit the most from reducing their salt intake. (Pear-shaped means that you carry most of your extra weight around your hips and thighs rather than your stomach.)

Many nutritional experts agree that the average diet shouldn't contain more than 3,000 milligrams (about one and a half teaspoons) of salt every day.

The following chart shows how much salt some popular foods from the different food groups contain:

Food groups	Quantity	Sodium (milligrams)
Bread, cereal, rice and pasta group		
Cooked cereal, rice, pasta, unsalted	1/2 cup	trace
Ready-to-eat cereal	1 ounce	100-360
Bread	1 slice	110-175
Vegetable group		
Vegetables, cooked without salt	1/2 cup	less than 70
Vegetables, canned, with sauce	1/2 cup	140-460
Tomato juice, canned	3/4 cup	660
Vegetable soup	1 cup	820
Fruit group		
Fruit, fresh, frozen or canned	1/2 cup	trace
Milk, yogurt and cheese group		
Milk	1 cup	120
Yogurt	8 ounces	160
Natural cheeses	1-1/2 ounces	110-450
Processed cheeses	2 ounces	800

Food groups	Quantity	Sodium (milligrams)
Meat, poultry, fish, dry beans, eggs and nuts group		
Fresh meat, poultry, fish	3 ounces	less than 90
Tuna, canned, water pack	3 ounces	300
Bologna	2 ounces	580
Ham, lean, roasted	3 ounces	1,020
Other		
Salad dressing	1 tablespoon	75-220
Ketchup, mustard, steak sauce	1 tablespoon	130-230
Soy sauce	1 tablespoon	1,030
Salt	1 teaspoon	2,000
Dill pickle	1 medium	930
Potato chips, salted	1 ounce	130
Peanuts, roasted in oil, salted	1 ounce	120

Other high-salt products include many canned vegetables, meats and soups; sliced sandwich meats; some ready-to-eat cereals; boxed macaroni and cheese; olives; meat tenderizer; and most fast foods.

Here are a few tips to help you cut down on your salt intake:

- ❏ Learn which food have a high-salt content. When checking ingredient listings, be on the lookout for the words salt, soda and sodium. Try to buy low-salt or salt-free products.
- ❏ Eat fewer salty foods or cut them out of your diet completely.
- ❏ Don't add extra salt at the table.
- ❏ Try using half the amount of salt a recipe recommends.
- ❏ Don't add salt to pasta or other starchy foods that will be topped with other foods. The toppings usually add enough flavor so that you don't even notice the missing salt.
- ❏ Balance your salt intake. If your breakfast is high in salt, eat low-salt meals for the rest of the day.

Medical Source ————————————————
The Food Guide Pyramid, United States Department of Agriculture

The road to better health

Armed with the latest information on food groups, serving sizes, calories, fat, sugar and salt, you're ready to start your journey to better health. Using the Pyramid's guidelines, decide what changes you can make for a healthier diet.

Make small changes at first, like switching from whole to 1 percent milk. Add bigger changes gradually to help make the transition to a new way of eating easier for you and your family.

The USDA's Human Nutrition Information Service offers additional information on healthy eating habits. For more information, write:

U.S. Department of Agriculture
Human Nutrition Information Service
6505 Belcrest Road
Hyattsville, MD 20782

You can also contact your local county extension office, public health nutritionist or dietician (at the local health department or hospital) for more information on improving your family's diet.

Medical Source —————————————————————
The Food Guide Pyramid, United States Department of Agriculture

Get your fill of fiber

Fiber — it's what we used to call "roughage."

By now, we all know that adding roughage to our diets each day can help keep us healthy.

Numerous studies have shown that a diet high in fats can increase your risk of colorectal cancer and that a diet high in fiber actually helps lower your risk. However, current studies show that most people aren't eating nearly enough fiber.

But exactly how much should you eat to lower your risk of developing colon cancer? Researchers recommend eating 39 grams of fiber each day. That probably seems like a lot, but consider the benefits: You may be able to reduce your risk of colorectal cancer by one-third.

If everyone ate more fiber, researchers estimate that as many as 50,000 fewer cases of colon cancer would be diagnosed in the United States every year.

However, the average person only eats about 23 grams of fiber a day.

But, what do you need to eat to make sure you get your daily 39 grams? The National Cancer Institute recommends five or more servings of a combination of fruits and vegetables, especially citrus fruits and green and yellow vegetables.

Also, increase your intake of starches and other complex carbohydrates (beans, peas, lentils, breads, rice and cereals) by eating six or more servings each day.

Complex carbohydrates are excellent sources of fiber and energy without providing extra, unwanted calories. (Carbohydrates have only four calories per gram; fat has nine calories per gram).

An average serving is approximately a half cup for most cooked or fresh vegetables, fruits, dry or cooked cereals and legumes (kidney beans, lentils, etc.), or one medium-sized piece of fruit, a slice of bread, a roll or muffin.

Medical Sources ————————————————————
Journal of the National Cancer Institute (84,24:1887)
Diet and Health, National Academy Press, Washington, D.C., 1989

Fiber facts

Fiber is the part of plants that your body can't digest because enzymes in the intestinal tract won't break it down. But, that's what makes it beneficial to you.

Dietary fiber helps move waste quicker through the intestines. This helps reduce levels of cancer-causing agents in the intestines and the bacteria that produce cancer-causing agents.

There are different kinds of fiber, including cellulose, hemicellulose, lignin, pectin and gums. Each one falls into one of the two categories of fibers — soluble and insoluble.

Soluble fibers are fibers that can be absorbed (pectin and gums) and help lower cholesterol. These fibers are digested slowly, and can help chronic bowel diseases such as Crohn's disease and ulcerative colitis, often characterized by acute diarrhea.

Insoluble fibers are fibers that can't be digested (cellulose, most hemicellulose and lignin) and help prevent constipation. Diarrhea symptoms may get worse if you take in too much insoluble fiber. Natural sources of soluble and insoluble fiber are listed below.

Natural sources of insoluble fiber
Lentils
Bananas
Potatoes
Brown rice
Corn
Brussels sprouts
Broccoli, spinach
Cauliflower
Wheat germ
Wheat bran cereal
Whole-wheat bread
Whole-wheat crackers
Pasta

Natural sources of soluble fiber
Oat bran, oatmeal
Barley
Berries
Apples
Apricots
Peaches, nectarines
Oranges, grapefruit, tangerines
Okra, cabbage, turnips, peas, sweet potatoes
Pinto, kidney, navy beans
Chickpeas, split peas, lima beans
Carrots, celery, zucchini

Medical Sources

Diet and Health, National Academy Press, Washington, D.C., 1989
Nutrition Prescription, Crown Publishers, Inc., New York, 1987
Eat Smart for a Healthy Heart, Barron's, Hauppauge, New York, 1987

Easy ways to eat more fiber

Besides lowering your risk of colorectal cancer, fiber works as a natural laxative to help keep you regular. It can be a real diet-booster as well. Loading up on fruits and vegetables can help you feel full so that you won't snack on high-calorie junk food.

You can eat a wide variety of fruits and vegetables and not use a bunch of calories for the day. Here are some easy ways to eat more fiber:

> ➤ Substitute whole-wheat flour for white. Use whole-wheat or spinach pasta instead of regular. Replace white rice with brown.
> ➤ Eat vegetables with their skins. The skins contain high levels of fiber.
> ➤ Eat fruits with seeds, such as blackberries, raspberries, strawberries and figs, which are all good sources of fiber. You should avoid fruits with seeds if you have diverticulosis.

Remember to drink plenty of liquids to help the fiber-filled foods pass through your body.

Medical Sources
Diet and Health, National Academy Press, Washington, D.C., 1989
Nutrition Prescription, Crown Publishers, Inc. New York, 1987

Get the most out of your fruits and vegetables

- ❑ Select produce that is not bruised or damaged.
- ❑ Choose dark green, orange and yellow vegetables and fruits — these are high in beta carotene.
- ❑ Pick fresh vegetables and fruits rather than canned.
- ❑ Try to shop on the first day your grocery store receives its produce for the freshest selection.
- ❑ Place your fruits and vegetables near a window to sun-ripen them.
- ❑ Avoid storing produce that has already been cut or sliced — exposure to air can destroy vitamins.

☐ Rinse your fruits and veggies with water just before you serve them.

☐ Don't soak your produce — it can remove valuable nutrients.

☐ Try not to remove the peelings or skins (nutrients are concentrated in the skins).

☐ Steam, stir-fry or microwave foods to preserve the most nutrients.

☐ Be sure not to overcook foods — you can lose vitamins and minerals.

☐ Don't deep-fry foods. You'll avoid unnecessary fat and calories.

☐ Don't cook vegetables with baking soda — it can damage the vitamin contents.

Medical Source ————————————————

American Institute for Cancer Research, 1759 R Street N.W., Washington, D.C. 20069

A number one disease fighter

You've heard of the concept of a handy man — a man who can do lots of different jobs around the house to make your life run more smoothly.

Well, yogurt isn't exactly a man, but it just might be the newest "handy-food" — it does all kinds of "jobs" in your body that make things run more smoothly.

Once known as "curds and whey," yogurt has been around for centuries. But, no matter what the name, its benefits are still the same.

Yogurt is a high-calcium, high-protein snack that is quick and easy to carry and eat and not too filling. Many kinds of yogurt are low in fat, which helps you to keep your fat intake low while satisfying those between-meal cravings.

The body uses the calcium in yogurt to build strong bones and teeth in children and adolescents. And it helps protect against osteoporosis, the brittle-bone disease, often caused by a calcium deficiency, especially common among postmenopausal women.

The protein in yogurt helps build a strong immune system to fight off disease. This vital protein is especially important for people who don't always get a well-balanced diet, such as elderly people and diet-conscious adolescents. It also promotes muscle development in adults and children, and it ensures healthy growth during pregnancy and childhood.

Another very "handy" thing about yogurt is that you can use low-fat yogurt to replace high-fat creams and sauces. For example, you can use yogurt instead of mayonnaise or sour cream when making salad dressings or sauces. You can also use it to top fruits and desserts instead of fattening whipped creams.

It won't fix your leaking roof, but it's still very useful to have around the house. Try adding some yogurt to your diet for a high-protein, high-calcium "handy-food" that works as smoothly as it tastes.

Medical Source ——————————————
FDA Consumer (26,5:27)

Yogurt: The great substitute

Low-fat yogurt makes a great low-fat substitute for many high-fat foods and recipes. Here are a few options you might want to try:

> ➤ Use low-fat yogurt in the place of milk or cream to add body and a slight tart flavor to soups and sauces. You may want to add a little cornstarch to prevent the yogurt from curdling if it overheats.
> ➤ Replace the sour cream in your favorite coffee cake with yogurt.
> ➤ Try topping your baked potato with plain low-fat yogurt and chopped chives.
> ➤ Low-fat frozen yogurt is a great alternative to ice cream.
> ➤ Make your own special low-fat "yogurt float" by pouring your favorite diet drink over a couple of spoonfuls of frozen yogurt. Yummy!

Try substituting yogurt in some of your own favorite recipes.

Medical Sources ——————————————
The Atlanta Journal/Constitution (Jan. 6, 1994, H9)
Hints from Heloise, Avon Books, New York, 1980

The healing powers of chicken soup

Chicken soup will cure what ails you — or so mom says, anyway. Not only does the steam and aroma help relieve a stuffy nose, but chicken soup also seems to work as an anti-inflammatory, relieving the aches and pains that make a cold so hard to bear.

According to new research, chicken soup seems to keep the white blood cells called neutrophils from moving into damaged tissue and adding to inflammation. Neutrophils are normally helpful cells that fight infection.

However, these white blood cells can get out of control. When they swarm into the damaged area, they make inflammation worse and they can actually attack human tissue.

A California researcher, Dr. Stephen Rennard, asked his wife to prepare her Lithuanian grandmother's favorite recipe for chicken soup. He took samples while she was cooking and put them in a plastic chamber with neutrophils on one side and substances that attract neutrophils on the other.

After his wife had added onions, parsnips, turnips, sweet potatoes and carrots, the soup started working against the neutrophils.

The chicken soup kept the neutrophils from traveling over into the other side of the plastic chamber. In the body, that would mean that chicken soup reduces inflammation.

The healing recipe Dr. Rennard's wife made is fairly simple:

- Put a stewing chicken in a large pot and cover with water. Bring to a boil.
- Peel and add 3 large onions, 1 large sweet potato, 3 parsnips, 2 turnips and 12 to 15 large carrots.
- Salt to taste.
- Cook 1 1/2 hours.
- Add 6 celery stalks and 1 bunch parsley.
- Cook 1 hour (or until all vegetables are very soft).
- Remove the chicken. You can use it for another recipe.
- Puree vegetables in food processor. Return them to broth and stir.
- If you'd like, you can chill the soup, skim off the fat and reheat.

Your own favorite chicken soup recipe should have healing powers, too.

Not all chicken soup measures up nutritionally, however. Dietitian Susan M. Kleiner, private nutrition consultant to the Cleveland Browns and the Cleveland Cavaliers, says that while soup can be nutritious, most soups alone don't constitute a complete meal.

When you combine your soup with salad and whole-grain bread, you have a wonderfully comforting meal that's also good for you.

Busy cooks find soups a time-saver, too, because a large pot can carry you through a whole week.

Suppose you don't have time to cook a pot of soup. You can just open a can of prepared soup for the same benefits, right? Not so fast.

You have to read the label first. Some soups are high in sodium — not good for people with high blood pressure and heart disease. Some canned soups even contain sugar or sweeteners, a no-no for diabetics.

You may be better off taking the time to put together your own soup, after all. That way, you control the ingredients. For a healthier homemade soup, try these nutritious tricks:

- ❏ Substitute skim or low-fat milk to cut fat in a cream soup.
- ❏ Substitute herbs for salt.
- ❏ Let your meat stock cool, then skim off the fat.
- ❏ Use a vegetable stock as the base for your soup.
- ❏ Combine green, orange and yellow vegetables for a soup that contains cancer-fighters like beta carotene and vitamin A.
- ❏ Add grains to your soup for iron, thiamin, niacin and riboflavin.
- ❏ Get the protein and carbohydrates you need from beans or peas.
- ❏ If you prefer a vegetarian soup, you'll need a side dish to complete your protein requirements. Grains, nuts or seeds complete a pea or bean soup, and dairy products or eggs add protein to vegetable soups. All of these soups will add fiber to your diet.

Athletes, take note: Soup transports well in a vacuum bottle, and it can replenish needed liquid as well as nutrients.

Soups are also great for jocks because they can be low in fat and easy to digest.

Bean and pea soups are so high in fiber that they are harder to digest, so you might want to avoid eating soups containing legumes before you work out.

Medical Sources ————————————————

    The Physician and Sportsmedicine (20,12:43)
    Medical Tribune (34,11:11)
    The Atlanta Journal/Constitution Food Pharmacy (Aug. 5, 1993, W14)

Healthy shopping: new food labels

If current food label lingo has you in limbo, there's light ahead. New labels are on-line.

In the past, one out of every five items did not carry a food label. Some of the ones that did have labels were so complicated you needed an interpreter to understand them.

The FDA set out to remedy this situation, and after more than two years of deliberation finally issued new label guidelines on Jan. 6, 1993. Over 300,000 food products will be affected and will cost consumers $1.4 to $2.3 billion over the next 20 years. The figures sound high, but each consumer will only be paying about 46 cents extra each year.

The new labels have a different focus from the old. These labels make it easier for people to use nutrition to avoid heart disease, cancer, osteoporosis, obesity, high blood pressure and allergic reactions to food.

Since most people now risk dietary excess rather than dietary deficiency, the labels will emphasize fat, sodium, carbohydrates and protein. Vitamins and minerals are listed, but they are not given the emphasis they had on past labels.

The label also has a new term, Daily Value (DV), to tell you how much of each nutrient you need.

Beside the listed nutrients, Daily Value tells you what percentage of each nutrient one serving provides. Amounts of nutrients are also listed in grams or milligrams. The recommended Daily Value is based on a 2,000 calorie diet.

Even if you don't eat exactly 2,000 calories a day, it's still easy to calculate how a certain food fits into your overall food intake. The Daily Values for sodium and cholesterol stay the same no matter how many calories you eat.

A chart appears at the bottom of each label listing the nutrients needed for a 2,000-calorie diet and a 2,500-calorie diet, making calculations easier. Most men over 50, women and children fall into the 2,000-daily calorie requirement.

The 2,500-calorie-a-day diet applies to younger men, teen-age boys and all very active people.

At the very bottom of the label is the reminder that one gram of fat contains nine calories, one gram of carbohydrate contains four calories and one gram of protein contains four calories.

All the new labels follow the same basic format.

□ SERVING SIZE — This appears at the top of the label. Serving sizes will now be the same for similar foods. To determine serving size, the FDA divided foods into 139 categories, including 11 infant food groups.

The FDA bases serving sizes on amounts normally eaten at one sitting. Same serving sizes for similar types of food will make it easier to compare nutrient values of different brands. The new regulations also prevent companies from making serving sizes smaller to "reduce" fat or other product nutrients.

□ FAT — The label lists total fat as well as saturated fat and the number of calories in the product that come from fat. Saturated fat raises blood cholesterol and increases risk of heart disease and stroke. Overall, fat should supply no more than 30 percent of your total calories. Saturated fat should make up 10 percent or less of your total fat consumption.

Meat labels may list stearic acid, a type of saturated fat, separately from other fats. It is rumored that stearic acid has possible health benefits, but researchers aren't definite. For now, simply consider stearic acid as a saturated fat.

On food labels for children under age two, information concerning calories and fat may not be provided. Fat is necessary during the first few years of life to ensure adequate growth and development. The FDA reasoned that including this data on labels of children's food might make parents think that fat intake for young children needs to be restricted, which is not the case.

- ☐ **CHOLESTEROL** — 300 milligrams is the maximum daily allowance.

- ☐ **SODIUM** — 2,400 milligrams is the maximum daily allowance.

- ☐ **CARBOHYDRATES** — The total number of carbohydrates one serving contains is listed. Total carbohydrates should supply at least 60 percent of daily calories. On a 2,000 calorie diet, carbohydrates should provide at least 1,200 calories. The carbohydrate category is broken down into the subcategories of Fiber and Sugar. About 280 of carbohydrate calories will come from fiber and sugar. The remaining calories fall into the subcategory of complex carbohydrates, which will probably not be listed on most labels. If these carbohydrates are listed, they may be included in the category of Other Carbohydrates.

- ☐ **FIBER** — At least 20 grams of fiber or 11.5 grams per 1,000 calories daily is probably necessary to stay "regular" and help reduce the risk of cancer and other diseases.

- ☐ **SUGAR** — This category includes sugars that occur naturally in food as well as added sugars. The FDA has not decided on a set amount of sugar to recommend. Some nutrition experts recommend 50 grams or less.

- ☐ **PROTEIN** — Daily Values of proteins are not required although some companies may choose to include them. Their percentage would be based on proteins providing 10 percent of a 2,000 calorie diet. That would mean about 200 of your calories would come from proteins.

Companies can now make claims about foods they distribute that "may" or "might" reduce risks of certain illnesses. Any product that promotes a health benefit must meet strict FDA guidelines.

Grain products, fruits and vegetables that contain at least .6 grams of soluble fiber per serving and are low in fat and cholesterol may reduce the risk of heart disease and cancer.

Adequate intake of calcium may help reduce risk of osteoporosis. Reduced sodium consumption may lower blood pressure and possibly decrease risk of stroke and heart failure.

If you have allergic reactions to food colorings, this FDA guideline may brighten your day. Any color additive now has to be referred to by name instead of just by the word "color."

Also, any flavorings or other ingredients that contain protein hydrolysates, many of which are high in sodium, have to be identified. These disclosures will be helpful for people on sodium restricted diets.

Restaurant foods, foods served on airplanes and foods produced by small businesses with sales of less than $50,000 a year are exempt from these new regulations.

Fresh meat, poultry, fish, fruits and vegetables are also exempt.

Labels are not required on plain coffee and tea or on products smaller than 12 square inches, such as a small candy bar, although manufacturers must provide an address or phone number so consumers can write or call for this information.

Most products, especially packaged foods, should be carrying these new labels already.

Medical Sources ─────────────────────
Wellness Letter (9,6:3)
Nutrition Action (20,2:7)
British Medical Journal (306,6870:83)
Tufts University Diet & Nutrition Letter (10,12:3)

Label claims: Can you trust them?

Low fat, low cholesterol, low sodium, low calorie. These are just a few of the eye-catching phrases manufacturers love to put on labels. In the past these claims differed from product to product and sometimes they were downright deceptive.

With the new label guidelines the FDA issued in January of 1993, these claims will be much more trustworthy than they have been.

Here are some of the claims you can expect to see. Some of the labels may still have loopholes, but if you know what to look for you won't be tripped up.

LOW CALORIE — A low calorie product has 40 calories or less per serving. A low calorie meal or main dish such as frozen dinners and entrees contains 120 calories or less per 100 grams — about 3.5 ounces.

LOW FAT — A low fat food must have three grams or less of fat per serving. On individual foods, low fat claims are trustworthy. However, on meals and main courses that claim to be low fat, make sure that there are no more than two grams of fat per 100 calories. Lobbyists for the dairy industry managed to bypass the regulation standard and get the low fat label put on 2-percent milk, which actually has five grams of fat per serving. Only skim or 1-percent milk has 3 grams or less of fat.

LOW IN SATURATED FAT — Saturated fat should make up no more than one gram of all the fat contained in a single serving. In meals or main dishes, less than 10 percent of the calories should come from saturated fat.

LOW CHOLESTEROL — A single serving of a low cholesterol product must contain 20 milligrams (mg.) or less of cholesterol. Saturated fat, which raises blood cholesterol, must not exceed two grams. A low cholesterol meal or main course should contain no more than 20 mg. of cholesterol for every 100 grams of food. A 10-ounce meal should contain about 60 mg. of cholesterol.

LOW SODIUM — A low sodium food contains 140 mg. or less of sodium per serving. Prepackaged meals should contain no more than 140 mg. of sodium per 100 gram serving. A 10-ounce meal would contain about 400 mg. of sodium. A 16-ounce meal should not exceed 600 mg. of sodium.

VERY LOW SODIUM — There should be only 35 mg. or less of sodium per serving.

LIGHT or LITE — These words have several possible meanings.

For foods that get half or more of their calories from fat like cheese and hot dogs, a light version of these foods contains no more than half the fat of the original product.

Less fatty foods can be called light if the fat content has been cut by half or the calories by a third. The label must tell you which has been done.

A main dish can be called light if it meets FDA regulations for being low fat or low calorie.

Light may mean the product has half its usual sodium content, but the label must say light in sodium.

If the food is already light or low calorie, then light can be used to mean the product contains half the normal amount of sodium. In this case, the word sodium does not have to be mentioned.

Light may be used to describe a product's color or texture, but the label must make this clear.

On foods like brown sugar, cream or molasses, the word light can be used without explanation if it has traditionally been part of their name.

LESS or FEWER — Foods that contain 25 percent less of some nutrient than a similar food can be labeled less or fewer.

REDUCED — A reduced product has been altered by the manufacturer and contains 25 percent less of a nutrient or calories than the regular product.

FREE — A serving contains none or only very small amounts of fat, cholesterol, sodium, sugar and/or calories.

PERCENT FAT FREE — This phrase tells what part of a food's weight is fat free. However, this label claim can be very tricky to interpret correctly. Percent fat free refers to the fat that makes up a food's weight, not how many calories fat contributes to a food's overall calorie total. For example, a food serving that weighs 100 grams can have two of those grams come from fat and legitimately claim on the label that the food is 98 percent fat free. If you figure the number of calories the fat grams contribute to total calories, the fat percentage is startlingly different. If one serving of this same food contains 75 calories, those two grams of fat make up 18 of the total calories. (Each fat gram contains 9 calories). Eighteen fat calories of a 75 calorie total means that in one serving of food, 24 percent of your calories will be coming from fat, not 2 percent as the label may seem to imply.

GOOD SOURCE OF — A product that claims to be a good source of certain vitamins, minerals, calcium, fiber or other nutrients must contain 10 to 19 percent of that item. A good source food contains at least 10 percent. A high source food contains at least 20 percent of the recommended Daily Value. A product can make a good or high source claim if it contains any food that meets these definitions.

If a label makes a claim that the product is a good source of calcium or other nutrients yet the item exceeds Daily Value recommendations for fat, saturated fat, sodium or cholesterol, the FDA requires a disclosure on the front of the product that says *See back panel for more information about saturated fat and other nutrients.* The disclosure is required when 30 percent of the Daily Value for these nutrients is contained in a main dish or 40 percent in a meal. Some nutritionists believe the disclosure should appear for foods with even less than these percentages of fat, sodium or cholesterol.

LOW — Product contains 5 percent or less of a nutrient.

MORE — A serving of a food labeled "more" contains 10 percent more of a nutrient than the regular product.

Food serving sizes of less than two tablespoons have to meet tighter guidelines to be labeled "low" in sodium, fat, calories or other nutrients. Most low foods can be eaten frequently without exceeding dietary guidelines.

The new regulations do not require companies to label fresh meat, poultry or seafood. However, for manufacturers who choose to label these products, the Department of Agriculture has created a few new terms to help consumers choose healthier cuts of meat. Few cuts of meat can be labeled low fat, but there will be categories of lean and extra lean. Keep in mind that manufacturers can take the fat and sodium counts from either fresh or cooked meat, depending on which makes the numbers lowest.

LEAN — Lean meat contains less than 10 grams of fat, four grams of saturated fat and 95 milligrams (mg.) of cholesterol per serving.

EXTRA LEAN — Extra lean meat contains less than five grams of fat, two grams of saturated fat and 95 mg. of cholesterol.

Some nutrition experts suggest that "low-fat" and "low in saturated fat" foods should be chosen to replace "lean" and "extra lean" whenever possible. They recommend no more than two grams of fat and less than one gram of saturated fat per 100 calories.

These new guidelines may not turn you into a label lover, but they can at least give you the reassurance that most label claims are reliable.

Medical Sources ───────────────────
Nutrition Action (20,2:8)
Tufts University Diet & Nutrition Letter (10,12:3)

Increase immune response with vitamin power

They are not "magic pills" that contain mysterious wonders that can prolong your life. But they may lengthen your years of illness-free living and cut your chances of getting sick by 50 percent.

Scientists have recently discovered that multivitamin-multimineral supplements can improve immune responses in elderly people. The researchers who conducted the vitamin-immune response study were concerned that many elderly people experienced more than their fair shares of illness because they weren't getting the proper nutrients in their diets.

Apparently, more than 40 percent of elderly men and women suffer from some type of vitamin and mineral deficiency. These deficiencies can weaken the immune system and increase the risk of minor and major illnesses.

In fact, only about 25 percent of elderly people have immune responses as vigorous and healthy as those of younger people.

A research team from Memorial University of Newfoundland enlisted 96 volunteers (all over the age of 65) to test the effects of vitamin and mineral supplements on immune response.

None of the volunteers had known illnesses or were taking other medications that might interfere with the study. However, some had slight vitamin deficiencies.

The group was randomly divided into two small groups. Group one received a daily placebo (fake pill). Group two received a daily supplement that contained several different vitamins and minerals. Each volunteer took the assigned pill once a day for 12 months.

Throughout the 12 months, researchers took blood samples at different times to measure the amounts of nutrients in the blood and to check immune responses. They also kept records of how often the volunteers suffered from illnesses. At the end of the 12 months, the researchers noted some remarkable results.

According to the study, the volunteers who took the placebo didn't show an improvement in their immunity against disease. But, the volunteers who took the vitamin-mineral supplements did show improved immune response.

Those suffering from vitamin deficiencies at the beginning of the study enjoyed an improvement in their nutritional status if they received the supplement pill. Those who had received the placebo still suffered from the same deficiencies.

Most significantly, volunteers in the supplement group enjoyed a 50-percent decrease in the number of infection-related illnesses compared to the placebo group.

The researchers stress that the supplements used in the study did not contain huge amounts of vitamins or minerals. Some supplements contain as much as 30 times the Recommended Daily Allowance (RDA). But the amounts of vitamins and minerals in the supplement were close to RDA for each of the nutrients.

Taking large doses of vitamins and minerals can actually impair immune responses. In other words, getting too much of the nutrients can be just as bad as getting too little.

Talk to your doctor about adding some vitamin and mineral supplements to your diet to help improve your immune response and cut down on your infection-related illnesses.

Medical Source ————————————————
> *The Lancet* (340,8828:1124)

Make vitamins easier to swallow

Your doctor has suggested that you take some vitamin supplements to help improve your immune response. You think the idea is great, but you dread the thought of taking the supplements.

You're not alone. People across the nation, both young and old, experience the same difficulty you do when trying to swallow pills of any size.

Below are six simple ways of swallowing pills that might make your vitamin supplements a little less threatening:

- ☐ Take a sip of water (or other liquid) and drop the pill in your mouth. Then hold your head back as if you were going to gargle. The water and the pill will fall towards the back of your throat, and you can swallow the pill easily with the water.

- ☐ Place the pill in a spoonful of soft food such as applesauce, ice cream, jello or yogurt. When you swallow the food, the pill goes with it.

- ☐ Cover the pill with a thin layer of butter or margarine to help the pill slide down your throat.

- ☐ Break large tablets in half. The smaller halves will be easier to swallow. Just remember to take both halves.

- ☐ Ask your pharmacist if the pill comes in liquid form.

- ☐ Ask your pharmacist if grinding the pill to a powder will affect the potency of the drug. Some pills are "time-released" and grinding them up will interfere with the activity of the pill. If the pharmacist says that grinding the pill is okay, place the pill in a zip-lock bag and crush it. Then put the powder in a teaspoon to take it. You can wash it down with some water, or you can mix it with a teaspoon of soft food (applesauce, etc.) to help swallow it.

Medical Source ————————————————
American Family Physician (47,1:103)

Water: The nutrient you can't live without

The human body is almost two-thirds water, so water is obviously an important part of your daily diet. In fact, if your body doesn't get enough water, your good health will literally "dry up."

Water makes up a large percentage of the fluid in the blood, and it accounts for a huge portion of the contents of every cell in your body.

Water works wonders in so many areas of the body that pharmacists would gladly bottle it up and prescribe it as a miracle drug if they thought they could get away with it! Here are a few of the wonders water works in your body:

- ❏ Water regulates your body temperature through sweat.
- ❏ Water helps keep you regular. It's one of the best natural laxatives around. Drinking lots of water helps keep stools soft and helps you avoid problems with constipation.
- ❏ Water carries medicine to its action sites and then helps flush away the break-down products after the drug has done its job.
- ❏ Water helps your body absorb and use the nutrients healthy meals provide. Then, it helps your body flush out wastes.

And that's not all! Here are a few extra benefits of drinking plenty of water:

- ❏ Water helps reduce wrinkles. "Well-hydrated" skin is much smoother than dry skin and is less likely to develop small, fine wrinkles.
- ❏ Water helps keep the urinary tract free from bacteria, which makes it less likely that you'll suffer from a urinary infection.
- ❏ Water can help you lose weight and keep it off. You might say water is the best "diet drink" ever created. This no-calorie beverage can help you feel full faster during meals, and it also gives you a feeling of fullness in between meals to help curb your appetite.

So, how much water should you drink every day? You need about four 8-ounce glasses of water for every 1,000 calories you use.

Most people use about 2,000 calories each day, so eight 8-ounce glasses is the magic number. Some people, however, may need more water than their calorie intake might indicate.

People taking diuretics, also known as water pills, often need to drink extra water. Unfortunately, many people taking diuretics drink less water in order to "help" the diuretics remove excess fluid from the body.

Not drinking enough water while you're taking diuretics may cause you to fall, affect your mental abilities or even damage your kidneys. If you're taking diuretics, ask your doctor how much water you need to drink every day.

Athletes who lose considerable water through sweat also need to drink extra water. If you tend to sweat heavily during your workout, weigh yourself before and after exercising.

Generally, one pound of sweat equals two cups of water. If you lose two pounds during an intense workout, drink four cups of liquid to replace that lost water.

Many physicians recommend drinking one to two cups before the workout, drinking liquid every 20 minutes during the workout, and drinking a few cups of liquid after the workout is over.

Athletes who work out more than one hour at a time need to consume fruit juices or sports drinks like Gatorade to replenish their energy as well as their water supply.

However, you don't have to drink just water. Other beverages, such as fruit juices and decaffeinated drinks, contain water and will help you meet your daily requirement.

But don't be fooled by caffeinated tea, coffee and soft drinks. The caffeine in those drinks causes you to go to the bathroom more often than normal. You'll actually have to drink more water to make up for the water you lost after drinking caffeine. Alcoholic beverages can also have a dehydrating effect on your body.

Medical Sources ————————————————
Senior Patient (1,4:26)
The Physician and Sportsmedicine (20,11:33)

How to recognize and treat dehydration

Dehydration is a condition that most people associate with illnesses that cause vomiting or with marathon runners after a long race.

But it's a condition that's far too common in everyday life. Children, teen-agers, adults and the elderly are all potential victims of dehydration, even during the course of normal, everyday activities.

Dehydration occurs when the body does not have enough water. This may be caused by not drinking enough water or by losing too much water (through sweat, urine, vomiting, etc.).

Dehydration can cause weakness and fatigue, increased heart rate and other physical symptoms. If left untreated, severe dehydration may lead to coma and death.

The easiest way to avoid dehydration is to drink plenty of fluids. This often means drinking well beyond the point of thirst (possibly a pint of water every hour during the heat of the day). If your urine is clear or very pale-colored and you make frequent trips to the bathroom, you're probably getting enough to drink.

One of the most dangerous aspects of dehydration is that most people don't even recognize that they are dehydrated, so they don't do anything about it. In order to avoid the problems that can come with dehydration, it is important to recognize the warning signs:

❑ Loose skin. When you pinch the skin on the arm, it doesn't spring right back—instead, it stays in the "pinched" position for a second or two.

❑ Slow capillary refill. When you push down on a fingernail, it takes more than a second or two for the pink color to return.

However, among elderly people, those indicators are not necessarily specific for dehydration.

Many elderly people have a decreased sense of thirst, so they often don't feel thirsty even when they need the fluid.

Also, most elderly people have loose skin normally, so that sign can't be used to indicate dehydration.

Some better indicators of dehydration in the elderly are:

> ➤ Tongue dryness
> ➤ Deep lines run along the length of the tongue
> ➤ Dryness of the gums and cheeks inside the mouth
> ➤ Unusual upper-body weakness
> ➤ Mental confusion
> ➤ Speech difficulty
> ➤ Sunken eyes

Here are some helpful remedies you may try at home to treat dehydration. Since dehydration can be serious and even life threatening, consult your doctor before attempting to treat yourself.

☐ Drink small amounts of clear liquids frequently. If dehydration has depleted your stores of salt and sugars, you may want to try an electrolyte solution. These are simple to make at home. Mix 1 pint of boiled water, 2 teaspoons of sugar and 1/4 teaspoon of baking soda.

☐ Rest quietly until you recover. You may read or watch television.

☐ Stay away from salty foods. They can make your dehydration worse.

Medical Sources —————————————————
Emergency Medicine (24,15:59)
Complete Guide to Symptoms, Illness and Surgery, 2nd edition, The Body Press, New York, 1989

Drinking water causes hip fractures?

You know you need to drink water for maximum health, but you may not know that the chemicals we use to purify our drinking water may put you at risk for bone fractures or worse.

Nearly 75 percent of the nation's public water systems use chlorine to kill impurities in the water. Many water systems also include fluoride to prevent tooth decay and bone degeneration.

Despite the benefits they provide, these chemicals may have some unpleasant side effects.

An overall look at water studies conducted between 1966 and 1991 indicated that people who live in communities where the water is heavily chlorinated have increased risks of developing bladder or rectal cancer.

Researchers suggest that the bladder and rectum develop more cancer than other areas of the body because they are exposed longer and more often to chlorination by-products, as the body stores waste containing these products, preparing to eliminate it.

Recently, doctors have turned to fluoride treatments as a way of treating osteoporosis, the brittle-bone disease. New research indicates that while fluoride may strengthen the spinal bone, it may also weaken the hips.

Researchers studied three communities in Utah. They found that the elderly people in the community with the highest fluoride levels had more hip fractures than elderly people in the other communities.

Even water fluoridated to one part per million (ppm), which is not a very high level of fluoridation, may pose a risk.

In Brigham City, Utah, where the water is fluoridated to 1 ppm, women ages 65 to 80 and men age 70 and above, had more hip fractures than people the same age who lived in Logan and Cedar City, which have lower fluoridation levels than Brigham City.

They had been exposed to the fluoridated water for approximately 20 years. This study was the first to document the risk in such low concentrations of fluoride, although other studies have found similar effects in communities with high levels of fluoride.

These findings don't mean that we should stop disinfecting our water. The risks from contaminated water, such as typhoid fever, are far greater than the suspected hip fracture or cancer risks. What we need to do is find safer ways of purifying our water.

One such method is called chloramination, which disinfects water by using a combination of chlorine and ammonia, which means smaller amounts of chlorine are used. Find out what method of water disinfection your community uses. You may want to suggest chloramination.

Besides talking to the water authorities in your town, here are safety steps you can take at home.

- ❑ Buy bottled water. Be sure to investigate the bottling company. Some merely package tap water.
- ❑ Purchase a charcoal filter for your home faucet. It will remove most of the chlorine compounds from your water, though not all other elements.

In spite of this news, don't stop drinking water! Your body needs plenty of it to function well, and the drawbacks of not getting enough water far outweigh the known risks of these additives.

Medical Sources ——————————————————

The Journal of the American Medical Association (268,6:746)
American Journal of Public Health (82,7:955)

WEIGHT CONTROL

Why traditional diets fail

Another year down in history, another New Year's resolution down the tubes. Did anyone get rid of those 5, 20 or 50 pounds they swore they'd lose last year?

Dieting is an "auld" acquaintance that most of us would dearly like to forget. Some doctors are saying we should forget it. After all, nine out of 10 people who lose weight gain it all back within five years.

People who manage to lose weight fast — three or more pounds a week — almost always gain it back within the next year.

We lose weight for a class reunion, gain it back, lose it again for a beach vacation and gain it back. That cycle, known as yo-yo dieting, is almost as bad for your health as being overweight. It puts you at risk for gallstones and heart disease, not to mention poor self-esteem.

So should you just forget counting calories, accept your body as it is and bring on the cookies and ice cream? Probably not. Traditional diets aren't working, but there's a middle ground between endless bouts of crash dieting and simply giving up.

It's called weight management, and it includes normal, healthy eating and moderate exercise.

Forget the old rigid diets that restricted you to a list of acceptable foods and an extremely low number of calories each day. With the traditional diet, you get so hungry and feel so deprived that you can't think logically about food.

You have uncontrollable cravings for high-fat foods, and you can't resist giving in to eating binges. After you go on an eating binge, you feel so guilty that you hardly eat anything for a couple of days and start the cycle all over again.

These starvation diets slow down your metabolism and make your fat cells more resistant to losing their stored fatty energy reserves.

With weight management, you learn how to create three healthy, low-fat, high-carbohydrate meals a day plus between-meal snacks. You won't feel deprived, hungry or anxious about the food you eat.

You can reduce the amount of fat in your food without bringing on an eating binge, and you'll still have enough energy to exercise.

Calorie-burning exercise is the only way to lose weight and keep it off. Exercise will give you more energy, boost your self-esteem and even reduce your desire for fatty foods.

Many crash dieters are "crash exercisers," too. Once they decide to exercise, they begin a tiring, demanding schedule that they just can't keep up. You may want to start off simply walking 10 or 15 minutes a day and build up to a 45-minute workout three times a week.

To get the most out of your work-out time, complete your 25 minutes of walking, biking or aerobic exercise with 20 minutes of weight lifting or muscle-building exercises, such as push-ups and leg lifts with ankle weights.

Lean muscles use more calories than other body parts, so you boost your resting metabolism when you build muscles. You'll burn extra calories even when you're just sitting around.

Hate exercise? Think of it this way: If you exercise, you can occasionally indulge in a bite-size chocolate bar or a small slice of thick and cheesy pizza without feeling guilty.

Once you've lost weight, don't let hard-to-lose pounds creep up on you. Get on the scales every morning. If you've gained an extra pound, don't crash diet, but cut back on calories for the day.

Medical Sources ————————————————
Journal of the American Dietetic Association (93,9:1007)
Postgraduate Medicine (93,1:082)
Nutrition Today (28,2:4)
The Physician and Sportsmedicine (21,6:45)

The 5-step eating plan that works

1) Get all the candy, potato chips and gooey cinnamon rolls out of your house and don't buy any more. If your kids can't live without them, tell them

to put them in their rooms under lock and key or stash them at a friend's house.

Fill your refrigerator with tasty fruits and vegetables to snack on. If you decide to eat a cookie or a cup of ice cream every once in a while, buy single servings.

2) Eat plenty of whole-grain breads, cereal, rice and pasta to get your fiber and B vitamins. Choose five to six servings of fruits and vegetables a day for vitamin A, vitamin C and fiber.

Go easy on dairy products, fats, sweets and meats. You shouldn't eat more than five or six ounces of meat a day. (A 3-ounce serving of meat looks about like a stacked deck of cards.)

This menu recommended by the American Dietetic Association provides all the necessary nutrients with only 1,983 calories:

Breakfast:
>   3/4 cup orange juice
>   1 bagel
>   1 tbs. light cream cheese
>   1/2 banana
>   1 cup 1-percent milk

Lunch:
>   1 bowl chili
>   1 baked potato with skin
>   1/2 cup low-fat cottage cheese
>   Salad — lettuce, 1/4 cup carrots, 1/4 cup green
>   pepper, 1/4 cup garbanzo beans
>   4 tbs. low-cal dressing

Dinner:
>   Chicken cacciatore — 3 oz. skinless chicken breast,
>   1/2 cup stewed tomatoes, 3/4 cup brown rice
>   1/2 cup steamed broccoli
>   1 slice French bread
>   1 tsp. margarine
>   1 pear

Snack:
  1 oatmeal raisin cookie
  1 medium apple
  1 cup 1-percent milk

Now that you know what a day's menu should look like, get creative. You can have cereal or oatmeal for breakfast, soup or a sandwich for lunch, and fish, lean hamburger or stir-fried chicken and vegetables for supper.

Remember to drink at least a quart of water a day, too.

3) Always look for foods low in fat:
  ➤ Choose lean meats, such as skinless, white poultry, pork loin, flank steak and ham.
  ➤ Bake or broil your meat instead of frying it.
  ➤ Steam your vegetables or sauté them in chicken broth instead of butter or oil.
  ➤ Flavor cooked vegetables and fish with lemon or lime juice and herbs instead of butter or margarine.
  ➤ Substitute these low-fat foods for high-fat foods:

High-fat food	Low-fat substitution
Mayonnaise	Mustard (or low-fat mayonnaise)
Sour cream	Nonfat plain yogurt
2 percent low-fat milk	1 percent low-fat milk
Margarine	Jam (or low-fat margarine)
Potato chips	Pretzels
Peanuts	Air-popped popcorn
Bran muffins	Bagel
Snack crackers	Water crackers
Bacon	Canadian bacon
Olives	Pickles
Ice cream	Low-fat frozen yogurt or Popsicles

4) There's no rule that says you have to eat a big lunch and dinner even when you're not hungry. If you satisfy your hunger pangs with a small, healthy snack when you get home from work, eat smaller portions for dinner. That's

what skinny people do. The same goes for your kids. Let them eat when they're starving (like right after school), and don't force them to clean their plates at mealtimes. Choose what they eat, but not when or how much.

5) Eat a healthy breakfast, a hearty lunch and a small dinner. You'll lose weight if you eat one 2,000 calorie meal a day in the morning, but you'll gain weight if you eat that meal at night.

Most binge eaters eat very little for breakfast and lunch, then stuff themselves in the evening. If you eat normally throughout the day, you won't feel so much like bingeing at night.

Medical Source ————————————————————————
Medical Tribune (34,2:4)

The root of the problem is denial

Despite a long history of dieting, some people never seem to lose weight.

"But I eat like a bird," you say. Eating like a bird could be your problem. Most birds seem to peck away at tidbits, but some actually consume their weight in food each day.

If weight loss continues to be a problem for you, you may be eating more and exercising less than you think.

After studying 90 obese people for 14 days, researchers found that all participants underestimated the amount of food they ate and overestimated how much they exercised.

As many as 80 percent of us underestimate the number of calories we eat, sometimes by as much as 800 calories a day. One possible reason for this is that some of us don't accurately judge how much food we put on our plates.

In the study, the "diet-resistant" participants (people who had a long history of dieting without losing weight) consumed nearly twice as many calories as they thought and exercised approximately one-fourth less than they estimated.

The root of the problem appears to be denial. Researchers speculate that denial may stem from pressures caused by a lifetime of unsuccessful dieting and from society's prejudice against people who cannot control their weight.

The pressure to fix their weight problem may have affected their ability to think objectively about calorie intake and output.

The diet-resistant participants also believed a genetic or metabolic abnormality was responsible for their weight problem. Although many had taken thyroid or other hormone-regulating medications to control their weight, scientific testing did not reveal genetic or metabolic disorders.

When some of the diet-resistant participants stuck with a truly low-fat diet, they lost weight.

Some critics of the study still contend that genetic factors influence the tendency to become obese. "It is possible," argue Drs. Elliot Danforth, Jr. and Ethan A.H. Sims, "that the level of physical activity, as well as that of food intake, is genetically determined." It appears that both genetics and behavior play a role in becoming obese.

If you are trying to lose weight, be sure to weigh and measure the food you eat, so you'll be able to accurately judge serving sizes. This is especially important for high-fat foods.

Keep a food log. Researchers say that those who kept track of what they were eating were more successful at losing weight than those who did not. It may also be helpful for you to keep an exercise journal.

There are factors that may conceal or slow your weight loss. Fluid retention can hide the loss of fat for up to 16 days. After you have dieted for several weeks, your metabolism may slow to the point that weight loss is almost unnoticeable — especially if you are not exercising.

An undiagnosed thyroid disorder or medicine that lowers your metabolism may also slow the rate of your weight loss. If you think you have a metabolic or genetic disorder that is interfering with your weight loss, see your doctor.

Medical Sources ————————————————
The New England Journal of Medicine (327,27:1893,1947 and 328,20:1494)
American Family Physician (47,4:898)

Is life getting shorter for women?

The scales of health may be slowly tilting in favor of men.

Right now, women seem to be the healthier sex. At least, they live longer. The average life expectancy for a woman is 80 years, five to nine years more than men can expect to live.

But women are getting fatter, and that puts them at greater risk of the five leading causes of death: heart disease, cancer, stroke, diabetes and atherosclerosis.

Overweight women are troubled by osteoarthritis, osteoporosis and menstrual irregularities. They are at higher risk of cancers of the endometrium, uterus, gallbladder, cervix, ovaries and breast.

Risk of heart disease doubles for women who have gained more than 20 pounds as an adult, and overweight women are three times as likely to get diabetes as women who are not overweight.

Weight problems have always been a greater health risk for men, especially because they tend to gain weight in their stomach and upper body more easily than women. Stomach fat significantly increases the risk of heart disease and diabetes. Now, women are gaining so much weight that stomach fat is a problem for them, too.

It's no wonder that more women have eating disorders than men. Women are valued by their appearance more than men and feel social pressure to be thin and beautiful. Underweight models present an unhealthy and unrealistic image for women to live up to.

More than half of all young girls in grades one through six develop a distorted body image and believe that they are fat. During puberty, girls naturally develop fat deposits, and many of them start to diet, exercise too much and compulsively overeat.

Some of them develop an eating disorder such as anorexia nervosa, an abnormal fear of gaining weight, or bulimia, where you overeat then vomit.

Almost three-quarters of all 14- to 21-year-old girls diet. Women never get a chance to develop normal, healthy eating habits.

If women want to maintain their status as the healthier sex, they need to strive for reasonable weight-loss goals with a sensible, low-fat, high-carbohydrate diet.

Medical Source ————————————————
Journal of the American Dietetic Association (93,9:1007)

Six diet tips for seniors

Older people get the fat end of the deal when it comes to food. You know you're not eating any more than you used to, but you keep putting on extra pounds.

You've got three strikes against you:

☐ The rate your body burns calories (your metabolic rate) decreases about 2 percent every 10 years.

☐ Your body makes less protein as you get older. Protein burns calories. Since your body is making less protein, you need less calories than before.

☐ You are probably less active and get less exercise than when you were younger.

It's O.K. to be a few pounds heavier than you were in your 20s. Many older people are too thin — that's also a health risk. If you're 40 or 50 pounds overweight, you're increasing your risk of heart disease, diabetes, cancer and arthritis. You'll really improve your health even if you lose only 10 or 15 pounds.

Special cautions for dieting seniors

☐ Limit your calories to about 1,200 a day. You may want to ask your pharmacist to help you choose a good multi-vitamin/mineral supplement.

☐ Try to get about 70 grams of protein a day. You can get this much from five or six ounces of lean meat and two large glasses of skim milk. Grains, fruits and vegetables are also good sources of protein.

☐ Make sure you take in 1,200 to 1,500 milligrams of calcium a day. Women over 60 and men over 70 often have trouble absorbing calcium. Older people often avoid dairy products because of lactose intolerance. (If you're lactose intolerant, dairy products may cause intestinal gas and stomach cramps.) You may need lactase-treated milk (Lactaid) or Lactaid tablets. You probably should take a calcium supplement if your multi-vitamin/mineral tablet doesn't provide calcium.

☐ Buy dairy products that have vitamin D added to them or help your body produce vitamin D by spending 15 minutes a day in the sun. Vitamin D helps your body absorb calcium.

☐ Drink plenty of fluids while dieting, especially if you're also taking diuretics.

☐ Exercise regularly to keep your muscles toned and your weight down. You don't automatically lose muscle and gain fat as you get older.

Good exercises for seniors include stretching, walking, low-impact aerobics, water aerobics, swimming and cycling. If you can't move very well, do leg lifts and arm exercises while you are sitting or lying down. Even if one arm or leg is painful to move, exercise the other one. It's best to exercise at your target heart rate for 20 minutes with a 10-minute warm-up and 10-minute cool-down.

To get your target heart rate, subtract your age from 220 to find your maximum heart rate (for example 220 - 40 = 180). Multiply by the rate you'd like to hit (80% of your maximum heart rate would be .80 x 180 = 144). Check with your doctor before you start exercising.

Medical Sources ————————————————
American Family Physician (47,5:1187)
Geriatrics (48,9:88)

Overweight teens face more health risks in later life

"He'll outgrow it — that's just baby fat."

You've hear that said countless times when mothers talk about their overweight adolescent children.

The problem is, if they don't "outgrow" baby fat relatively quickly, they could be taking years off their lives. Recent studies show that adults who were overweight adolescents suffer from increased risk of heart and blood vessel diseases, cancer, arthritis and gout.

Researchers from Tufts University studied 238 people classified as obese adolescents (more than 20 pounds above their ideal weight) and 270 people who were classified as lean teen-agers.

After 55 years of follow-up, researchers found that the men and women who were overweight as adolescents suffered from an increased risk of illness and death compared to the men and women who were lean adolescents.

Men who were fat teen-agers were 2.3 times more likely to die of heart disease than men who had been lean teen-agers. They also suffered from increased risk of gout and colon and rectal cancers.

Both sexes who had been overweight as teens were more likely to suffer from blood vessel diseases, such as atherosclerosis. The American Heart Association explains that the blood vessels of obese teen-agers change from flexible tubes into hardened pipes that carry less blood.

Apparently these changes can be reversed by losing weight while still in the teen-age years. Waiting until adulthood to try to lose weight and reverse the hardening of the vessels is less successful.

The Tufts University researchers also found that women who had been overweight adolescents were 1.6 times more likely to develop arthritis compared to women who had been thin as teens.

And the formerly overweight women who did not develop arthritis still reported increased difficulty in walking and climbing stairs compared to the formerly thin women.

Men and women who had been overweight teens also suffered an increased risk of hip fracture compared to the men and women who had been lean adolescents.

According to the study, up to 25 percent of all adolescents in the nation are overweight and are at risk for developing the adult consequences of adolescent obesity. Preventing or resolving teen-age obesity seems to be the most effective, and possibly only way to reduce the risk of these consequences.

Check with your pediatrician to see if your children are classified as overweight. If they are, the doctor will be able to place them on a safe and healthy diet to help them lose the appropriate amount of weight for their heights and ages.

Do not try to place your children on diets without a doctor's advice. Children need a healthy, well-balanced diet for proper growth and development. "Homemade" diets run the risk of being poorly balanced in essential nutrients, which could be more damaging to a child than obesity.

Medical Sources ————————————————

The New England Journal of Medicine (327,19:1350)
Science News (142,20:326)
American Heart Association news release (June 5, 1992)

Choosing a weight-loss program

Statistics indicate that as many as one-quarter to one-third of all Americans are overweight, and many of them experience discouraging results from diet attempts. A large number of people either fail to lose weight or fail to keep it off for a few simple reasons:

- ❏ Set unrealistic goals and get discouraged early on and give up.
- ❏ Use unsafe, crash-diet methods of weight loss that do not involve any kind of long-term maintenance programs.
- ❏ Fail to get support from friends and family or from local diet support groups that offer encouragement through slow periods of weight loss.
- ❏ Start easing up on new diet habits after losing some weight, and end up putting the weight back on.

These factors might sound unimportant, but they seem to have a serious impact on the success or failure of a weight-loss program. Researchers suggest that successful weight-loss programs should include the following elements:

- ❏ Realistic goals. Your doctor can help you determine how much weight you should safely lose, and how long it should take you.

- ❏ New habits. Choose a weight-loss program that stresses developing a new mind-set on eating and exercising. Try to form some new habits that will stay with you long after you lose your weight. Avoid short-term gimmicks that leave you with the same old bad habits after you lose weight.

- ❏ Support. Talk with your family and friends about how they can help encourage and support you as you try to lose weight. If possible, get involved with a support group (weight-loss support group, nutritionist or doctor) to help you deal with your weight loss. They can also be great sources of information on health and nutrition.

Losing weight is never easy, but taking a few simple steps to avoid the common pitfalls of weight-loss programs will help improve your chances of success.

Medical Source ―――――――――――――――――
Nutrition Today (27,4:27)

Evaluating weight-loss programs

Weight-loss programs can be enormously successful and life-changing, but you need to consider several things before you enroll.

First, decide what will work best for you: a program that meets three days a week or just once a month; a program that meets in the mornings or evenings; an inexpensive program or a costly one, and so on.

One rule-of-thumb to remember is this: Don't judge a weight-loss program based on the "success" stories that they publish or advertise. These success stories don't always reflect the true success of the program as a whole.

Instead of listening to success stories, try to get the following information:

☐ How many people who enroll in the program actually complete it?
☐ How many of the people who enrolled and finished the program lost the amount of weight they wanted to?
☐ How many who lost their desired amounts of weight kept it off for one, two and five years after the program?
☐ Have many people experienced any kind of emotional, mental or physical problems related to the program?
   If the program you are looking at does not have this information available, you might be able to find it in some published studies. Ask your local librarian to help you locate this information.
   After getting the answers to those first questions, it's time to begin

looking into the more specific details of the program. Take time to find out about the following:

☐ Does this program require that you buy and use its food, or can you prepare your own meals using food you buy at the grocery store?

☐ Does the exercise program require you to use specialized equipment from its program, or can you learn the proper exercises and then do them at home or at your own private health club?

☐ How does this program blend together a mix of diet, exercise and behavior modifications? Is there a good mix of all three, or are one or two areas stressed more than the others?

☐ Does this program combine counseling with the weight-loss program? If so, is it a group setting or individual counseling? If it is group counseling, will there be open or closed groups? (Open groups allow people to drop out or join randomly. Closed groups start with a small group of people and don't add newcomers, even if some drop out.)

☐ If this program does provide counseling, how are the counselors trained? Are they professionals with the appropriate educational degrees, or were they "trained" at a weekend seminar?

☐ Does this program offer any type of continuing education — for example, classes on nutrition, preparing healthy meals, exercise safety, etc.? If so, are the teachers properly trained?

☐ Does this program stress long-term behavior changes that will help you keep the weight off and live a healthier life, or does it focus on quick weight-loss gimmicks?

☐ Do you set your own weight-loss goals, or do program directors help you decide how much weight to lose?

Take time to ask questions. Each of these factors will impact the success or failure of your weight-loss plan. It's important to get all the information you can on the program you're thinking of joining.

You might want to ask your doctor or pharmacist about the weight-loss plan you're considering. They can look at the information you have gathered and give you a "professional" opinion on the program.

Professional weight-loss programs are certainly not the only way to effectively lose weight and keep it off. However, if a professional weight-loss program is the route you choose to follow, make sure you've done your "homework."

Getting the facts before you start the program will help you make the right decision on the best program to suit your needs and improve your chances of creating a new, slimmer you.

Medical Source ——————————————————
  Nutrition Today (27,4:27)

Weight loss dangers

Losing weight the natural way is a great and healthy concept, unless the "natural way" includes herbal tea made from the herb germander. Seven people who drank the natural herbal tea to help them lose weight ended up battling a dangerous illness.

Folk medicine has suggested that the herb germander can help with weight loss. Available in herbal tea bags, herbal liquors and even capsules, germander preparations were considered harmless. The latest evidence suggests otherwise.

After about nine weeks of drinking the tea, these people went to their doctors complaining of abdominal bloating and pain, unusual tiredness, vomiting, nausea and jaundice (yellowing of the skin and whites of the eyes). Jaundice is caused by problems with the liver.

The doctors realized that the people were suffering from hepatitis (inflammation of the liver). If not treated properly and quickly, hepatitis can be life-threatening.

Fortunately, the doctors treated the hepatitis successfully, and the illnesses and symptoms cleared up after a few months. The doctors told the seven people to avoid the herbal tea.

If you have been drinking herbal teas, germander herbs or any other herbal preparations and notice suspicious symptoms, discontinue use of the product immediately and contact your doctor.

Medical Source ——————————————————
  Annals of Internal Medicine (117,2:129)

EXERCISE AND FITNESS

Fight colds and flu with exercise

Can moderate exercise boost your immune system? Most people who exercise will agree that it makes them feel healthier.

But can regular exercise actually strengthen your immune system to help fight off colds and flu? While studies are ongoing, some researchers now believe that moderate exercise can help boost your immune system — if you enjoy it.

If exercising is stressful, chances are it could have negative effects on your immune system. But if exercising is a joy — researchers believe it is probably beneficial in helping your immune system fight off infections.

Researchers believe that moderate exercise helps increase the activities of natural killer cells which can help fight off viruses and other illnesses.

Other studies show that even if you develop a cold — regular, moderate exercise can lessen the severity of your cold and make it go away quicker.

Try these other natural ways to avoid infections:

- ❏ Never share your water bottles with anyone.
- ❏ Wear shower shoes if you shower where you work out, and don't share your soap with anyone else.
- ❏ Wash your hands often.

While moderate exercise can help boost your immune system, studies show that long, intense exercise may have the opposite effect. It can actually leave you more prone to infections. It increases the output of adrenaline and cortisol which can lower your immune defenses.

What if you have an upper respiratory infection — is it safe to exercise? If you have symptoms above the neck, such as a runny nose, sneezing or scratchy throat — you can go ahead and exercise with caution.

Begin slowly, and if you start to feel weak, develop a headache or just don't feel well, stop exercising and rest a few more days. However, if you have a fever or symptoms below the neck, such as muscle aches, a hacking cough, vomiting or diarrhea — don't work out.

You need to wait until these symptoms have disappeared before you get back into your workout routine.

General exercise tips:

❑ Remember to gently stretch your muscles before and after your workout.

❑ Drink plenty of water while exercising. This rule applies in cold weather as well as hot.

❑ Wear a hat and gloves while exercising outdoors in cold weather to avoid losing body heat.

❑ Slow down a little and take a few deep breaths if you get a cramp in your side.

❑ Stop exercising and call your doctor immediately if you have severe chest pain, shortness of breath, dizziness or vomiting.

Medical Source —————————————————————
The Physician and Sportsmedicine (21,1:125)

Staying fit for a healthy heart

If you've been putting off exercising because it seems to take too much effort, take heart.

Researchers now say that you don't have to be extremely fit to lower your risk of heart disease. And this is just one of the benefits of moderate aerobic exercise.

Regular walking, swimming, jogging, biking or other aerobic activity can increase your life span, keep your weight and blood sugar under control, and may reduce your risk of cancer.

One way of determining your exercise rate is to measure how quickly you use oxygen during exercise. An easy way to measure exercise intensity at home is to measure your heart rate with an electronic heart monitor.

Your doctor, as well as many current fitness books, can provide charts showing what your heart rate should be for your age and fitness level. They can also tell you what your heart rate should be to improve fitness. But what is moderate, you ask warily.

Moderate means that while exercising, you maintain your heart rate at 40 to 60 percent of your maximum heart rate.

Researcher Steven N. Blair, of the Cooper Institute of Aerobics Research, maintains that how much you exercise is more important than how hard you exercise.

He believes that 30 to 40 minutes of walking or other exercise equivalent to that, if done regularly, will improve the average person's fitness level and result in important health benefits.

Is vigorous exercise, or exercise in which you maintain your heart rate above 60 percent of your maximum, better? It depends on your situation, but probably yes. More vigorous activity seems to result in increased cardiovascular benefits.

In a study of Harvard alumni, heart-disease risk was reduced more significantly among people who played vigorous sports as opposed to those who participated in less strenuous activities.

Studies have also indicated a relationship between higher energy output and longer life spans. Additionally, if you are already active or are trying to improve athletic performance, you will have to exercise more intensely to achieve significant results.

The bottom line is that people who do a little bit of exercise are better off than those who don't do any exercise. And those who do a little more are even better off.

Although higher levels of exercise will result in greater benefits, the important thing is to exercise regularly.

According to Dr. John Cantwell, a cardiologist at Georgia Baptist Medical Center, taking up some form of exercise that you enjoy doing for a long period of time is usually better than getting into an activity that puts you at risk for injury and causes you to drop out in just a few weeks.

So, find an exercise you like and stick with it. With so many benefits from even a little exercise, what are you waiting for?

Medical Source ——————————————————
The Physician and Sportsmedicine (20,12:123)

Measuring your heart rate

The simplest way to find your target heart rate is to follow this formula:

> ➤ **Subtract your age** from 220 to find your maximum heart rate (for example 220 - 40 = 180).
> ➤ **Multiply by the rate** you'd like to hit (80% of your maximum heart rate would be .80 x 180 = 144).
> ➤ **Take your pulse** during exercise. You'll find it by placing your fingertips near the base of your thumb on the palm side of your hand, or on your throat next to your Adam's apple. Count the beats for 15 seconds, and then multiply by 4. (Or count for 10 seconds and multiply by 6. If you're 40, your target heart rate for 10 seconds would be 24.)

The higher your target heart rate during exercise, the more fit you will be and the shorter your workout can be.

After you've exercised for several weeks, you may need to increase your level of intensity to maintain the heart rate you want.

Consult your doctor before beginning an exercise program.

Medical Source ─────────────────
The Physician and Sportsmedicine (21,3:227)

Burn more fat with moderate exercise

In the struggle to fight off fat, "no pain — no gain" used to be the battle cry for fitness buffs.

But as the fitness boom comes of age, sportsmedicine specialists realize that a longer, less intense workout is actually more effective than a short, tough exercise routine.

According to some authorities, your body can only burn off fat when you exercise aerobically or "with air." In other words, your activity should raise your heart rate from 60 to 80 percent of its maximum rate.

After exercising at this level for 20 minutes, your body will begin to consume fat for fuel.

On the other hand, if your workout pushes your heart rate above 85 percent of the maximum level, this is considered anaerobic or "without air" exercise.

At this point, your body automatically switches over to the higher test fuels, carbohydrates and protein, leaving the fat right where you don't want it!

Here are some tips to help you get the most out of your aerobic workout:

- ❏ Establish a target heart rate using the guidelines given on the previous page.
- ❏ Check your heart rate regularly during your workout.
- ❏ Exercise aerobically three to five times weekly for 20 to 60 minutes each time.
- ❏ Include your arms in your workout, but don't raise them over your head.
- ❏ Be sure to involve the muscles of your legs, stomach and chest.
- ❏ If your heart rate gets too high, lower the intensity of your workout by keeping your arms down and your feet close to the ground or floor.

Finally, keep in mind that length, not intensity, is the factor that assures you of a workout that benefits your heart and burns off fat at the same time.

Medical Source ————————————————
Cardiac Alert (14,12:5)

The practical fat-burning exercise

Need to exercise but can't afford an expensive health club membership or a complicated piece of computerized machinery? Try shoveling snow. If done correctly, shoveling snow can give you a good workout — but don't overdo it — or you could end up with an aching back or worse.

Besides being totally free and very practical, snow shoveling can be a great aerobic exercise. Briskly shoveling light snow can burn as many calories as playing a tennis match.

Several aspects of snow shoveling make it an excellent aerobic workout. For example, using both your arms and legs to lift the weight of the snow increases your heart rate and works the muscles.

Also, just being outside in the cold winter air makes you breathe faster and your heart pump harder to circulate warm blood through your body.

Be sure to check with your doctor before you decide to shovel your driveway. It can be very dangerous for people with heart problems.

Here are some tips on getting the best workout from shoveling snow from Dr. Barry A. Franklin, director of Cardiac Rehabilitation and Exercise Laboratories at William Beaumont Hospital in Royal Oak, Michigan:

☐ Keep your knees slightly bent as you lift your shovel. By using both your arms and legs, you will increase the aerobic aspect of your exercise and decrease the risk of straining your back.

☐ Don't try to lift too much snow at one time. Shovel small loads.

☐ If possible, push or sweep snow. Don't lift heavy snow if you don't have to.

☐ Go at your own pace. You are the best judge of your ability, so listen to your body and take a break when you need one.

☐ Don't eat a big meal or drink alcohol before going out to shovel snow. Contrary to popular belief, alcohol will not keep you warm. It adds to the workload for your heart and circulatory system.

☐ Dress warmly in several light layers. As you warm up, you can easily remove a layer or two and maintain a comfortable temperature.

By following these helpful hints and being careful not to overdo it, you can get a great workout and clear your driveway at the same time.

Medical Source ———————————————————
The Physician and Sportsmedicine (21,1:177)

Why jog when you can walk?

Does the regular jogger who also lifts weights five times a week get more cardiovascular benefits than the regular walker who follows a moderate exercise program?

A National Exercise for Life Institute report says that although the person who exercises heavily might be more fit, the "light" exerciser gets exactly the same cardiovascular benefits.

That means if you are a walker, you can lose body fat and improve your "good" HDL cholesterol levels just as a jogger can. According to some fitness experts, your body burns the most fat and achieves the best aerobic conditioning when you exercise at low to moderate intensity.

That's important news for couch potatoes because the Centers for Disease Control in Atlanta reports that an inactive lifestyle causes more deaths each year than high blood pressure, diabetes or smoking.

You say you don't have enough time to begin a regular exercise program? The National Exercise for Life Institute estimates that most Americans have 15 to 18 hours of free time every week, some of which we could use to get in shape.

The Institute suggests that many people keep exercise painless by scheduling workouts in one of these ways:

> Skip the commute and walk, jog or bike to work.
> Create your own home gym.
> Take advantage of a corporate fitness program and work out during your workday.
> Pick up the pace on daily activities like yard work, housework or grocery shopping.
> Remember that whether you enjoy a heavy workout or just a brisk walk, whatever elevates your pulse rate will help your heart stay healthy!

Medical Source ————————————————
Aviation Medical Bulletin, May 1992

Healthy heart habits are important for women, too

Women start out with a lower risk of heart disease than men because young women have lower blood pressure and higher levels of "good" cholesterol (HDL). However, as women approach menopause, hormone changes begin to cancel out that advantage.

Older women tend to be more depressed and to have lower levels of HDL cholesterol. They also often gain weight, which can trigger high blood pressure.

All of these factors add up to a higher risk of heart disease and stroke.

But researchers believe that women can use exercise to put the brakes on these changes.

After studying over 500 middle-aged women, they report that the healthiest women were those who continued or began to exercise regularly.

These active women gained less weight, reported less stress and depression and showed a slower decline in HDL cholesterol than the nonexercisers.

Older women can easily get the protection exercise offers without making dramatic changes in their lives.

For example, walking only 20 minutes three times a week uses 300 calories per week, and the results are worth it. You can lose weight, maintain your levels of HDL cholesterol, and keep your spirits up at the same time.

Medical Source ───────────────────────
Circulation (85,4:1265)

Are morning or afternoon workouts better?

The peak time for heart attacks and other serious cardiac events occurs between 6:00 a.m. and 12:00 noon. More people suffer from heart attacks and other life-threatening cardiac events during that time period than any other time of day or night.

The factors behind the large number of morning cardiac events are interrelated and include the following: increases in heart rate and blood pressure, greater "stickiness" of the platelets in the blood that can lead to clots, and greater surges of hormones that can trigger a cardiac event.

Given the fact that morning is the most dangerous time for people with high risks of heart attacks or other life-threatening cardiac events, many people wonder if they should avoid exercising in the mornings to lower their risk of having a heart attack. The answer is no, according to one medical study.

A group of scientists from the Bowman Gray School of Medicine at Wake Forest University in Winston-Salem, N.C., evaluated cardiac events in two groups of people with known heart disease who exercised either in the morning or the afternoon.

The group of volunteers who exercised in the mornings was made up of men and women with an average age of 63 years. Seventy-six percent of the group were men.

The evening-exercise group contained 83 percent men, and the average age of the entire group (men and women) was 61 years.

The exercise sessions lasted for one hour per day, with a 10-minute warm-up phase, a 40-minute exercise period, and a 10-minute cool-down phase. The volunteers exercised three days each week.

The morning exercise group worked out from 7:30 to 8:30 a.m., and the afternoon exercise group worked out for one hour anytime between 3:00 and 5:00 in the afternoon. The aerobic exercise included walking, jogging, swimming or bicycling.

During each morning and afternoon exercise session, physical therapy staff members and an internist or a cardiologist were present to determine which time of day would be the safest for the heart muscle.

After monitoring 168,111 hours of patient exercise in the morning hours and 84,491 hours of afternoon exercise, the scientists gathered the records they had made and compared results.

They found that morning exercise resulted in about three cardiac events per 100,000 hours of exercise. Afternoon exercise resulted in about 2.4 cardiac events per 100,000 hours of exercise.

In other words, the number of serious cardiac events in people with heart disease undergoing regular exercise was very low, whether the person exercised in the morning or in the afternoon.

The time of day of the exercise session did not seem to have a significant effect on the number of cardiac events that occurred during exercise. The scientists suggested that regular exercise for people with heart disease is very safe and very desirable, whether in the morning or the afternoon.

If you are suffering from heart disease and your doctor has recommended that you exercise regularly to strengthen your heart, you are safe to exercise any time of the day that happens to be convenient for you.

Always check with your doctor to make sure your exercise plan is not too strenuous for your heart — too much exercise during any time of the day could be hazardous to your health.

Medical Source ————————————————
Archives of Internal Medicine (153,7:833)

How to choose a workout time

If your heart doesn't care when you exercise, is there a prime time of day to work out? The best time of day is whatever works best for you. Here are a few points to consider:

Morning workouts

☐ Morning workouts can help you feel ready to face daily stress.
☐ In general, morning workouts are better on your lungs, but your body might not be as flexible as in the evening.
☐ Some studies suggest that early-bird exercisers are most likely to stick with a workout program.

Evening workouts

☐ Evening workouts may be better if you need to unwind and forget about the day's frustrations.
☐ According to Peter Raven, professor of physiology at the Texas College of Osteopathic Medicine, work out in the afternoon if you are trying to lose weight — your body temperature and, subsequently, your metabolism rate go up then.
☐ If you really want to lose weight, John Duncan, exercise physiologist and associate director of the Cooper Institute for Aerobics Research in Dallas, believes exercise right before dinner can act as an appetite suppressant.

Medical Source ————————————————
The Atlanta Journal/Constitution (March 9, 1992, B5)

Worst time for angina sufferers to work out

Remember when your mother used to warn you never to swim right after you ate?

You would always roll your eyes, wait your designated 30 minutes, then get back into the pool with no problem.

Now researchers believe that waiting for just 30 minutes after eating to exercise could be very hazardous to your health — if you suffer from angina, that is.

Angina is the medical term for chest pain that occurs when parts of the heart muscle aren't getting enough oxygen. It is not the same thing as a heart attack, and the chest pains usually go away when you sit and rest awhile.

There are millions of people across the nation who suffer from angina, and a good portion of those people exercise regularly. But scientists are now recommending that those people with stable angina who exercise regularly should wait at least five hours after a meal before beginning their exercise session.

The scientists made this recommendation after reviewing the results from a study designed to test the cardiac effects of exercising 30 minutes after a meal.

The scientists recruited 20 volunteers for the study. The average age for the volunteers was 59 years (range 47 to 70), and each one suffered from stable angina.

The scientists put the volunteers through two treadmill exercise tests to determine how the heart responded in the two different situations. For the first test, the volunteers were allowed to eat a small breakfast.

Then, five hours later on an empty stomach, they each got on the treadmill and walked until exhausted or until their chests began to hurt (angina). The scientists monitored their hearts during the treadmill test to determine how they were responding.

For the second treadmill test, the volunteers received a 1,000-calorie meal to eat before exercising. Thirty minutes after the meal, they started the treadmill test and walked until they were exhausted or until the angina was too bad to go on. Again, the scientists monitored the heart during the exercise period.

After comparing the information from the two treadmill tests, the scientists found that exercising only 30 minutes after a meal caused an average 12-percent increase in heart rate compared to exercising on an empty stomach.

Exercising on a full stomach also resulted in a 20-percent reduction in the time it took for the heart to begin suffering from a lack of oxygen, and it caused a 15-percent reduction in the amount of time before angina started.

What these results really mean is that exercising only 30 minutes after a meal causes the heart to work harder, get less oxygen and hurt more quickly compared to exercising on an empty stomach.

Exercising on an empty stomach allowed the volunteers to exercise longer before they had to stop and rest because of chest pains.

The scientists recommend that people suffering from stable angina not exercise right after a meal. Instead, they should wait at least five hours after eating to begin exercising to get the best results and put the least amount of stress on the heart.

People with unstable angina could be in danger of a heart attack if they exercise, so scientists recommend that people with unstable angina (or other serious heart conditions) talk with their doctors before beginning an exercise program.

If you suffer from chest pains, you should check with your doctor right away to make sure your heart is healthy. And be sure to ask your doctor if exercising is safe for you. If it is, plan your daily exercise session for a time of day at least five hours after your last meal for the best and safest results.

Medical Source ————————————————————
Journal of the American College of Cardiology (21:1052)

Can you exercise too much?

Exercise is good for the heart. We've heard this fact all our lives. Yet medical science still doesn't know how much exercise is beneficial.

And now a recent report indicates that too much exercise can have a harmful effect on your heart. How much is too much, you ask. Obviously, your physical condition plays a role in your overall risk. But even if you are in superb condition — that is no guarantee that you won't have heart problems.

Endurance athletes have been stricken by fatal heart attacks even in the absence of prior heart disease. Autopsies have revealed injury and scarring to the muscle of the heart without any evidence of coronary artery disease to explain why this injury would have occurred.

Normally, such scarring is the result of fatty blockages in the major arteries of the heart. If there is no blockage in the arteries of these athletes, there must be some other cause. But what?

The answer may lie in the body's manufacturing of adrenaline. Very long endurance exercise raises levels of adrenaline. Excessive levels of adrenaline can cause arteries to constrict. Spasm of the coronary arteries can result in low blood flow to regions of the heart and cause permanent injury.

What should be done to prevent this type of cardiac injury? One recommendation is to limit participation in long endurance events such as the ultra-marathon to no more than every three months.

If you plan to participate in such an event, realize that factors such as cold, heat, altitude, dehydration and electrolyte (salts, fluids and potassium in the body) depletion can also play a role.

Medical Source ─────────────────────
The Lancet (340,8821:712)

Staying young

So you're getting older ... does that mean you should hang up the sneakers, forego the weights and forget flexibility?

Absolutely not, says Dr. Henry C. Barry, assistant professor in the Department of Family Practice at Michigan State University.

If you once believed that the risks of vigorous exercise outweighed the benefits for seniors, don't buy that myth any longer.

Doctors are now saying that if you don't use it, you lose it. In other words, being a couch potato can lead to sugar intolerance, lower resistance to infection, heart trouble and deterioration of your bones, among other problems.

On the plus side, doctors now believe that exercise helps older people stay active and independent longer and can even prevent cancer. Strength training and flexibility can help prevent falls, the leading cause of death from injury for people over age 75.

In addition, exercise clearly helps seniors recover from these typical problems of age:

> Fractures   > Arthritis
> Stroke   > Depression

Don't worry that you might not be able to get fit again. Older bodies seem to adapt to exercise in the same way that younger bodies do. All it takes is about one hour three times a week.

But before you join a bench-aerobics class, ask your doctor's advice about a program that's right for you. Heart trouble, breathing problems like emphysema or chronic bronchitis, uncontrolled diabetes, seizures or arthritis prevent some people from starting or maintaining an exercise program. Certain medicines can also affect your ability to exercise.

When you do get the O.K. from your doctor, design your exercise program with these three goals in mind:

- **Flexibility** — Be sure you learn to stretch properly. Since men tend to be less flexible than women, stretching is especially important for them.

- **Increased strength** — Weight lifting helps you avoid joint and muscle injury and prevents bone thinning (osteoporosis), a serious problem for many women.

- **Cardiovascular endurance** — This should be your most important goal. You can reach this goal by swimming, walking, rowing, biking, doing water aerobics and other low-impact activities.

Whatever exercises you choose, you'll find it's easier to stick with your program if you enjoy the activities and find an exercise group or a setting that you like. Here are a few helpful hints to make your exercise program a success:

- Limit the expense of your exercise.
- Exercise with friends for added fun.
- Build variety and pleasure into your routine.

- ☐ Avoid accidents by exercising during the bright part of the day.
- ☐ Drink water before, during and after exercise to avoid dehydration. This is especially important for seniors because they have less total body water than younger people.
- ☐ Layer your clothing so that you can adapt to varying temperatures.
- ☐ Wear cotton sports socks and shoes that fit well.
- ☐ Personalize your exercise goals so they are realistic and you will be able to reach them.

A word of caution: Stop exercising and call your doctor if you experience any of these symptoms:

> ➤ Chest pain
> ➤ Shortness of breath
> ➤ Pain in neck or jaw
> ➤ Faintness or dizziness
> ➤ Excessive fatigue
> ➤ Nausea or vomiting
> ➤ Heart racing
> ➤ Extreme muscle or joint pain

Even if you have a very limited capacity to exercise, your activities can improve your quality of life.

Medical Sources ———————————————
Geriatrics (47,8:33)
The Physician and Sportsmedicine (21,2:124)

If the shoe fits ...

The shoes you wear while walking or playing your favorite sport are more than just a fashion statement. Look at your sneakers not just as an accessory, but as a part of your basic exercise equipment.

Does this mean that you need a special pair of shoes for each sport you play: one for walking, one for basketball, another for tennis and still another for your aerobics class? If you walk or engage in a sport at least three times a week, you probably need a shoe designed for that sport.

For example, running shoes are more flexible around the toe area than walking shoes. Aerobics shoes provide extra cushioning around the ball of the foot, and shoes designed for racquet sports are built to provide side-to-side stability. If you play two different sports on the same surface, you might be able to wear the same shoes for both sports.

But how do you go about finding the right shoe among the hundreds lined up on the store wall? Here are some guidelines for choosing well-fitting, comfortable sports shoes:

- Visit the shoe store in the afternoon or after your workout — when your feet are the biggest.
- Wear the socks you normally wear to exercise. And don't forget to wear socks every time you exercise. They help absorb perspiration and can help prolong the life of your shoes.
- Try the shoe on your largest foot.
- Be able to fully extend your toes in the shoe when you stand up.
- Make sure you have at least a thumbnail's length between your longest toe and the end of the shoe.

- Choose shoes that give you plenty of room in the toe area, especially if you have bunions.
- Check out the men's shoes. Men's shoes are built wider than women's shoes. A woman with wide feet might try a man's shoe two sizes smaller than the size she wears in women's shoes.
- Try to buy a well-known brand. However, the highest-priced shoe may not necessarily be the best shoe for you. Tom Brunick, footwear editor of *Runner's World* magazine, recommends choosing a shoe in the $50 to $80 price range. Cheaper shoes are often made from poor quality materials and have a shorter life span.
- Choose shoes that are comfortable from the moment you put them on.

Once you've found the perfect shoes and you're enjoying wearing them, how often do you need to replace them?

Dr. Francesca Thompson, head of the adult orthopedic foot clinic at St.

Luke's-Roosevelt Hospital Center in New York City, says that while most sports shoes are good for about 300 to 500 miles, you may need to change sneakers as often as every three months.

The midsole (the wide area between the toe and the heel) of the shoe is the part you should watch for wear; it cushions your foot and prevents it from rolling too far to the inside or outside. While the rest of the shoe may still look good — a worn midsole can cause shin splints and foot, ankle and knee troubles.

To determine if your midsole is worn out, place your sneakers on a table and examine them from eye level. If either shoe doesn't sit evenly or looks lopsided, it's time for you to get a new pair.

Medical Sources
The Physician and Sportsmedicine (21,3:204)

Home gym hazards

In increasing numbers, exercisers are bringing the gym home instead of going to the gym.

And as the number of home stationary bikes, rowing machines and treadmills increases, the number of injuries from these machines is on the rise as well.

Injuries from exercise machines fall into two categories:

> ➤ Injuries that result from allowing children to play around the machines unsupervised.
> ➤ Injuries that result from incorrect use.

Stationary bikes can be particularly dangerous for children. When the wheels of a bike are turning, the spokes seem to disappear.

Children who stick their fingers between the spokes or who get fingers stuck in the chain and sprocket assembly have actually amputated their fingers.

The dangers for adults are more likely to arise from improper use of a device. For example, if the resistance is set too high on a rowing machine, you may injure your joints or ligaments or the muscles of your lower back.

If you are thinking about buying home exercise equipment, consider these helpful tips:

- ☐ Remember that quality is more important than cost in the long run, and you usually get what you pay for.
- ☐ Choose a machine that is built solidly, with no exposed cables or chains to injure little fingers. Many exercise bikes are now built with spokeless wheels.
- ☐ Look for comfort and a good fit. If it's not comfortable, you won't use it!
- ☐ Try the machine out for a few days before buying it if the dealer allows.
- ☐ Get instructions on how to use the machine properly.
- ☐ Don't get features you don't think you will use or need.
- ☐ Get a warranty on your machine.
- ☐ Don't allow children to play unsupervised on exercise equipment.

Medical Source ───────────────────────
The Physician and Sportsmedicine (21,2:59)

Exercise without fear of Fido

You're out for a jog or bike ride, minding your own business, your mind a thousand miles away. Little did you know, you've just invaded the territory of the giant dog across the street. You're on his turf, and now you're wondering if you'll make it home in one piece.

Unfortunately, the boundaries of a dog's territory are invisible, and can extend well beyond the dog's own yard. When you're out running, you're on a dog's turf before you know it, and he feels threatened.

Movement can compound the problem too. After all, you're just as much fun to chase as a squirrel, only you're bigger. And if Fido is a natural herder like a border collie, your motion might even trigger his instinct to "herd" you back into his territory.

In the face of a fearsome display of canine courage, what can outdoor exercisers do to ensure safety? Body language is the key to dealing with angry dogs:

☐ Watch ahead for free-range dogs. If the dog has picked you up on his radar, he will be standing, looking at you with ears erect.

☐ When you see a potentially dangerous pooch ahead, do an about face or move to the other side of the street. Slow or maintain your speed.

☐ Avoid eye contact. Dogs see stares as a challenge.

☐ Walk with your own canine companion. Dogs with long legs and short hair make the best running companions. Your exercise mate should also be a mature, leash-trained dog whose overall health is good.

In case of a dog attack, you can minimize your danger by freezing immediately. Then you have a few choices:

☐ Face the dog, so that you look bigger, and firmly command, "No," "Sit," "Stay," or "Go home." Of course, this direct contact could backfire and enrage the dog more.

☐ Imitate the submissive behavior you've seen some dogs use. Turn sideways and lean away from the dog with your hands across your chest or at your side.

☐ Don't look at the dog and don't scream.

☐ If you are riding a bike, put the bicycle between you and the dog.

When the dog retreats, the time has come for you to sidestep slowly away.

If a dog attacks and knocks you to the ground, curl in a ball with your hands in fists covering your ears (fingers and ears are the most likely targets in a dog attack).

If you can, "feed" your jacket or other piece of clothing to the dog, so the dog will bite it instead of you.

You should thoroughly wash any dog bite with soap and water, and check with your doctor to see if you need antibiotics, tetanus or rabies shots.

Finally, report the offending canine to the police. Although many communities do not strictly enforce leash laws, heightened awareness can be your first step to better animal control.

Medical Source ————————————————————
The Physician and Sportsmedicine (21,4:142)

Exercise and diarrhea: What you can do to stop the trots

You're in the middle of your daily walk when suddenly the urge to have a bowel movement hits you right in the gut.

This troublesome tendency can range from cramping and diarrhea to the urge to have a bowel movement during your exercise. It can even mean having bloody diarrhea after strenuous exertion.

But if you plan ahead, you can avoid exercise-induced stomach pain and cramping, nausea, gas, diarrhea, heartburn and rectal bleeding, says Dr. Bryant Stamford, director of the Health Promotion and Wellness Center and professor of allied health, School of Medicine, University of Louisville, Kentucky.

When you exercise vigorously, your body automatically reduces activity in your digestive system. This is due to our built-in "fight or flight" mechanism that says exercise (being able to run away or fight) is more critical to survival than digestion.

Suppose you've just eaten dinner, and then you go out for a jog. Both digestion and exercise require a huge blood flow, but your body simply can't serve two masters at one time. Your working muscles take priority and most of the blood flow is diverted away from your digestive system, resulting in intestinal discomfort.

Dr. Stamford says that gastrointestinal problems like diarrhea can also occur for any or all of these reasons:

❏ Working out can disrupt the normal function of hormones and nutrients that aid in the absorption of nutrients.

❏ Moving and breathing vigorously can agitate and squeeze the digestive system, forcing food through the intestines too quickly. Exercises that jar your body, such as running, are most likely to cause frequent bowel movements.

❏ Taking anti-inflammatories like aspirin and ibuprofen before or during your workout can cause bleeding in your stomach.

❏ Sweating and diarrhea can cause dehydration, which lowers the amount of blood in your body. You can actually sweat two to eight cups of water an hour if you're working out strenuously on a hot day.

☐ Anxiety during exercise can trigger diarrhea.

☐ People who are allergic to insect stings or who break out in itching hives while exercising tend to get diarrhea.

☐ Various dietary factors, including high-fiber diets, milk intolerance and some of the sugars found in fruits, can set off bowel disturbances. Sometimes problems of this sort resolve themselves as you become more fit.

Stomach upsets may persist even after you stop exercising, because it takes your body several hours to readjust after a hard workout.

Postponing your workout for two to three hours after a meal will help solve some of your GI problems. But you don't have to give up the idea of exercising after eating.

A brisk walk not only speeds the passage of food through the GI tract, it also relaxes the mind, and your body digests food better when your mind and body are relaxed.

Try these tips to avoid stomach problems while exercising:

☐ Wait two to three hours after a meal to begin exercising. Liquid meals can help you avoid diarrhea.

☐ Choose foods that are high in carbohydrates, not in fat or protein.

☐ Go to the bathroom just before exercising.

☐ Avoid dairy products, fruits and products sweetened with sorbitol and mannitol.

☐ Avoid gassy foods like broccoli and beans.

☐ Drink water or low-sugar sports drinks to avoid dehydration.

☐ Reduce the need for nonsteroidal anti-inflammatory drugs, or NSAIDs (aspirin, ibuprofen, etc.). Warm up before you exercise and reduce the intensity of your workout. If you must use NSAIDs, take them after you exercise.

☐ If you'll be participating in a particular event, train at the hour of day the event will start to allow your body to get accustomed to exercising at that time.

By planning ahead, you should be able to exercise without worrying about embarrassing or uncomfortable tummy troubles.

If the problem persists, check with your doctor to make sure there is no other health problem causing the diarrhea.

If all else fails, ask your doctor about trying a diarrhea medicine containing dioctahedral smectite. These products seem helpful in preventing diarrhea.

Medical Source ────────────────────
The Physician and Sportsmedicine (20,10:63 and 20,11:163)

When exercise is a pain in the ... knee

It may hit you during exercise or afterwards; it can make your knee swell, and it can make sitting in a car, riding a bike or going up and down the stairs a real pain in the ... knee.

Patellofemoral syndrome (pain behind the kneecap) is one of the most common injuries among runners. But regardless of when it starts, knee pain can really throw your exercise routine off track.

Dr. Thomas Rizzo, a consultant to the Department of Physical Medicine and Rehabilitation at the Mayo Clinic in Rochester, Minn. and codirector of the Mayo Sports Medicine Center, says patellofemoral syndrome results when the kneecap fails to move in a straight line up and down at the end of the thigh bone.

Certain people are more likely to develop this disorder:

> ➤ Youngsters who are still growing
> ➤ Runners, basketball and tennis players
> ➤ Women (because of the angle at which the thigh and knee meet)
> ➤ People with flat feet

Of course, you can't change some of these characteristics, but Dr. Rizzo has a few suggestions for preventing and reducing behind-the-kneecap pain:

❏ Avoid a sudden, large increase in the speed and distance of your daily run.

☐ Replace worn running shoes.

☐ Stop activities that cause knee pain.

☐ Change to an activity that doesn't make the kneecap hurt. Swimming using the flutter kick can strengthen your thigh muscles, too.

☐ Take aspirin or ibuprofen to reduce inflammation (unless you have stomach problems or ulcers).

☐ Use ice packs for 20 minutes daily to relieve pain.

☐ Stretch your hamstring muscles and strengthen your thigh muscles. Stretching your hamstring muscles can reduce pressure on the underside of the kneecap.

Hamstring stretch

Sit on the floor. Extend your left leg straight out in front of you. Place your right foot against the inside of your left knee. Lean forward toward your ankles until you feel a stretch in your left thigh.

Hold for 30 seconds to three minutes. Repeat the exercise for the right leg. Do your hamstring stretches twice a day.

Thigh muscle stretches

These exercises work well to strengthen thigh muscles. Stop the exercises if you feel any pain.

1) Stand with your back to a wall. Your feet should be 1 1/2 to 2 feet from the wall. Lean against the wall. Slowly lower your body until your thighs are parallel to the floor. Hold this position for 10 seconds. Repeat three times. Stop the exercise if you feel pain.

2) Strap on a pair of ankle weights. (Ask your doctor what size would be best for you.) Place a large, soft pillow or firm ball under the sore knee. Recline on your back. Prop yourself up with your elbows. Raise your ankle, tightening the muscles on top of your thigh, until your leg is extended straight out. Hold this position for 10 seconds. Repeat the exercise three times.

3) Recline on your back. Prop yourself up with your elbows. Squeeze a pillow between your knees. Hold for 10 seconds. Repeat this exercise three times.

You may need to do these exercises for four to six weeks before the pain lessens. Continue these exercises even after the pain is gone.

Medical Sources ────────────────────

American Family Physician (47,1:185)
The Physician and Sportsmedicine (20,12:141)

Running, jumping and shin splints

Running might not be considered a contact sport — but just tell that to your legs!

The stress of regular running and jumping can inflame the muscles and tendons on the front of your leg above the ankle so badly that you're actually unable to run.

Runners call this condition shin splints because it hurts along the shinbone, but the real name for this injury is medial tibial stress syndrome. It is the most common of all running injuries.

If you run two miles daily, you're taking more than 3,000 strides. For each step you run, your leg absorbs two to three times your body weight. So it's easy to understand how almost 20 percent of all runners get this painful injury at one time or another.

Fortunately, there are steps you can take to prevent shin splints:

❏ Stretch carefully before running.
❏ Warm up and cool down slowly.
❏ Wear the right shoes. Some runners believe the shock-absorbing power of running shoes wears out after 300 miles.
❏ Alternate two different brands of running shoes to give your feet and legs a break.

Shin splints often start as pain that accompanies the beginning of your workout and then disappears during your run. If your shin splints get worse, you may feel the pain throughout your workout and into the cool-down.

At their worst, the pain of shin splints will persist into your everyday routine, and the front of your leg above the ankle will feel tender to the touch.

Changing your routine for a couple of weeks can help you recover from shin splints:

- ☐ If pain doesn't prevent you from running, continue your workouts, taking special care to warm up and cool down slowly.
- ☐ If pain persists throughout your run, give your legs a rest from running. Change to no-impact activities like riding a stationary bicycle, using a stair-climbing machine or swimming.
- ☐ Massage your shins with ice for eight to 10 minutes three times daily, especially after your workout.
- ☐ Take an anti-inflammatory, such as ibuprofen.
- ☐ As your shin splints improve, move up to treadmill running or running on a flat, even surface.
- ☐ Stretch your leg muscles carefully (if it doesn't cause any pain).
- ☐ Ease back into your running routine by running every other day or alternating running with a no-impact activity.

You'll probably be able to start running regularly again about four to eight weeks after your injury.

Dr. Daniel S. Fick, a member of the departments of family practice and orthopedic surgery at the University of Iowa Hospitals and Clinics in Iowa City, recommends that you follow the rule of the "toos" to prevent shin splints or to avoid reinjury: don't run too much, too soon, too fast.

See your doctor if pain persists.

Medical Source ───────────────────────
The Physician and Sportsmedicine (20,12:105)

When running is out, try cycling and water workouts

Running — it's good for your heart and a balm to your soul, say fitness buffs.

Unfortunately, more of it may not always be better. Run too much too often, and before you know it you have an overuse injury that could sideline you for up to six weeks.

So you have to back off on running for a while. But just three weeks of being a couch potato and your cardiovascular fitness goes down the tubes.

However, a team of researchers from Brigham Young University have discovered that you can maintain a high level of fitness by changing activities during your healing period.

The goal of their study was to discover whether healthy runners could switch from jogging to deep water running or cycling for six weeks and maintain the same performance on a two-mile run and a test of oxygen use.

During the study, one-third of the participants ran, one-third cycled and one-third jogged in deep water wearing flotation vests.

At the end of the six-week period, all three groups slightly improved their performances in the two-mile run and showed similar changes in their oxygen use.

Water aerobics and water walking are excellent alternative ways to exercise. They help ease the jarring and pounding muscles and joints experience during a run.

Medical Source ————————————————
American Journal of Sports Medicine (21,1:41)

Health risks

Quitters are winners

"Better late than never."

This time-tested cliché has never been more true than it is with smoking — better to stop smoking late in the game than never at all.

Unfortunately, many people who have smoked cigarettes for 20 years or more think that stopping smoking after that much time is really pointless. "The damage is done now — stopping won't help anything," is their common excuse.

The good news is that it will help. The lungs start healing almost immediately after you quit smoking. Researchers conducted a five-year study on 7,181 elderly men to test the effects of smoking cessation after many years of smoking, and the results were encouraging.

Men who were current smokers experienced twice the rate of dying from smoking-related illnesses, such as heart attack, cancer, etc., compared to people who had never smoked.

However, former smokers (those who quit smoking) experienced the same low rate of dying from heart problems as people who had never smoked. In other words, the former smokers had no greater risk of dying from heart problems than people who had never smoked.

And those results were true for people who stopped smoking 20 years ago, or for those who stopped smoking two days before the study began. No matter how old you are or how long you have smoked, you can still cut your risk of dying from heart disease or cancer if you quit smoking.

Every year, as many as 17 million people try to quit smoking, reports the Food and Drug Administration. Unfortunately, only about 1.3 million succeed.

Try these helpful hints to make your journey to a smoke-free life easier:

☐ Keep track of the times and situations that make you want to smoke. For example, do you smoke only when you are tense or nervous? Do you smoke when you get bored? Do you smoke only when you talk on the phone? Or only after meals?

☐ Fill in the times and situations that make you want to smoke with other activities. For example, exercise or go for walks when you get nervous. Remove ashtrays from phone areas, and limit your phone conversations to minimize your temptation to smoke. Sit in the nonsmoking section of restaurants to avoid smoking after meals.

☐ Cut down a little at a time. For example, don't smoke the whole cigarette—smoke less of each cigarette you light. Try inhaling less deeply or not inhaling every time you put a cigarette in your mouth. Also, consider switching to a low-tar, low-nicotine brand of cigarettes.

☐ Keep a diary of how many cigarettes you smoke and how much money you spend on cigarettes each day. Document each day that you smoke fewer than the day before. Don't get discouraged and give up if you "slip" sometimes. Just do better the next day.

☐ Enlist the help and support of family and friends. Ask them to help you resist temptations, and encourage them to be patient during the times that nicotine withdrawal makes you nervous and irritable.

☐ Don't be discouraged if you gain a few pounds as you quit smoking. The weight gain is usually only a small one. Starting a regular exercise or walking program will help you burn off those extra calories and will also help you occupy your time and energy so you won't be as likely to smoke because of boredom.

☐ Plan to avoid places where smoking is accepted and even encouraged, such as lounges or break rooms at work, smoking sections in restaurants, etc. Ask other friends or family members not to smoke around you to help you resist the temptation.

☐ Join a local support group for moral support. The American Lung Association, the American Cancer Society and the American Heart

Association can give you names and addresses of groups meeting in your area.

☐ Talk to your doctor about a nicotine-replacement program, such as nicotine gum or nicotine transdermal patches. Nicotine gum is just like regular chewing gum except that it contains nicotine, the addictive substance in cigarettes that makes the smoking habit so hard to break. The transdermal patch is a Band-Aid type patch that contains nicotine. It delivers nicotine to the blood through the skin.

The trouble most people have when they try to quit smoking is nicotine withdrawal. They suffer from irritability, anger, anxiety, headaches, hunger, restlessness and the inability to concentrate as their bodies "withdraw" from their daily doses of nicotine.

Nicotine gum and nicotine transdermal patches replace the nicotine while the person cuts down on cigarettes. Later, that person can gradually lower the doses of the nicotine from the gum or patch and soon be nicotine- and cigarette-free.

Cigarette smoke contains more than 4,000 chemicals that can possibly harm the body, and each year smoking is blamed for countless cases of lung cancer, heart attacks and other serious health problems. Breaking the cigarette habit greatly reduces the risk of those dangerous illnesses.

Medical Sources ———————————————————
Emergency Medicine (24,14:26)
Geriatrics (47,12:57)
FDA Consumer (26,10:16)

Unexpected risk from quitting smoking

Exchanging a bad habit for a healthy habit is often the way people quit smoking.

But, for one 55-year-old man, his new habit eventually put him in a life-threatening situation. The man quit smoking after suffering a heart attack, and he began chewing gum to ease the difficulty of kicking the smoking habit.

At a routine check-up a few months later, his doctor noticed that the man's blood pressure was a little high, so he prescribed some medicine and sent the man home. The medicine seemed to work fine in controlling his blood pressure.

A few years later, however, when the man came in complaining of stomach pain, his doctor found that his blood pressure was up again and the level of potassium in his blood was too low. (Potassium is an important mineral in the blood — too much or too little can cause life-threatening heart problems.)

The doctor soon discovered that the man had been chewing two packs daily of a type of gum known as Stimerol since he quit smoking four years ago.

The gum contained glycyrrhizinic acid, which causes the body to retain sodium and lose potassium, resulting in high blood pressure. Licorice contains this same chemical.

The doctor advised the man to stop chewing gum, and four weeks later his health improved. Fortunately, he suffered no serious consequences from the gum.

If you use special brands of chewing gum to break the smoking habit, talk to your doctor or pharmacist about possible side effects. Follow any instructions carefully to avoid potential problems.

Medical Source ————————————————
The Lancet (341,8838:175)

Kicking the habit may be easier if you're black

If you are trying to kick the smoking habit, your chances of success are better if you are African-American.

Black smokers find it easier to quit smoking than white smokers because they are generally less addicted to nicotine than their white smoking counterparts.

An incredible 98 percent of black former smokers are able to quit smoking without any outside help or intervention. However, only 85 percent of white former smokers are able to quit on their own.

Black smokers also seem less addicted to nicotine than white smokers.

Apparently, black smokers find it easier to refrain from smoking in nonsmoking areas or situations than the white smokers in the study.

Black smokers also reported smoking fewer cigarettes each day compared to white smokers, and they waited longer in the mornings before having their first daily cigarette.

These results indicate that African-American smokers usually have a lower level of nicotine dependence than white smokers, which makes it easier for them to quit smoking altogether.

Medical Source ————————————————————
American Heart Association news release (Nov. 18, 1992)

Children's behavior up in smoke

Your child's behavior seems out of control. You never know what to expect next — disobedience, depression or cruelty to other children. Debating the problem, you reach for a cigarette to calm your nerves.

Before you smoke it, consider this: It may be your smoking habit that has sent your child's behavior problems skyrocketing.

Researchers investigated 2,256 children from ages 4 to 11 and found a direct link between moms who smoked and children with behavior problems. After questioning the moms, who ranged in age from 21 to 29, investigators found that smoking during pregnancy, only after pregnancy or both significantly increased the risk that their children would have behavior problems.

Misbehavior seems to worsen with the number of cigarettes smoked. Smoking more than a pack of cigarettes a day increased the risk of behavior problems 1.54 times; smoking less than a pack a day increased this risk 1.41 times.

Children born with certain characteristics, such as low birth weight and asthma, often have increased risks of behavior problems. Smoking appears to multiply these risks.

For example, a male child with an extremely low birth weight whose mother smokes a pack or more of cigarettes per day is eight times more likely to have extreme behavior problems than other children. If the child also has asthma, his risk of extreme behavior problems is increased more than 19 times.

Researchers have several theories to explain the apparent link between maternal smoking and children's behavior disorders.

Children regularly exposed to smoke, either during or after pregnancy, may have alterations in brain structure or function which lead to behavior problems.

Another possibility is that smoking alters the mother's behavior, causing increased behavior problems in her children. It may simply be that smoking lowers a mother's tolerance level so that she interprets normal childhood behavior as a problem.

This study adds yet another item to the growing list of adverse conditions found in children whose mothers smoke. Low birth weight, higher rates of infant death, more respiratory and ear infections, asthma and even a slightly lowered IQ have all been linked to maternal smoking.

The bottom line is this: To improve your child's behavior and overall health, give your smoking habit a kick in the butt.

Medical Source ————————————————
Pediatrics (90,3:342)

Smoking and cancer: More than your lungs are at risk

Cigarette smoking puts more than your lungs at risk of cancer. It may increase your risk of cervical cancer, too.

Some scientists noticed that a large number of women who had cervical cancer also smoked and had an infection from the sexually transmitted virus known as the human papillomavirus.

So, a group of researchers from the University Hospital in Groningen, Netherlands, recruited 181 women to participate in a study to determine the link between cigarette smoking, cervical cancer and the human papillomavirus.

Each of the 181 volunteers had experienced two abnormal Pap smears in the previous year. The abnormal Pap smears indicated the possibility of cervical cancer.

To determine whether there was a link between smoking, human papillomavirus (HPV) and cervical cancer, the researchers performed several tests to gather the necessary information for the study.

They had the women fill out detailed questionnaires that contained vital information about smoking history, age of first sexual encounter, the number of sexual partners in their lifetimes and other medical questions. (The younger the age of the first sexual encounter and the greater the number of sexual partners, the higher the risk of contracting the human papillomavirus.)

Then, the scientists performed biopsies of the abnormal cervical cells to look for cancer and other abnormalities.

The scientists also performed routine laboratory tests to determine if any of the volunteers suffered from an infection with the human papillomavirus.

After gathering all the necessary data, the researchers studied the information and came up with some interesting results.

They found that cigarette smoking is not directly related to cervical cancer. Smoking doesn't seem to directly increase the likelihood of a woman developing cervical cancer.

However, the scientists discovered that smoking seems to damage the body's natural immune response to viruses, making a woman who smokes more likely to become infected with the human papillomavirus than a woman who does not smoke.

The smoker's immune system can't fight off the virus as well as the nonsmoker's can.

The scientists also found that infection with the human papillomavirus seems to increase a woman's risk of getting cervical cancer. Therefore, smoking seems to indirectly be related to cervical cancer. Smoking results in a weaker immune response to the human papillomavirus, which increases the risk of developing cervical cancer.

If you smoke, talk to your doctor about your risk of developing cervical cancer. Then talk about breaking the smoking habit. Getting rid of that bad habit may help reduce your risk of developing a life-threatening disease.

Medical Source ————————————————————
British Medical Journal (306,6880:749)

Smokers, you may be missing an important nutrient

"Kissing someone who smokes is like licking an ashtray," is a common complaint among people who date or are married to smokers.

But bad breath should be the least of a smoker's worries. Smoking depletes the level of an important nutrient in the cells that make up the lining of the mouth — the cells that are directly exposed to the cigarette smoke.

The important nutrient is folic acid, also known as folate or folacin. Folic acid is an important B vitamin that aids the development of new cells. New cell development in the mouth is especially important because of all the abrasions the mouth suffers from chewing during meals.

New cells and cell layers are constantly produced in the mouth to maintain the protective lining of cells in the mouth. Low amounts of folic acid in these cells could interfere with their normal production, as well as predispose them to cancerous changes.

Folic acid is also an important cancer-fighting nutrient in the body. People who eat diets rich in folic acid enjoy lower risks of developing different types of cancer, especially colorectal cancer.

The bad news for smokers is that smoking not only lowers the amount of folic acid in the cells of the mouth, but it also lowers the amount of folic acid that circulates in the bloodstream.

To demonstrate the negative effects smoking has on folic acid concentrations in the body, a group of researchers recruited 59 volunteers to participate in a scientific study. Twenty-five of the volunteers were smokers, and 34 were nonsmokers.

Each of the volunteers completed detailed questionnaires on their dietary habits, alcohol intake and health history. Then the researchers took blood samples and samples of the cells in the lining of the volunteers' mouths, and they analyzed both for folic acid levels.

After carefully analyzing the results of the blood and cell samples from the smoking and nonsmoking volunteers, the researchers discovered that the volunteers who smoked had significantly lower levels of folic acid in the lining of their mouths than the nonsmokers.

And, although the smokers' blood folic acid levels were within the "normal" scientific range, they were significantly lower than the blood levels in the nonsmoking volunteers. The results from the questionnaires indicated, however, that both the smokers and nonsmokers consumed about the same amount of folic acid in their diets.

In other words, the smoking somehow seemed to be depleting or destroying the vital nutrient. These results suggest that a typical dietary intake of folic acid is insufficient to provide and maintain an essential level of folic acid in smokers.

Medical Source ———————————————————
International Journal of Cancer (52,4:566)

Drinking and breast cancer

"I'll have a glass of wine and a deadly case of breast cancer to go with my dinner, please." — It's a ridiculous statement, of course, but the words are not far from the frightening truth.

Women who drink more than two alcoholic beverages per day have anywhere from a 40 to 100 percent increased risk of developing breast cancer compared to women who don't drink.

Scientific studies have demonstrated the risk over and over again. A recent study of nearly 14,000 women found that women over the age of 40 who drink two alcoholic beverages a day are at least 50 percent more likely to get breast cancer than women who drink less.

Although scientists have known about the dangers of women drinking too much alcohol, they haven't been able to determine how alcohol increases the risk of breast cancer. Until now.

A new study suggests that drinking alcoholic beverages elevates the level of hormones in the bloodstream, which can contribute to the development of breast cancer.

A group of researchers from the National Cancer Institute in Bethesda, Maryland, recruited 34 young women to participate in a study to test the effects of alcohol on hormone levels.

For six months (six menstrual cycles), all the women ate the same food provided by the researchers to make sure that any differences in hormone levels were not due to different diets.

During the first three menstrual cycles, half the women consumed no alcohol. The other half drank approximately 30 grams of alcohol (about two drinks) per day just before going to bed.

During the last three menstrual periods, the researchers reversed the alcohol consumption of the two groups: The women who had drunk no alcohol started drinking it, and the two-drinks-a-day group stopped drinking.

The researchers took regular blood and urine samples to compare hormone levels in the women during the different stages of the study. They found that the women had elevated levels of different hormones when they were drinking alcohol every day compared to normal hormone levels when they weren't drinking.

In other words, drinking 30 grams of alcohol per day caused an increase in the production of hormones. These hormones (from the "estrogen family") influence the growth and development of breast tissue.

Elevated hormone levels in the blood could increase the risk of breast cancer — by as much as 40 to 100 percent.

Women with a family history of breast cancer have a greater risk of developing breast cancer than those without such family history. Unfortunately, this risk factor cannot be changed.

However, a woman can change her drinking habits. Cutting down to fewer than two alcoholic drinks per day could slash a woman's risk of breast cancer in half.

Medical Sources ————————————————
Medical Tribune (33,13:1)
Journal of the National Cancer Institute (85,9:722)

Easy way to slash your blood pressure

Your doctor has warned you that if you don't stop drinking he's going to have to put you on blood pressure medication to keep you from having a stroke or a heart attack.

But, you just don't want to give up your daily drinks.

Well, you may not need to give up drinking altogether to lower your blood pressure.

A group of researchers recruited 54 male volunteers to participate in a study that would test the effects of reducing daily alcohol consumption on blood pressure. After collecting information over a six-week study period, the researchers discovered some encouraging results.

They found that when the men cut their alcohol consumption in half, they experienced a drop in blood pressure, compared to the men who did not cut their alcohol intake. The men's blood pressure went back up when they resumed their old drinking habits.

The researchers reported that all the volunteers cut their alcohol intake in half without any apparent problem. This indicates that many social drinkers with mildly elevated blood pressure could lower their alcohol intake each week (not give it up altogether — just cut back the number of drinks each week) and reap the benefits of lower blood pressure.

Lowering blood pressure (to below 140/90) helps reduce the risk of developing heart and blood vessel diseases, kidney problems and strokes.

The scientists report that they aren't sure what the long-term (greater than six weeks) effects of alcohol reduction on blood pressure are. They are currently planning studies to test those effects.

Medical Source ——————————————————
Hypertension (21,2:248)

What causes the beer belly

The next time you start to propose a toast, take a look at your bulging belly — the two are closely related.

The "beer belly" that is staring back at you was probably caused by drinks just like the one you are about to drink. And it's not just the extra calories in the drink that cause you to get fat. The alcohol actually changes your metabolism.

Apparently, people who don't drink alcohol (or drink very little alcohol), burn a certain number of "fat" calories and a certain number of "healthy" calories every day. The difference between the number of "fat" calories and "healthy" calories that each person burns off each day is balanced so that people can maintain their weight.

The problem with drinking a lot of alcohol is that the alcohol causes the body to "shift" its metabolism. Instead of burning as many fat calories, the body starts burning off healthy calories.

As long as you burn calories, what does it matter? you ask.

Well, to keep from getting fat, the body needs to burn more of the "fat" calories. The fat calories that are not burned off are converted to body fat. The change in metabolism tips the body's balance toward fat storage. And people who burn less fat, get fat.

The extra calories in alcoholic beverages don't help, either. A couple of drinks with dinner can turn an 1,800-calorie day into a 2,500-calorie day in a matter of minutes.

The following chart lists a few examples of how many calories some popular drinks contain:

Beverage	Calories
Beer, 12 fluid ounces (one can)	150
Wine, dry, 5 fluid ounces	115
Liquor, 1-1/2 ounces	105

And remember that any additional soda or fruit juices added to a drink add even more calories. If you are trying to lose weight or just want to maintain your current weight without gaining, you should cut down on the amount of fat in your diet and drink less alcohol.

Plus, drinking more than two drinks a day can multiply your risk of developing dangerous diseases, such as cancer.

Medical Sources —————————————
The New England Journal of Medicine (326,15:983)
The Food Guide Pyramid, United States Department of Agriculture

When a healthy diet is useless

You eat a well-balanced diet, get plenty of fresh fruits and vegetables and have a couple of occasional "social" drinks.

You should be pretty healthy, right? Wrong!

The anti-cancer effects that those fruits and vegetables could have in your body are wasted — if you drink too much alcohol, that is.

Fruits and vegetables have very strong protective effects against colorectal cancer, the second leading cause of death from cancers in the United States today.

However, drinking too much alcohol each day seems to "cancel out" the protective effects of the fruits and vegetables.

Scientists studied the diets of thousands of people without colorectal cancer and compared them with the diets of people with colorectal cancer. Results showed that the vitamin folic acid (also known as folate or folacin) provides protection against developing colon polyps that could turn into colorectal cancer.

Folic acid is found in fruits and vegetables, and the people in the study who ate large amounts of folic acid-rich fruits and vegetables had a significantly lower risk of developing colorectal cancer compared with people who did not eat a folic acid-rich diet.

Based on the study results, women who had high intakes of folic acid experienced a 34-percent-lower incidence of colon polyps when compared with women who had low levels of folic acid in their diets.

And the men who ate large amounts of folic acid experienced a 37-percent-lower incidence of the colon polyps compared with the men who ate small amounts of these foods.

But that's where the good news stopped. The scientists also discovered that the men and women in the study who drank too much alcohol actually increased their risk of developing colorectal cancer, even if they ate folic acid-rich diets.

Compared with the people in the study who did not drink alcohol, the men and women who drank more than 30 grams of alcohol every day (about two drinks) had a significantly greater risk of colorectal cancer.

The women in the study who drank more than two drinks per day had an 84-percent-increased risk of developing precancerous colon polyps compared with nondrinking women. And the drinking men experienced a 64-percent-greater risk of colon polyps compared with nondrinking men in the study.

To maximize the protective, anti-cancer effects of fruits and vegetables in your diet, you might need to cut back on the number of alcoholic drinks you have each day. If you don't, you're back at square one, with no extra protection against cancer.

Medical Source ————————————————————
Journal of the National Cancer Institute (85,11:875)

Is your food 'intoxicating' you?

You don't allow your young children to drink alcoholic beverages, but you serve them chicken baked in a wine sauce without batting an eye.

"The alcohol is burned off," you explain.

Guess again.

People all across the continent have always heard, and believed, that the actual alcohol in cooking liquors is burned off during the cooking process, but that theory was never scientifically tested.

Until now.

A team of researchers recently prepared six recipes, each recipe calling for some type of cooking liquor, and measured the amount of alcohol that remained in the entrée after the preparation. The results were quite dizzying.

The following recipes were prepared for the test: pot roast Milano, orange chicken burgundy, scalloped oysters, brandy alexander pie, cherries jubilee, and Grand Marnier sauce. The different liquors that were used in the various recipes included burgundy, dry sherry, brandy, creme de cocoa and Grand Marnier.

The researchers followed the recipes carefully to make sure no measurement errors were made, and they prepared two samples of each dish to make sure the results were the same.

After each of the recipes was prepared, the researchers measured the amount of alcohol that remained in each sample.

The pot roast Milano still contained 4 to 6 percent of the alcohol that had been used in the recipe. The orange chicken burgundy contained up to 60 percent of the original amount of alcohol used.

The scalloped oysters retained up to 49 percent of the original alcohol amount, and the brandy Alexander pie kept up to 77 percent of the recipe's amount.

The cherries jubilee and the Grand Marnier sauce retained up to 78 and 85 percent of the original amount of alcohol from the recipes.

Researchers were astonished at these results, especially because all but one of the recipes had been "cooked" in some manner.

The pot roast had been simmered at 185 degrees Fahrenheit for two and a half hours.

The oysters had been baked at 375 degrees for 25 minutes, and the cherries jubilee had been flamed for 48 seconds. Yet, in spite of the cooking, a great deal of alcohol had not been "cooked off."

After studying the results of the recipe tests, the researchers made some important discoveries about preparing foods with alcohol:

They found that the longer a recipe is cooked, the more alcohol is cooked off; and the larger the surface area of the cooking pan, the more alcohol evaporates during the cooking process.

However, all cooks should be aware that even after cooking a recipe for a long time in a large pan, some alcohol might still be present in the food.

The next time you serve your child chicken with wine sauce, think about how much alcohol might still be in the dish.

Medical Source ————————————————
Journal of the American Dietetic Association (92,4:486)

Living in harmony with the environment

Allergies
Infections
Mother Nature
Food poisoning
Chemical
 poisoning

ALLERGIES

Surviving the 'air attack'

One out of every four Americans suffers from the constant itching, running nose, scratchy throat, sneezing, post-nasal drip, cough, headache, earache and red eyes that come with hay fever, or allergic rhinitis.

Hay fever may feel like a cold, but it's completely different. You can't catch it from a friend. Hay fever is an allergic response to an allergen or irritating substance.

Your body's immune cells mount an attack on the invading substance, trying to counteract the allergen's effect.

One of the body's cells that plays a central role in this attack is known as the mast cell, which releases the chemical "histamine" to fight irritating substances.

Other substances, like prostaglandins, thromboxane, leukotrienes and cytokines, are also released into the bloodstream to counteract the allergen.

Unfortunately, these substances, which are released into the bloodstream to help you, also cause many of the symptoms associated with an allergic reaction (stuffy nose, teary eyes, wheezing, etc.)

The symptoms of the allergic reaction show that the body is trying to get rid of something (such as pollen, mold, dust, chocolate or a chemical) that it believes shouldn't be there.

Occasionally you can identify an allergy sufferer by the appearance of his face.

Some children with allergies get dark circles under their eyes called allergic shiners, and many people get a red crease across the bridge of their noses called an allergic salute.

The crease is caused by constantly rubbing your nose to stop it from running or itching. These marks aren't permanent, but they are a sure sign of allergic rhinitis when they are combined with cold symptoms.

"Rhinitis" means the mucous membranes of the nose are inflamed and swollen, making it painful and hard to breathe.

This swelling can be accompanied by congestion, dryness of the membranes in the nose and extra mucus.

The culprits you breathe that cause all the trouble are known as "inhalant allergens," and they can cause seasonal or perennial allergic rhinitis. Seasonal allergies, the most common type, is usually caused by pollen, such as ragweed.

Most people are familiar with the fine yellow dust that covers cars, yard furniture and other outdoor objects during the early spring.

This yellow dust is from pine trees and is just one of the many types of pollen that saturate the air.

In most parts of the nation, late spring to mid-summer heralds the peak of grass pollen season.

And pollen from weeds begins sometime in the spring, reaching the peak of the season in late summer and early fall.

Contrary to popular belief, pollen from spring flowers are not among the list of worst allergy offenders. These pollen are spread by insects and not by wind currents, so there is hardly ever any flower pollen "floating around" that will aggravate your allergies.

On the other hand, tree, grass and weed pollen are carried through the air on gusts of wind and are frequently inhaled.

Perennial allergies are those that occur throughout the year for years at a time. Some of the most common perennial allergens are:

☐ **Dust mites**
Dust mites are tiny insects, related to spiders, which live in bedding, mattresses and carpets. They eat small pieces of dead, sloughed-off human skin cells and produce waste material (feces) which is coated in enzymes from the mite's intestines.

This enzyme coating is mainly responsible for triggering the allergic reaction. The fecal balls the mites produce are heavy, compared to other types of allergens, so they don't float around in the air very long.

When you change the sheets or vacuum, the mite feces blow around in the air for 30 minutes or so before settling down. During the period in which the mite feces are airborne, you can inhale the allergen and suffer from an allergic reaction.

❑ **House dust**
House dust is really a mixture of lint, dust mites, mite feces, animal fur, insect parts, fibers and other small particles.

❑ **Cat allergens**
Cat allergens come from the household cat's fur, skin and saliva. These allergens are lightweight and are constantly floating about in the air in homes where there are household cats.

❑ **Dog allergens**
Dog allergens are not made up of dog hair, like the cat allergens. Instead, the problem substances are found in the saliva, skin and urine from "house" dogs. Since dog hair is not the offender, long-haired dogs cause no more allergic rhinitis symptoms than short-haired dogs.

❑ **Cockroaches**
The common household cockroach triggers an allergic reaction in many people.

❑ **Orris root**
Orris root is a compound that has been widely used in making cosmetics. Its presence in some cosmetic products today accounts for some allergic reactions.

❑ **Pyrethrum**
Pyrethrum is an insecticide which is produced from plants related to ragweed.

❑ **Cottonseed and flaxseed**
Cottonseed and flaxseed are substances that can be found in animal food products, fertilizers, some inexpensive upholstery, hair-setting formulas and even in some foods.

❑ **Vegetable gums**
Vegetable gums are present in some denture adhesive powders, tooth powders, hair-setting preparations and cosmetics.

❐ **Fungi or molds**
Fungi and molds are especially offensive allergens because they can be found everywhere. They can grow both indoors and outdoors. Smut and rust fungi are commonly found near granaries. *Penicillium* and *Aspergillus* are two common molds that are frequently found in basements, bedding and other damp areas inside the house.

Although the source of the offending allergen is different, seasonal and perennial allergic rhinitis cause similar signs and symptoms.

Some of the most common symptoms include episodes of sneezing; itching of the eyes, nose, throat and top of the mouth; runny or stuffed-up nose; swelling around the eyes; and "postnasal drip" or drainage.

An allergic reaction might even cause reddened, itching or scaly skin. Sometimes fluid builds up in the middle ear, which can lead to decreased or dulled hearing ability.

A person ailing with allergic rhinitis may have fever, swollen lymph nodes, a sore throat or even bronchitis.

People suffer with varying degrees of allergic rhinitis. Ragweed might cause occasional sneezing in one person, while it causes severe symptoms in the next person.

But, no matter what the degree, the treatment is basically the same — avoid the offending allergen and provide relief for the symptoms.

Ways to control your allergies

Anyone who suffers with the sick-all-over feeling of allergies wishes for the magic cure. While there is no special potion, there are some steps you can take to keep your allergies under control:

❐ **Determine what you are allergic to — pollen, dust, mold, etc.**
Consult your doctor. Most family doctors are equipped to help isolate the source of your allergies.

❐ **Avoid what makes you sneeze and itch.**
This may mean changing the time of year for enjoying your favorite activities. If ragweed is your personal enemy, you should stay away

from open fields during the late summer and early months of fall. Go hiking during the late fall, winter and early spring before the pollen count gets so high.

Avoid activities such as raking leaves and mowing grass if you are allergic to molds.

You don't need to give away the cat if you're allergic to cat dander, but you might need to put the cat outdoors or keep the cat confined to one part of the house. That way you have a smaller area to keep free of cat dander and you can avoid the other areas on days when your allergies are acting up.

☐ Start allergy control in your bedroom — if you spend more than eight hours there.

➤ Cover mattress, box springs and pillows with air-tight plastic casing.

➤ Wash your bed sheets, comforters and mattress pads in very hot water every week to kill the dust mites that live there.

➤ Vacuum or dry clean bedding that can't be washed.

➤ Avoid using feather pillows on the beds. Use synthetic pillows instead, which you can throw in the washer every now and then to get rid of the mites. The same is true for down comforters.

➤ Keep furry pets out of your bedroom. Even if you're not allergic to the pet, its fur can carry pollen into your room.

➤ Use window shades or washable curtains.

➤ Remove stuffed toys, wall pennants, silk flowers and wicker baskets. They collect dust.

☐ Drive in an air-conditioned vehicle with the windows closed, especially during high-pollen season and during the day, when trees and grasses pollinate. This reduces your exposure to allergens.

☐ Keep the house air-conditioned and windows closed for the same reason. And, if you can't air-condition the whole house, try to cool one room (like the bedroom). This one area of the house can serve as a retreat on the days when your allergies are severe.

☐ Reduce the amount of dust, pollen and other air-borne allergens in the air in your house with a high-efficiency air filter. They are especially effective for smaller spaces, such as the bedroom. However, before buying one and having it installed, consider renting an air filter unit for a while to see if you can tell the difference in the air.

☐ Use a professional exterminator to rid your home of any cockroaches or other insects that could be aggravating your allergies.

☐ Switch brands of cosmetics, hair products or denture products if you show any allergic reactions. There are now many "hypoallergenic" formulas for common household products — using these products might reduce or even eliminate the severity of your reactions.

☐ Use a surgical mask, to cut down on the allergens you inhale, if you must perform chores that aggravate your allergies (such as mowing the lawn or fertilizing the garden).

☐ Steam-clean your carpet occasionally to kill the dust mites living there.

☐ Dust the house regularly, preferably by a member of the family who isn't bothered by allergies. Use a wet dust cloth that will pick up the dust instead of just stirring it around.
Cut down on the number of dust-collecting surfaces in your home. For example, replace venetian blinds on your windows with shades.

☐ Consider getting rid of the carpet if you have hardwood floors under it. Carpet provides a place for dust mites to live, and it collects dust. Although hardwood floors also collect dust, they are easier to clean. Area throw rugs can be cleaned in the washer or at the local cleaners.

☐ Do not allow smoking in the house. Do not use wood-burning stoves, fireplaces or kerosene heaters in the house. These things can aggravate allergies.

☐ Paint your basement walls with water-tight sealant to minimize the amount of moisture and dampness in the basement and cut down on the growth of molds.

☐ Fix leaky pipes and faucets around the house to eliminate the growth of molds.

☐ Clean the shower stalls and curtains with a bleach mixture regularly to prevent the growth of molds.

☐ Keep the window and door frames well-caulked and sealed to prevent moisture accumulation and mold growth within the house.

Soothing your allergy symptoms

☐ Use over-the-counter antihistamines. Antihistamines block the release of histamine from mast cells, those cells that are responsible for the body's allergic response to foreign substances (like pollen). However, remember that antihistamines can cause sleepiness or drowsiness. Do not use them when you want to be alert, and especially when you'll be driving or operating machinery.

☐ Use over-the-counter decongestant medications to help clear up your stuffy or runny nose. These come in the form of tablets, liquids or nasal sprays. A word of warning: Using a nasal spray for more than three days in a row will create more problems than it solves. Although the nasal spray does its job as a decongestant for the first few days, after about three days of continuous usage, it begins to cause congestion.
So, stop using the nose spray after a few days and try the liquid or tablets instead. After a week or so, you can safely use the nasal spray again.

☐ Drink lots of liquids during the day to "wash out" the congestion.

Warm liquids might soothe your sore throat and help "loosen up" any mucus or phlegm in your lungs to make it easier to cough up.

❏ Drink plenty of liquids and get plenty of rest if you have a fever accompanying an allergy. The fever is another indication that your body is fighting off the irritating substance you inhaled.

❏ Stand in a hot shower or sit in a steamy room to help clear up your congested nose, head and lungs.

❏ Use throat lozenges to help soothe your irritated throat. They won't get rid of any symptoms for long, but they will give a little relief from a dry, sore throat.

If you can't seem to find relief from your case of allergic rhinitis, you might need to call your doctor.

He can prescribe some stronger medication to help relieve your symptoms, and he might recommend a series of allergy shots to help your body respond more agreeably to allergens.

Medical Sources ───────────────────
The Journal of the American Medical Association (268,20:2807)
Postgraduate Medicine (91,4:215)

Is your comforter making you sick?

Those probably weren't the doctor's exact words, but they contain the right message for one 31-year-old Dutch lady who went to the doctor complaining of fever, breathing problems and coughing up thick sputum.

According to her doctor, the lady developed a lung illness known as alveolitis. This is a condition in which the tiny sack-like compartments in the lungs known as alveoli become inflamed and irritated.

Apparently, she developed an allergy to her goose feather comforter that she had used for several years without any problem. The doctor tested his diagnosis by removing the goose feather comforter.

The lady's symptoms cleared up. Later, the doctor returned the comforter, and the lady came down with the same symptoms.

If you are suffering from lung problems and you own a goose down comforter, don't throw it out too quickly. The comforter the lady was allergic to was made with goose feathers. Most comforters in America are made with goose down.

People who experience allergic reactions to goose down comforters are probably allergic to dust mites and not the goose down.

Medical Source ————————————————
   Medical Tribune (33,23:14)

Food allergy: When the foods you love don't love you

You think it might be a brain tumor — you've been suffering from horrible headaches once or twice a week for several months, and nothing seems to make them go away.

The headaches come on so unpredictably that you've ruled out stress and other common causes of headaches

Well, before scheduling an appointment with a neurosurgeon, try looking for the answer in your refrigerator. Your favorite food or midnight snack might be the culprit. And it might also be causing your chronic cough, your joint pain and your skin rash.

The problem could be a food allergy.

Food allergies occur when the body "mis-identifies" something that you eat. The body "thinks" the food is harmful instead of nutritious, and so the body reacts to the food. Unfortunately, this reaction can cause some pretty serious health problems.

For example, certain nutritious grains can cause severe joint pain. When researchers put a group of arthritis-plagued men and women on a four-week special diet that did not contain wheat, rye, oats or barley, their arthritis symptoms improved. They had fewer tender and swollen joints, less stiffness and more grip strength. These benefits were still present a year after the diet ended.

The following symptoms and diseases can be caused by or related to food allergies:

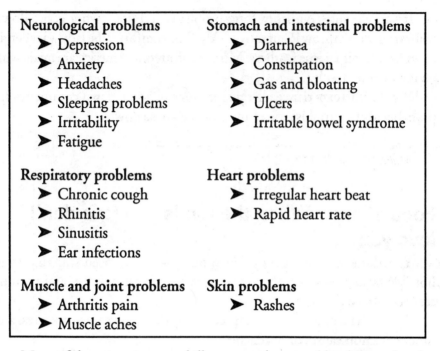

Neurological problems
➤ Depression
➤ Anxiety
➤ Headaches
➤ Sleeping problems
➤ Irritability
➤ Fatigue

Respiratory problems
➤ Chronic cough
➤ Rhinitis
➤ Sinusitis
➤ Ear infections

Muscle and joint problems
➤ Arthritis pain
➤ Muscle aches

Stomach and intestinal problems
➤ Diarrhea
➤ Constipation
➤ Gas and bloating
➤ Ulcers
➤ Irritable bowel syndrome

Heart problems
➤ Irregular heart beat
➤ Rapid heart rate

Skin problems
➤ Rashes

Many of these symptoms and illnesses can be caused by things other than food, such as viruses, bacteria, tension, and so on. But when those "other things" have been ruled out by your doctor, food allergies could be the source of the illness.

The problem is that many people (including doctors) do not think of food as a possible cause of a health problem, so the problems often go untreated for long periods of time.

One 72-year-old woman suffered from a chronic cough for 10 years before doctors discovered that the cough was caused by a food allergy. The lady was allergic to wheat, and when she stopped eating wheat food products, her 10-year cough disappeared.

If you are suffering from an illness that you think might be related to a food allergy, try keeping a food diary. In a small notebook, write down your suspicious symptoms, how often they occur, and how severe they are. Then, make a small chart to keep track of what you eat and when the symptoms occur (before or after a meal, for example).

Keep this food diary for at least two weeks before your next doctor's appointment, and then take the diary with you to the doctor. The doctor may suggest an "elimination diet" to determine if the suspected foods really are the problem.

A food allergies elimination diet means you'll quit eating some common allergy-causing foods to see if those foods are causing your problems. After a while, the doctor will begin adding foods back into your diet, usually one at a time, and carefully monitoring your reactions.

When you prepare your food diary, take special notice of the effects of the following foods. They are some of the most common allergy-causing foods.

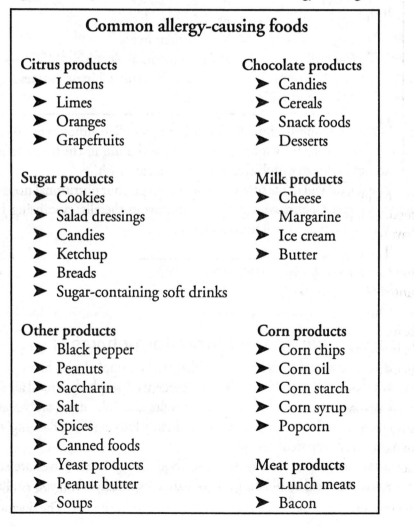

Common allergy-causing foods

Citrus products
➤ Lemons
➤ Limes
➤ Oranges
➤ Grapefruits

Chocolate products
➤ Candies
➤ Cereals
➤ Snack foods
➤ Desserts

Sugar products
➤ Cookies
➤ Salad dressings
➤ Candies
➤ Ketchup
➤ Breads
➤ Sugar-containing soft drinks

Milk products
➤ Cheese
➤ Margarine
➤ Ice cream
➤ Butter

Other products
➤ Black pepper
➤ Peanuts
➤ Saccharin
➤ Salt
➤ Spices
➤ Canned foods
➤ Yeast products
➤ Peanut butter
➤ Soups

Corn products
➤ Corn chips
➤ Corn oil
➤ Corn starch
➤ Corn syrup
➤ Popcorn

Meat products
➤ Lunch meats
➤ Bacon

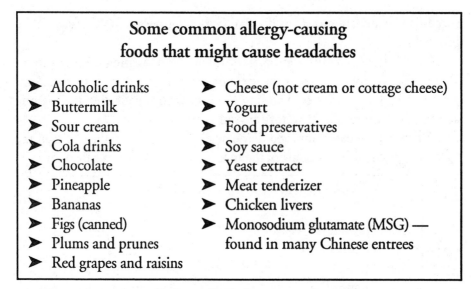

Some common allergy-causing foods that might cause headaches

➤ Alcoholic drinks
➤ Buttermilk
➤ Sour cream
➤ Cola drinks
➤ Chocolate
➤ Pineapple
➤ Bananas
➤ Figs (canned)
➤ Plums and prunes
➤ Red grapes and raisins

➤ Cheese (not cream or cottage cheese)
➤ Yogurt
➤ Food preservatives
➤ Soy sauce
➤ Yeast extract
➤ Meat tenderizer
➤ Chicken livers
➤ Monosodium glutamate (MSG) — found in many Chinese entrees

Do not attempt to eliminate foods from your diet without your doctor's advice. Eliminating the wrong foods can cause vitamin and nutrient deficiencies and cause greater problems than you started with.

The doctor will make sure your diet meets all your nutritional needs and help you plan a permanent diet that will avoid the allergy-causing foods without sacrificing overall nutritional value.

Medical Sources ————————————————
American Family Physician (46,5:775)
The Lancet (338,8772:899)

Common causes of food-allergy hives

If you have food allergies, you're likely to be troubled with hives. In fact, hives and other skin problems affect 65 percent of people with food allergies.

Breaking out in swollen, red, itchy welts is usually more embarrassing than dangerous. There's nothing like suddenly looking like a flashing, neon tomato for no apparent reason.

Children are particularly prone to food-allergy hives. Hives are sometimes accompanied by bloating and diarrhea, especially when you're allergic to milk or eggs.

These are the most common culprits of food-allergy hives:

> Eggs
> Peaches
> Hazel nuts
> Sunflower seeds
> Peanuts
> Lentils
> Cow's milk
> Fish

Although hives are usually caused by eating or touching something you're allergic to, if you're prone to hives, you can also break out when you get hot, stressed, tense or even when you just scratch yourself.

Medical Source —————————————————————
American Family Physician (45,6:2727 and 46,5:775)

Dry skin? Maybe it's your allergies!

Itch. Itch. Itch. All you do all day is scratch. Has your doctor diagnosed your dry, red, irritated skin as allergic contact dermatitis — your skin's angry reaction to something you've touched? Here are some tips on what you can do at home to bring relief to your itching skin.

Find out what's irritating you. It looks like poison ivy, it swells and blisters like poison ivy, and it even itches like poison ivy. But your rash could actually be allergic contact dermatitis.

Clothes

It's not uncommon to be allergic to your clothes. The formaldehyde compounds present in permanent press fabrics seem to cause allergic skin reactions in certain people.

The rash that comes with allergic contact dermatitis is usually confined to areas on your body that are covered by clothing. It may be worse in areas where your clothing is tighter (waistband, etc.).

The head and neck are rarely involved, except in the most extreme cases.

Some people may be bothered by severe itching while others are troubled by blistering, cracking or reddened skin.

What should you do if you suspect you are allergic to permanent press fabrics? Less drastic measures than becoming a nudist are available.

Your dermatologist can perform "patch tests" that show how a small area of skin responds to chemicals and irritants.

If you or someone you know is allergic to formaldehyde — simply avoiding permanent press clothing yields excellent results.

Athletic equipment

People who exercise regularly have particular trouble with their athletic equipment. The culprit could be the rubber, epoxy or resin in the following sports gear:

> ➤ Sneakers ➤ Support stockings
> ➤ Masks ➤ Tape
> ➤ Wet suits ➤ Shoe inserts
> ➤ Goggles ➤ Mouthpieces

You can also get contact dermatitis from rubbing your sore muscles with creams or ointments that contain methyl salicylate, the active ingredient in oil of wintergreen.

A word to the wise: If you have an allergic reaction to one of these ointments, avoid aspirin and other oral medicines that contain salicylates. The presence of aspirin in your system can trigger a recurrence of the original rash.

Contact dermatitis usually clears up when you stop using the equipment causing the trouble. If your rash is more serious, your doctor can prescribe corticosteroid pills to relieve your discomfort.

To avoid a return of contact dermatitis, try changing your equipment. Look for sneakers made from polyurethane instead of rubber, swim goggles made from neoprene, and athletic tape made with acrylate instead of resin.

You should be able to find equipment that will protect you during your activity yet won't irritate your skin.

Don't scratch! Scratching will instantly make an itch feel better, but can actually make your itching worse. Itching occurs when the skin releases histamine, and scratching usually stimulates the skin to release more histamine. Instead of scratching:

❐ Place a cool, moist washcloth on the area that itches.

❐ Apply pressure with the palm of your hand.

❐ Smooth moisturizer into your skin.

❐ Rub bath oils directly on your skin.

❐ Consider taking antihistamines. It's best to try this treatment at night since antihistamines will make you drowsy.

Soothe your nerves and your skin with herbal teas. Tea made with various herbs is an old Chinese remedy for dermatitis. People with dermatitis report that they itch less and sleep better when they drink herbal tea regularly.

To check out this news, researchers asked 40 people with dermatitis to drink tea containing 10 herbs every day for eight weeks. The herbal tea remedy worked! It reduced everyone's red, dermatitis-affected skin by an average of 50 percent.

A word of warning about herbs: Don't try to treat yourself with herbs if you're pregnant, and don't give any herbal mixtures to babies. Not enough tests have been done on the effects of herbs, so don't risk your infant's health.

Some herbs are known to cause liver damage. Here are some to avoid:

➤ Valerian	➤ Germander
➤ Comfrey	➤ Asafetida
➤ Hops	➤ Skullcap
➤ Gentian	➤ Senna fruit
➤ Mistletoe	➤ Chaparral leaf

If you can't stop itching, you may need to talk to your doctor. Causes of itching can be as diverse as kidney failure, thyroid problems, HIV, iron deficiency, infections, fungi and even parasites.

Medical Sources ————————————————

Postgraduate Medicine (92,7:34)

Medical Tribune (33,15:10)

The Physician and Sportsmedicine (21,3:65)

Journal of the American Academy of Dermatology (27,6:962)

INFECTIONS

Travelers, is airplane air making you sick?

"Something in the air is making me sick" has become a common complaint of brain-weary office workers.

Many people think that the air-conditioned, stale air they share with their co-workers saps their powers of concentration, causes infections, fatigue and headaches.

But if workplace air is harmful to your health, imagine what the air on a eight-or-more hour airplane flight could do to you! Flight attendants and other airline workers are convinced that recirculated cabin air is a serious health hazard.

In the past, the air on a passenger flight was completely replaced with fresh air every three minutes. Now, many airlines save about $60,000 per plane every year by combining recirculated air with fresh air.

The recirculated air is full of bacteria and viruses, and can cause outbreaks of the flu, measles and even tuberculosis. The nausea and headaches you call jet lag after a long flight are probably the result of airplane air.

Until airlines see the error of their ways, there isn't much you can do about recirculated air on flights. Try to schedule at least one stopover for very long trips. When a stop is very short and it seems like too much trouble to get off the plane, do it anyway. You need the fresh air.

One plane bound for Alaska in 1979 was held on the ground for three hours with the air-circulation system shut off. Soon after they arrived at their destination, three-fourths of the passengers came down with coughs, fevers, headaches, sore throats and fatigue.

If a plane is held over on the ground for thirty minutes or more, insist that you be let off. Perhaps flight attendants, feeling ill themselves, will be cooperative.

Medical Source —————————————————
Medical Tribune (34,16:7)

Swollen lymph nodes? Your cat may be the reason

Your kids begged for weeks, and you finally gave in and got them the kitten they've been longing for. Now, three weeks and a few accidental cat scratches later, one of the kids is complaining of a sore neck and some swollen knots under his arm.

He could be suffering from "cat scratch disease."

It's an illness that was described more than 40 years ago, and it usually is quite harmless. In most cases, cat scratch disease follows just what you'd expect — a scratch or bite from a cat or kitten. Usually it causes nothing more serious than some swollen lymph nodes, especially under the arms and on the neck. Occasionally it can lead to serious problems.

Not long ago two elementary school children from Connecticut were hospitalized with life-threatening infections that developed from cat scratch disease. Both children recovered without any problems.

There are more than 22,000 cases of cat scratch disease diagnosed every year in the United States, with more than 2,000 hospitalizations resulting from the disease.

Studies suggest that the bacteria *Rochalimaea henselae* might be responsible for the disease, and the bacteria can be transmitted from a cat scratch, bite or even flea bites.

Currently, there is no vaccine that you can give to your cat to prevent infection with the bacteria. However, since cat scratch disease is rarely serious, most doctors and veterinarians are not concerned.

The most common symptoms of cat scratch disease include swollen lymph nodes, mild fever, a lesion where the cat bit or scratched you, and possibly some general "under-the-weather" feelings. The symptoms usually clear up in a few days without any medication or further trouble.

However, if the mild symptoms seem to get worse, call your doctor right away. Remember that some cases can become serious. Is cat scratch disease a reason to get rid of your cat or kitten (or avoid getting one)?

Probably not. Just be aware of the possibility of developing cat scratch disease after a scratch or bite during a play session with your feline. In the mean time, enjoy your family pet.

Medical Source ────────────────────────
   The New England Journal of Medicine (329,1:8)

Pelvic infections from the family pet

Cats and dogs can transmit another type of bacteria to humans that causes infections in women only. Women who are bitten or scratched by a cat or a dog can get a pelvic infection.

They have pain in the lower right side of the body, the stomach and the back; cramping; stomach tenderness; fever; and vaginal discharge.

The bacteria that causes the pelvic infection is called *Pasteurella multocida* and, as far as we know, is only passed from animal to human, never from one human to another. Cat bites and scratches cause the most infections even though dog bites account for 80 percent of bite wounds.

If you have the symptoms of a pelvic infection, see your doctor immediately. He will probably check for some of the more common causes of pelvic infections, such as sexually transmitted diseases or the use of an intrauterine device (IUD).

Be sure to mention any recent exposure to pets and any bites or scratches you may have received. This information may alter the way your doctor treats the infection and lead to a shorter healing time.

Pelvic infections are commonly treated with the antibiotics gentamicin and clindamycin. However, infections that may be related to injury from a pet should be treated with a wide-spectrum antibiotic — one that is effective against many different types of bacteria.

Untreated pelvic infections can damage the female reproductive tract and may even lead to fallopian tube and ovary removal.

Medical Sources ────────────────────────
   American Family Physician (47,2:318)
   The New England Journal of Medicine (327,19:1395)

Everything you need to know about Lyme disease

Lyme disease is the most common insect-borne disease in the United

States today. The tick-borne illness plagues the Northeastern Coast, the Midwest and the West Coast, and has caused more than 40,000 cases of infection since 1982.

Lyme disease is caused by the bacteria *Borrelia burgdorferi*, which is passed to you when you're bitten by certain ticks from the Ixodes family. These ticks have been found on at least 30 kinds of wild animals and on 49 different species of bird, but they are most commonly found on white-tailed deer.

The bacteria infect the Ixodes tick and live within the insect its whole life. The ticks live for two years, with three different life stages. During the larva stage, the ticks feed in the late summer.

The ticks then pass into the nymph stage, feeding during the following spring and early summer. The adult ticks feed mainly in the autumn.

The ticks are most likely to transmit the bacteria to humans when they are in the nymph stage of life. Since the nymphal ticks feed mostly during the spring and early summer months, that's when most people get infected — May, June and July.

Not everyone who gets a tick bite comes down with Lyme disease. In fact, the probability of getting Lyme disease after a tick bite in an area where Lyme disease is common is only 1.2 to 5 percent.

For the people who do get infected, however, the illness usually occurs in stages which are marked by certain symptoms.

The stages of Lyme disease

Stage One: The most characteristic feature of stage one is the "bull's eye rash" which usually appears three to 32 days after you're bitten by the tick. The medical name for the rash is "erythema chronicum migrans."

The rash usually begins as a small, red, raised dot that spreads slowly to form a large circular rash with a bright-red outer border and a lighter-colored center.

The area tends to be feverish, warm to the touch and very painful. Most tick bites and rashes are on the thigh or groin area, but they can be found anywhere.

Some Lyme disease rashes have very red centers that don't look like bull's eyes at all. Don't be fooled by a rash that looks a little different than the typical bull's eye. Also, 20 percent of the people with Lyme disease don't even develop a skin rash.

Stage Two: During this stage, the bacteria spread through the blood to other sites in the body. Common symptoms of stage two include mild to severe headache, mild neck stiffness, fever, chills, muscle and joint aches, fatigue and an overall sick feeling. Many people compare it to having the flu — you just feel bad all over.

Less common symptoms are swollen lymph nodes, swollen spleen, sore throat, dry cough, swelling of the testicles in men and eye irritation.

The stage two symptoms often come and go randomly, then disappear altogether after several weeks. However, several weeks to months later, about 15 percent of the people with Lyme disease develop problems with the nervous system, including meningitis.

Another eight percent develop heart abnormalities. These usually last only a few days to a few weeks, but they can sometimes be life-threatening.

Other people feel pains in their joints, tendons, muscles and bones that may last hours or several days at a time. The pains sometimes disappear and then reappear weeks later in a different spot in the body. Some people even develop arthritis.

Stage Three: The final phase of Lyme disease occurs two to three years after you were bitten by the tick. Arthritis is one of the most common long-term complications of Lyme disease.

Joints may be painful and stiff for months at a time instead of weeks, as they were in stage two. Some people also suffer from long-term nervous system problems, such as memory loss and altered mood and sleep patterns.

A skin disorder can appear years after the tick bite, too. A small area of redness and swelling appears, then gradually fades. The skin begins to waste away over time, and eventually you're left with an area of skin that is wrinkled and worn, like cigarette paper.

Treatment for Lyme disease

The most common treatment for the early stages of Lyme disease is the common antibiotic Doxycycline. Amoxicillin, another commonly pre-scribed antibiotic, is also an effective therapy.

One study suggests that the most safe and cost-effective way to prevent the complications of Lyme disease is to take antibiotics if you're bitten by a tick (in the areas of the country where Lyme disease is most common), even before any symptoms arise.

People who live in areas of the country where Lyme disease is rare don't need the preventative antibiotic therapy.

Although Lyme disease seems like a terrible disease to contract, treating it right away with antibiotics is very successful. A tick bite should not cause panic — only a small number of people who get a tick bite actually get the infection, and of the ones that do, antibiotic therapy works wonders.

The best way to avoid Lyme disease is to avoid getting tick bites.

Tips to lower your risk of tick bites and Lyme disease

Tip #1   Avoid wooded or grassy areas that are heavily populated by white-tailed deer during the early spring and summer. The ticks catch onto branches and grass from the deer and wait for another unsuspecting target to bite, such as you or your dog.

Tip #2   Do a thorough "tick check" of yourself and your dog after being in a wooded or grassy area. Fortunately, the ticks usually crawl around for several hours before they bite into the skin.

Tip #3   Always wear shoes, long pants and long sleeves if you have to go into a possible tick-infested area. Tuck your pants legs into your socks to prevent the ticks from getting on your socks and crawling up into your pants legs. Also tuck your shirt into your pants and wear a fairly tight belt to keep the ticks from getting in at the waistline.

Tip #4   Use insect repellent, especially formulas that contain the chemical DEET. Spray the insect repellent on your shoes, socks, pants, belt line, shirt, working gloves and hat. Before applying the repellent directly to your skin or hair, read the instructions carefully. Some repellents cause skin rashes and shouldn't be applied directly to the skin.

Tip #5   Remember that insect repellents on your skin are diluted and washed off if you sweat, swim or shower. Reapply the repellent as needed.

Tip #6   Wear light-colored clothing of tightly woven material when you go into wooded or grassy areas. This makes it easier to see the ticks on your clothes and harder for the ticks to grab on.

Tip #7   Check your pets for ticks regularly. Ticks often find their ways into homes by riding on dogs and cats. Use tick collars or sprays and wash pets regularly.

How to remove ticks

If you find a tick on yourself or a family member, the first thing to remember is not to panic. Only a very small number of people get Lyme disease from tick bites. Then, very calmly, remove the tick:

- ☐ If the tick hasn't attached itself to the skin yet, simply remove it with some tissue paper or tweezers and drop it into the toilet and flush.
- ☐ If the tick has already attached itself to the skin, use a pair of fine-tipped tweezers to grab the tick's mouth parts as close to the skin as you can. Pull the tick out in a steady, firm motion. Make sure you didn't leave parts of the tick's mouth in the skin. If you jerk the tick out, you'll probably leave some of it behind.
- ☐ If you don't have tweezers, use a piece of tissue to pull the tick out. Again, grasp the tick as close to the skin as you can.
- ☐ Tape the tick to an index card with clear Scotch tape. Write down the date of the tick bite, the location of the tick bite (ankle, right shoulder, etc.) and where you probably picked up the tick (wooded area next to your house, etc.). This information might be useful to the doctor if you develop symptoms later.
- ☐ Wash your hands and the area around the tick bite and apply antiseptic cream or spray. This will reduce your risk of infection with the Lyme disease bacteria or other bacteria.
- ☐ If you live in an area where Lyme disease is common (Northeastern Coast from Massachusetts to Maryland, Wisconsin, Minnesota, California and Oregon), call your doctor for some antibiotics to prevent Lyme disease from ever developing. If you live in an area where Lyme disease is rare, you don't need to contact your doctor unless you develop a rash or other symptoms of Lyme disease.

To get more information on Lyme disease, contact the Lyme Disease Foundation, P.O. Box 462, Tolland, Connecticut, 06084. You can call the foundation at (203) 871-2900.

Medical Sources ───────────────────
Emergency Medicine (24,11:28)
The New England Journal of Medicine (327,8:534)

The tick bites again: Human ehrlichiosis

You get it from tick bites, but it's not Lyme disease and it's not Rocky Mountain spotted fever.

It's a "new" tick-borne disease that was first described in the United States in 1986. Human ehrlichiosis (pronounced er-lick-ee-o-sis) has caused more than 215 cases since 1986. Some of those cases were fatal.

The bacteria that causes human ehrlichiosis is known as *Ehrlichia canis*, and it is related to the bacteria that is responsible for Rocky Mountain spotted fever.

Between 63 and 88 percent of the people who develop symptoms of human ehrlichiosis report that a tick bit them about three weeks before the symptoms started.

This indicates that the bacteria are passed by ticks, but scientists aren't sure which ticks carry these bacteria. Most cases of human ehrlichiosis occur in the mid-Atlantic and south-Central states during the spring and summer.

People who develop human ehrlichiosis after a tick bite usually begin to experience symptoms one to 21 days after the bite. The illness seems to start suddenly with a headache, fever, chills and an overall flu-like feeling.

A rash develops in over a third of the people with the illness. The rash can be either "maculopapular" or "petechial." A maculopapular rash is one that is discolored and raised above the normal skin surface.

A petechial rash is made up of pinpoint-sized, flat, perfectly round, purplish-red spots.

The rash, more common in children than adults, is often found on the arms and legs, but it can be anywhere on the body.

Other symptoms of human ehrlichiosis include vomiting, diarrhea, abdominal pain and cramping, confusion and sore throat.

Blood tests show that people with human ehrlichiosis suffer from abnormally low levels of white bloods cells, red blood cells and platelets.

These are very important components of the blood, and abnormal levels can cause serious medical problems. If not treated quickly, these problems can cause long-term complications, and even death.

Human ehrlichiosis responds easily to common antibiotics, so you can avoid long-term health problems by taking antibiotics.

Below is a chart that compares the symptoms of human ehrlichiosis, Lyme disease and Rocky Mountain spotted fever. Anyone who suffers a tick bite and begins to have any of the symptoms should seek medical help immediately.

Characteristic	Ehrlichiosis	Rocky Mountain spotted fever	Lyme disease
Cases per year	More than 50	More than 600	More than 1,500
First described	1986	1906	1975
Common location	Mid-Atlantic, South-central states	Mid-Atlantic, Central states	New Jersey to Maine, Wisconsin, Minnesota, California and Oregon
Peak season	spring & summer	spring & summer	spring & summer
Fatality rate	1 percent	5-15 percent	very rare
Rash	33-47 percent	74 percent	60-83 percent
Fever	85-100 percent	88-100 percent	59 percent
Joint pains	28-37 percent	rare	48 percent
Headaches	70-94 percent	85 percent	64 percent
Abdominal pain	19-38 percent	34-52 percent	8 percent
Anemia	33-62 percent	5-24 percent	12 percent

Medical Source ————————————————
American Family Physician (46,1:199)

Avoiding infections from a trip to the doctor's office

You go to the doctor for treatment and come home with an infection.

What are the chances of this happening to you? It can depend on how your doctor cleans routine examination equipment.

Stethoscopes. Doctors and other medical personnel typically wash their hands between visits, yet many neglect to clean their stethoscopes as often.

There are still no standard guidelines for cleaning stethoscopes, although studies done 20 years ago showed that these instruments can retain the *staphylococci* bacteria.

This bacteria may cause food poisoning, boils, severe skin blistering and internal abscesses.

It seems many doctors may not bother cleaning their stethoscopes at all. Out of 29 doctors interviewed, two cleaned their stethoscopes periodically and another had cleaned his once. Twenty-six of the 29 stethoscopes carried bacteria, and on five of the stethoscopes the bacteria was infectious.

Ask your doctor: Cleaning the stethoscope with a cotton ball soaked in alcohol reduces bacteria by approximately 97 percent. Ask your doctor about her stethoscope cleaning methods if she regularly treats *staphylococcal* infections or if you feel you are at increased risk of getting these infections.

Otoscopes. The instrument your doctor uses for examining your ears, the otoscope, can also transmit infections.

Examination of the otoscopes of 44 doctors in North England showed that 93 percent of the earpieces on these otoscopes harbored bacteria. In 32 percent of these cases, the bacteria was potentially infectious.

The ear has several natural defenses against bacteria, but it can be highly susceptible to infection if its defenses have been previously weakened by other bacteria, heat, moisture, injury or antibiotics.

Eighty-five percent of doctors responding to a questionnaire concerning their otoscope cleaning habits said that they believed serious infection could occur through contaminated earpieces. Yet 78 percent did not clean their earpieces after examinations. Lack of time and inconvenience are two reasons given for this contradiction between belief and action.

Ask your doctor: Does your doctor use disposable earpieces? If not, request that he clean the earpieces by boiling in water for five minutes, sterilizing with steam heat, or by immersing in 70-percent alcohol or other appropriate disinfectant.

Finger-stick devices. One group of people contracted hepatitis, a serious illness involving inflammation of the liver, from a simple device at the doctor's office.

Several common blood tests, such as cholesterol, hematocrit (to test for anemia) and blood sugar (to test for diabetes), are now performed with a single drop of blood.

Spring-loaded finger-stick devices have been developed to make blood collection easier. These devices are now widely used in doctor's offices and hospitals.

They are relatively safe if used properly, but, for a group of 26 people who contracted acute hepatitis B virus infection in a California hospital, these simple devices were doing more than collecting blood.

A review of the nursing procedures at the hospital revealed that the bottom of the finger-stick device platform had not been routinely changed after each use and became contaminated. The contaminated platform allowed the hepatitis virus to be transmitted to any person who used the finger-stick device.

Ask your doctor: Request sterile, pre-packaged, disposable finger-stick devices to eliminate any further transmission of illnesses. The California hospital switched to eliminate contamination with the finger stick device.

Diabetics should be especially aware of the need for clean finger-stick devices because they receive so many blood tests. These devices may also be used at cholesterol screening programs.

Instrument cleaning procedures vary from doctor to doctor. The best way to protect yourself against infection is to keep your eyes open and ask questions.

Medical Sources —————————————————

British Medical Journal (305,6868:1571 and 1573)
The New England Journal of Medicine (326,11:721)
Medical Tribune (33,6:4)

Kitchen remedies prevent infections

Ulcers and wounds can be a feeding ground for infections, especially in underdeveloped countries. Normal medicated wound dressings are simply not available everywhere. But now doctors have some cheap, easy solutions that may be beneficial here in the United States.

Salt. A simple solution of salt and water applied to sterile gauze, then placed over the wound, works to speed healing and prevent infection. Add approximately 3/4 teaspoon of salt (sodium chloride) to 3 pints of sterile water for the best mixture.

Honey. It eases your sweet tooth and flavors your tea — and now honey could achieve a higher status in your medicine cabinet — beside the hydrogen peroxide and bandages.

Doctors in New Zealand are testing a theory Egyptian mothers formulated over 2,000 years ago. The Egyptians discovered that applying honey to minor cuts actually helped the healing process.

Sugar. A paste of sugar and hydrogen peroxide applied to a new cut seems to halt the growth of bacteria. Researchers believe that sugar (and honey) work against bacteria by removing water from around a wound. Since bacteria require water to grow, honey or sugar can offer sweet relief from the growth of bacteria — and allow your cut to heal naturally.

New evidence suggests that honey is an even better deterrent to infection than sugar. Researchers believe that the flowers visited by bees contribute agents that actually fight certain bacteria.

In particular, honey from the New Zealand manuka flower shows promise in fighting *staph* infections and *E. Coli* bacteria that causes stomach upsets. Honeys derived from other flowers seem to be natural enemies to *strep* and *salmonella* bacteria.

Don't empty the medicine cabinet yet, though. Honey does show promise as an infection fighter, but its use as an antibacterial agent is still in the testing stage. Also, some honey may contain bacteria and pesticide residues.

Medical Source ⸺⸺⸺⸺⸺⸺⸺⸺⸺
   The Lancet (340,8831:1351 and 341,9:90)

MOTHER NATURE

Allergic to the cold?

Imagine this. You return from a 30 minute outdoor run during a cold, windy day and you begin to itch all over. You break out in hives and start to feel dizzy and anxious.

Although few of us recognize these symptoms, you are experiencing a form of physical allergy called cold urticaria.

Exercise in combination with certain foods can also cause the same itchy reaction, and so can heat, exercise and emotions.

Usually, cold urticaria occurs just in areas that are exposed to the cold, such as the head and neck. It is generally not dangerous and does improve with time.

However, cold urticaria can cause more serious and even life-threatening reactions in some people.

The most extreme reactions are angioedema and anaphylaxis. Angioedema means swelling around the lips and eyes that can spread to the neck and obstruct breathing. Anaphylaxis is a reaction that can lead to shock because it dilates the blood vessels so that blood pressure drops dangerously low.

Doctors test for cold urticaria by using, guess what? An ice cube held against the skin for up to 10 minutes. If you get hives under the ice cube, you're prone to develop cold urticaria.

Take these precautions to help avoid the itch of cold urticaria:

- ❏ Avoid being out in the cold for extended periods of time.
- ❏ If you desire to exercise in the cold, take an antihistamine before exercising.
- ❏ Those who have severe reactions to cold should exercise with a buddy who knows how and when to give them an epinephrine shot in case of anaphylaxis or angioedema.

Medical Source ————————————————
The Physician and Sportsmedicine (20,12:73)

Take the bite out of frostbite

When Christmas carolers sing "Jack Frost nipping at your nose," some cold-climate dwellers and winter-sports freaks get the shivers.

A nip or a bite from Jack Frost can mean serious injury to, or even loss of, the nose, toes, ears, fingers and cheeks of the hapless wanderer in a Winter Wonderland.

Frostbite is your body's natural reaction to cold weather. Struggling to keep the center of your body warm, your blood vessels narrow and shut down circulation to your limbs and outer surfaces.

Without a proper blood supply, your tissues start to die. In extreme cold, even the water in your body starts to freeze.

You can get frostbitten in less than a minute, especially if you're holding on to a metal tool or a ski pole with a bare hand, but it's more likely that frostbite will develop over several hours or several days.

Don't ignore the warning signs. With frostnip — the first stage of frostbite — your toes, fingertips or a patch of skin on your cheek will get cold, pale, firm and dry and will feel prickly or numb.

Always ski, hike or work outside with a buddy, so he can look at your white-patchy face and tell you to warm up or go inside.

When Jack Frost is out with a vengeance, take these steps to reduce your risk of frostbite:

❐ **Get out of the wind.** Besides cold temperatures, high wind and humidity are the two main weather risk factors for frostbite. Wind makes you lose heat five times faster than still weather, and rain or snow will chill your body 25 times faster than dry skies.

❐ **Drink plenty of water and other liquids.** Dehydration is by far the number one bodily cause of frostbite, say nurses in an Alaskan hospital's thermal unit.

❐ **Don't strain too hard and take regular breaks** when working, playing or seeking shelter from the cold. Fatigue and sweating raise your risk of frostbite.

❐ **Avoid alcohol and cigarettes.** Alcohol makes you think you're warm when you're not, so your body doesn't shiver. Shivering is a natural way to produce heat. Smoking makes frostbite more likely because it shrinks your outer blood vessels.

☐ **Be extra cautious in cold weather** if you have any injury or illness or are simply out of shape. Even a common cold makes your body less able to generate and conserve heat. Medication you might be taking for an illness can make circulation worse, too. Some conditions that particularly raise your risk of frostbite are:

➤ Raynaud's syndrome (An illness where your blood vessels in your hands and feet close up too much in response to cold weather or stress. Your fingers turn pale and tingly or numb.)

➤ Diabetes

➤ An old or new bone fracture

➤ Previous frostbite

➤ Head injury

➤ Heart disease

➤ Lung disease

➤ Kidney or liver disease

☐ **Make sure your clothes are well-insulated, dry and not too tight.** You need to be able to move freely. Don't forget your hat and scarf — 80 percent of your body heat is lost from your head and neck.

You're more likely to get frostbitten when you're used to milder winters and your body isn't adjusted to freezing temperatures. You're also at high risk for frostbite if you're so used to the cold that you ignore it.

Eskimos have an old tradition of exposing their ears on purpose so that they'll acquire frostnip. Frostnip can actually make you more sensitive to the cold and better able to avoid frostbite.

Be proud if you're sensitive to cold weather — you've got a built-in frostbite warning system.

First aid for frostbite

Your goal in treating frostbite is to thaw your frozen fingers, feet and ears as quickly as possible in warm water.

First, make sure refreezing isn't a risk. It's better to keep walking on a frozen foot than to stop and thaw it before you get to permanent shelter. Tissues that have frozen, thawed and refrozen probably won't recover.

Make sure the frostbitten person doesn't have hypothermia (extremely low body temperature — around 90° F instead of the normal 98.6° F). A person with hypothermia should never be soaked in warm water.

If a person can talk clearly and answer questions logically, he probably doesn't have hypothermia.

On the other hand, a person whose body core is too cold will seem extremely lethargic — on the verge of unconsciousness. Wrap him in blankets and get him to a doctor as quickly as possible.

Follow these steps to thaw frozen parts of your body:

- ❏ Soak in a tub of warm water — 100° F to 106° F. If possible, use a thermometer to check the temperature so you won't burn your numbed body. Since frostbitten skin is prone to infection, put a solution such as Hibiclens (an anti-infection solution) in the bath water.
- ❏ Thaw frostbitten ears with soft towels soaked in warm salt water.
- ❏ Don't try to thaw yourself with dry heat. Campfires and car heaters are likely to burn your tender, numb skin, especially since you won't be able to feel how hot that air is.
    You'll know you are thawed when your skin turns pink or red — the blood is flowing back in the frozen tissues. Gently rinse the frostbitten parts with clean water, then pat dry or allow to air-dry. Cover loosely.
- ❏ Don't burst any blisters. Apply burn ointment such as Silvadene or Thermazene to open wounds and wrap loosely with sterile gauze and bandages.
- ❏ Drink fluid. The more fluids you drink, the faster your body will heal. Avoid caffeine and smoking because they cause blood vessels to narrow — the last thing you want to happen.
- ❏ Make sure you eat meals high in protein, calories, vitamins and minerals.

❏ Take aspirin to ease pain.

❏ Exercise and stretch gently several times a day to help blood
circulate in damaged feet and hands. Also, take warm 20-minute
baths with an anti-infection solution, such as Hibiclens, twice a
day to help blood flow to damaged tissues.

If your frostbite is severe, make sure you contact your doctor as soon as
possible. You may need professional treatment.

Medical Source ————————————————
American Journal of Nursing (93,2:59)

Tingling hands in the cold may be Raynaud's syndrome

Does a late fall football game bring back memories of high school and hot
chocolate, or are you focusing on how bad your fingers are hurting from the
cold? Come to think of it, do your fingers begin to hurt and change color
when you get food from the freezer, too?

If these things happen to you, chances are you could be suffering from
Raynaud's phenomenon.

It is a condition in which the small blood vessels in your hands and feet
get smaller and the circulation becomes decreased in response to cold. It is
caused by poor blood flow to your extremities.

During attacks of Raynaud's, you may feel pain, numbness, tingling or
burning. It can happen in young, healthy people, and it is much more
common in women than in men.

Usually your fingers or toes turn white as they first react, they may then
turn a bluish color due to a deficiency of oxygen in the blood, and as they
recover the skin turns red. The causes of this reaction include:

> ➤ Exposure to cold
> ➤ Drugs that cause blood vessels to narrow
>   (vasoconstrictors)
> ➤ Emotional distress

What parts of your body are affected?

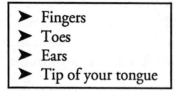

> Fingers
> Toes
> Ears
> Tip of your tongue

Tips to help minimize the effects of Raynaud's phenomenon include:

☐ Avoid the cold whenever possible.
☐ Wear thick gloves and socks even in moderately cold weather.
☐ Try heated gloves and socks (available at sporting goods stores).
☐ Keep a pair of gloves by the freezer to wear when you take out frozen foods.
☐ Don't hold cold beverages.
☐ If you are severely affected, you might want to consider moving to a warmer climate.

There are also several types of drugs that you should avoid:

> Tobacco
> Caffeine
> Amphetamines
> Cocaine
> Pseudoephedrine
> Phenylpropanolamine
> Ephedrine
> Phenylephrine
> Ergotamines. (These are found in some prescription migraine medications.)

Most of these drugs are commonly available, and many of them occur in over-the-counter medicines, so check the labels on any medications you take.

You can dramatically improve your symptoms if you eliminate all of these. If you smoke, eliminating tobacco is the best thing you can do to get better.

If you have Raynaud's phenomenon occurring more often than you can tolerate, or if you start to develop sores on the affected parts, see your doctor immediately.

Medical Source ——————————————————
 American Family Physician (47,4:823)

Hypothermia — a cold weather hazard

Even when the worst of our winter weather is nearly over, danger from the cold still lingers.

In fact, even spring-like temperatures of 50° F to 60° F can bring on hypothermia. This condition develops when the temperature at the center or core of your body falls below 95° F.

Normally, your body core temperature ranges from 96.8° F to 99.5° F. But prolonged exposure can cool your body to a dangerously low temperature. Most often this happens accidentally, when a person stays outdoors too long. In addition, hypothermia often results from a dip in cold water, or when alcohol or other drugs have lowered body temperature or caused a person to forget about the cold.

These medical conditions and chronic diseases also increase the risk of hypothermia:

> ➤ Hypothyroidism
> ➤ Hypopituitarism
> ➤ Hypoadrenalism
> ➤ Anorexia nervosa
> ➤ Head injury
> ➤ Stroke
> ➤ Extensive burns
> ➤ Sepsis
> ➤ Tumors of the hypothalamus
> ➤ Some spinal cord injuries

However, the people who are most likely to develop hypothermia are babies and older people. Infants' core temperatures fall rapidly because their small bodies simply cannot generate enough heat to keep them warm when they are exposed to cool or cold temperatures for a long time.

Older people are particularly vulnerable to hypothermia because they often have poor circulation.

Also, older bodies no longer regulate temperature well, and they sometimes lose the ability to shiver. Shivering can actually increase by five times the amount of heat your body produces. Seniors also run the risk of hypothermia if they fall and are unable to move from a cold to a warm environment.

You should suspect a person has developed hypothermia if he:

> is confused
> slurs speech
> acts irrationally (begins taking off clothes, etc.)
> becomes uncoordinated
> becomes rigid

If the body's core temperature falls as low as 86° F, the person will lose consciousness, and at 68° F, the heart stops beating.

Doctors sometimes find it hard to diagnose hypothermia because regular thermometers don't register low enough to accurately read a low body temperature.

The only sure way to assess core temperature is to get the person to a hospital, where the proper equipment can measure internally how cold someone really is.

If you suspect that someone is suffering from hypothermia, immediately follow these steps to rewarm him passively:

❏ Remove the person from the cold to a warm environment.
❏ Wrap the person in dry, unheated blankets.

As soon as you have begun passive rewarming, consult your physician about what to do next.

A person with hypothermia probably needs additional help that can only be given safely by medical personnel.

Medical Source ————————————————
Postgraduate Medicine (92,8:47)

'Lime disease' — a painful mix of margaritas and sun

You may have heard about Lyme disease — the flu-like illness you get from ticks, but did you know that lime juice and sun may be linked to a new "Lime disease" called phytophotodermatitis?

A 30-year old man discovered the painful effects of "Lime disease" when he mixed too many margaritas (containing lime juice) with too much sun.

After squeezing five dozen limes in the preparation of margaritas, the man proceeded to sunbathe for the rest of the afternoon. Two days later, he went to the hospital because his left hand (the hand he used to squeeze the limes with) had become severely burned, swollen and blistered.

Doctors were baffled by this isolated flare-up, until the man recalled his recent activities.

The physicians conducting the examination quickly diagnosed his condition as an extreme case of photodermatitis — a skin reaction caused by contact with large amounts of a substance that makes you sun-sensitive combined with prolonged exposure to the sun's rays.

Oranges, grapefruits and other citrus fruits, as well as celery, are prime photosensitizers or foods that can make your skin super-sensitive to sunlight if contact occurs.

Previously, photodermatitis has been known only as an occupational hazard among citrus workers and celery harvesters. However, other cases have been reported in isolated incidences including a group of day camp kids who were making pomander balls from limes, and a toddler who spilled lime juice on his chest.

If you're going to be mixing citrus or celery juice with the sun, be sure to use gloves on your hands for protection as well as sunscreen.

Medical Source ————————————————
The New England Journal of Medicine (328,12:891)

Sun sense means cancer prevention

"Slip! Slop! Slap!" is a popular Australian slogan these days. With one of the highest cancer rates in the world, many Australians are following the timely advice to "Slip on a shirt. Slop on some sunscreen. Slap on a hat."

The only known way to reduce your risk of skin cancer is to reduce your exposure to the ultraviolet rays of the sun.

As the ozone layer continues to deteriorate and ultraviolet rays become more intense, the Environmental Protection Agency predicts that cancer rates will continue to rise. Protecting yourself against the sun's rays therefore becomes more and more important, cautions medical experts.

Each time you expose yourself unprotected to the sun, you raise your risk of developing skin cancer. A history of repeated sunburns or even just one massive sunburn can increase this risk.

And, surprisingly, winter sun can be just as damaging as summer sun. Ultraviolet A (UVA) rays, that cause skin aging, stay constant throughout the year while Ultraviolet B (UVB) rays, which cause sunburn and tanning, are most intense during the summer. Both types of ultraviolet rays cause cancer.

Sunscreens can be very effective in shielding you from the sun's harmful rays whether you're swimming at the beach or snow skiing.

Below are a few tips to help you choose a sunscreen.

☐ Look for a sunscreen labeled "broad spectrum," which means that it protects against both Ultraviolet A and Ultraviolet B rays. Sometimes a sunscreen may simply say "protects against UVA and UVB."

☐ Check the Sun Protection Factor (SPF) on the label. The higher the factor number, the greater protection the sunscreen offers against burns. The lighter your skin and the longer you plan to be in the sun, the more protection you need.

Although SPF only measures a sunscreen's effectiveness against Ultraviolet B rays, a broad spectrum sunscreen protects against both Ultraviolet A and B. At this time there is no known way to rate a sunscreen's effectiveness against Ultraviolet A rays.

The Food and Drug Administration (FDA) has proposed that since an SPF of 30 appears to be the limit for sunscreen effectiveness that sunscreens with an SPF over 30 be removed from the market.

❏   Look for a sunscreen that provides protection when you perspire or swim. Water-resistant sunscreens provide in-the-water protection for as long as 40 minutes of swimming. Waterproof sunscreens provide in-the-water protection for as long as 80 minutes.

❏   Pick up some lip balm that contains sunscreen since the lower lip is a common site for skin cancer. Lip balm with sunscreen can also protect against cold sores, which may be triggered by ultraviolet radiation.

❏   Choose a tanning lotion that contains dihydroxyacetone if you insist on tanning. Creams containing this chemical only affect the dead cells of the skin's outermost layer.

Tips on how to apply sunscreen:

❏   Apply sunscreen evenly. This will help ensure a uniform tan.
❏   Apply 30 minutes before dressing to give your skin time to absorb the sunscreen. This will help prevent fabric staining also.
❏   Apply sunscreen two hours before exercising to avoid sweat streaks that could lead to a streaky tan.

If you do get burned, here's a special remedy for soothing a sunburn. Mix a 3-ounce bottle of Mennen's Afta aftershave with a 1-ounce tube of .5 percent hydrocortisone cream.

Apply to sunburned areas. Repeat after 30 minutes. Treatment is very effective and will also prevent blistering.

Despite all its bad rap, sunshine exposure has some good points. Time spent outside in the sun raises people's spirits and contributes to their sense of well-being.

Sunshine also stimulates the body's production of vitamin D, which strengthens bones and teeth. Some researchers suggest that vitamin D also protects against colon cancer. Five minutes of sun a day will help your body produce all the vitamin D it requires.

So, if you plan to be out in the sun longer than five minutes, remember the Australian "Slip! Slop! Slap!" slogan and "Slip on a shirt. Slop on some sunscreen" and "Slap on a hat."

You'll save your skin and maybe even your life.

Medical Sources ————————————————————
Medical World News (33,2:19)
The Physician and Sportsmedicine (21,3:30)

Take the sting out of sunscreen

Sometimes the sunscreen you use to prevent sunburn can cause you to break out in an irritating, itchy, blistering rash.

The rash may appear 30 to 60 minutes after applying the sunscreen or it may show up several days later as a part of your body's immune response to some ingredient in the sunscreen.

The rash usually lingers for several days, then turns scaly and gradually disappears.

There are two types of sunscreens — chemical and physical. The active ingredients used in chemical sunscreens protect against sunburn by absorbing ultraviolet radiation. These types of sunscreen generally cause the most reactions.

A sunscreen will not usually indicate whether it is chemical or physical. A glance at the active ingredients will tell you.

>   **Para-aminobenzoic acid (PABA)**, PABA derivatives and benzophenones are the active ingredients responsible for the majority of reactions. PABA offers long-lasting sunscreen protection, yet permits tanning.
>
>   However, the alcoholic solutions in which para-aminobenzoic acids are dissolved often cause drying, tightening and stinging sensations. Since many people have reactions to PABA, its use as an active sunscreen ingredient is declining. PABA can also leave permanent yellow stains in cotton and synthetic fabrics, such as nylon and polyester.
>
>   **PABA derivatives**, broadly grouped as para-aminobenzoic acid esters are generally replacing PABA as the active ingredient in many sunscreens. They are widely known as Padimate A and Padimate O. These derivatives are less irritating than PABA and do not stain

clothing. People seem to be the least sensitive to Padimate O, now the biggest selling sunscreen chemical in the United States.

Cinnamates are also commonly used sunscreen ingredients that may cause skin irritation. If you are allergic to perfume, you may also be allergic to cinnamates. Avoid sunscreen with cinnamates as well as perfume, medicine and toothpaste that contain cinnamates if you discover a cinnamate sensitivity.

Benzophenones are often used in combination with other sunscreen chemicals, especially cinnamates, to give complete sunscreen protection. Recent European studies indicate that reactions to benzophenones, particularly oxybenzophone, seem to be on the rise.

Salicylates and anthranilates are generally very mild sunscreen ingredients. Salicylates are considered to be among the safest of all sunscreen chemicals. In addition, salicylates soften the skin and won't come off easily in water.

Anthranilates are usually combined with some other sunscreen substances to give complete sunscreen protection.

Active ingredients used in physical sunscreens are not usually very troublesome. The size of the particles that make up the sunscreen and the thickness of the ointment itself provide protection by reflecting ultraviolet rays.

Zinc oxide seems to be the most effective of all physical sunscreen ingredients. Neither zinc oxide nor titanium dioxide cause reactions.

Physical sunscreens sometimes come in bright colors, which is often pleasing to young children. They do not wash off easily and they provide excellent protection for easily burned areas, such as the nose and mouth.

You may want to use these sunscreens if you're taking medications that cause you to be sensitive to light or if you work outdoors, such as lifeguards, sailors, farmers and construction workers.

Physical sunscreens do tend to melt with the heat of the sun, limiting protection to a few hours, and they are messy and visible. They can also block skin pores, hair follicles and sweat glands.

Sometimes dermatitis is not caused by the sunscreen ingredients that actively protect against the sun, but is a reaction to sunscreen preservatives. Alcohol, propylene glycol, dyes, lanolin and carbowax may also be the source of a skin rash.

To avoid skin rashes from sunscreen, read labels and avoid those creams you think could be a problem. Keep in mind that manufacturers may change ingredients from time to time with no label indication or change in product name.

If you generally have sensitive skin or suspect that you may be allergic to a particular sunscreen, test a small amount of sunscreen on your elbow before applying it to the rest of your body.

Apply sunscreen to that location for a minimum of three days, then expose the test area to strong sunlight for a while. Your skin may react almost immediately after you apply the sunscreen, or it may react a few days later or only when you expose the test area to the sun.

If you have a sunscreen reaction, discontinue use immediately and treat the affected area with hydrocortisone cream. If treatment does not relieve the rash, see a doctor.

If sunscreens cause an unpleasant stinging sensation but don't make you break out, try applying 1 percent hydrocortisone cream the night before you apply sunscreen.

Don't stop using sunscreens just because you experience discomfort. Keep searching until you find the sunscreen that's right for you. The protection sunscreens offer are well worth the effort.

If you develop a rash and suspect your sunscreen is the cause, try to identify the quilty ingredient and substitute another brand which uses a different active ingredient.

Medical Sources —————————————————
Cutis (50,3:190,4:253,5:331 and 6:397)

FOOD POISONING

Dodging food poisoning

If the "diarrhea dash" has you running, you may be one of the estimated 80 million Americans who suffer from food poisoning each year. Symptoms may appear as quickly as 30 minutes after you eat the contaminated food, or they may not develop for several days.

Discomfort normally only lasts one or two days but can persist for 10 days and may include:

➤ Nausea	➤ Stomach cramps
➤ Headache	➤ Diarrhea (may be bloody)
➤ Vomiting	➤ Chills
➤ Fever	➤ Exhaustion

However, by properly handling and preparing foods at home, you can cut your risk by as much as 85 percent.

Grocery store shopping tips

Preventive measures against food poisoning begin at the grocery store. Follow the tips listed below to help protect you and your family against food poisoning.

☐ **Examine packaged and canned foods** before putting them in your cart and pick them up first when you shop. Don't buy food in bulging cans or jars that have loose or swollen lids.

☐ **Check expiration labels.** Never buy outdated food. When buying dairy products, such as cottage cheese, cream cheese, yogurt, sour cream, milk, etc., buy the products that have the longest time left before they expire.

☐ **Choose Grade A refrigerated eggs.** Check the eggs to make sure none are cracked, broken or leaking.

☐ **Buy frozen foods, meat, poultry and fish last.** Carry plastic bags to hold your meat items, so if they drip they won't contaminate other items in your shopping cart.

☐ **Check for cleanliness at the meat and fish counter and at the salad bar.** When choosing fish, keep the words of a famous chef in mind: "Fish should smell like the tide. Once they smell like fish, it's too late."

It's OK if fish smells like seaweed, but it should never smell like ammonia. Make sure the store has fish types separated. For example, cooked shrimp on the same bed of ice as raw fish could become contaminated.

☐ **Buy shellfish from state-approved vendors only.** Don't buy shellfish from roadside stands or the back of a truck. If you catch your own shellfish, make sure the water is not contaminated.

☐ **Take an ice chest to store your perishable foods** if the grocery store is more than an hour from your house.

Food storage checklist

Properly storing foods at home is an important step in preventing food poisoning. Follow these steps for food storage:

☐ **Refrigerate or freeze perishable foods** immediately.

☐ **Check periodically to make sure your refrigerator temperature** is 40 degrees Fahrenheit or less and that your freezer temperature stays at zero degrees Fahrenheit. The only way to get an accurate temperature reading of your refrigerator or freezer is to use a refrigerator-freezer thermometer. These are available at hardware or discount department stores for about $5.

☐ **Don't store poultry or meat in the refrigerator for more than two days.** Keep the meat in its original wrapper. Make sure no juices can escape and contaminate other foods.

☐ **Don't store eggs in the refrigerator door** or leave loose in an egg

box. It's best to leave eggs in their carton, where they stay cooler and have less chance of cracking. To maintain flavor and freshness, use raw eggs within five weeks of purchasing them. Store hard-boiled eggs in the refrigerator until needed. You can store them up to 10 days.

❑ **Keep seafood in the refrigerator or freezer** until ready for use.

❑ **Don't cram your refrigerator or freezer full of food.** Air needs room to circulate.

❑ **Tightly wrap foods** destined for the freezer.

❑ **Keep mayonnaise and ketchup in the refrigerator after opening.** Some spices should also be refrigerated. Smoked, vacuum-packed or cured foods may need to be refrigerated. Check labels if you're unsure about refrigerating an item. If you forget to refrigerate an item, throw it out. Foods left sitting at room temperature for two hours or more should be thrown away.

❑ **Check for mold on cheese.** Cheese with mold does not have to be thrown away. Trim away the visible mold and a one-inch area around the mold to eliminate any invisible mold roots. Throw away molded cottage and cream cheeses and moldy bread.

❑ **Don't rely on your nose to detect food poisoning.** The bacteria that cause illness do not cause any odor or change in color.

❑ **Put newly purchased canned items behind older canned products,** so you'll use the older cans first. Check all cans for leaks. Return any new cans that are leaking to the store.

❑ **Don't store potatoes and onions under the sink** because pipe leakage could damage them. Store potatoes in a cool, dry place — not the refrigerator.

❑ **Never store foods near household cleaning products and chemicals.**

Protection from kitchen bacteria
Another way to prevent food poisoning is to keep your cooking area clean and clutter-free. Here are some simple ways to keep bacteria at bay:

☐ **Always wash your hands with hot soapy water** before cooking and before you eat, especially after visiting the bathroom. You should also wash your hands after you handle raw meat or poultry.

☐ **Cover long hair** with net or scarf.

☐ **Cover any open sores or cuts on the hands.** Stay out of the kitchen if any of these sores are infected.

☐ **Don't smoke while cooking.**

☐ **Wash utensils used on raw meat before using them on other items.** Don't put cooked meat on a plate that has held raw meat.

☐ **Clean cutting boards thoroughly after each use.** Wooden cutting boards harbor less bacteria than other types.

☐ **Wash lids of canned foods before opening.** This prevents any dirt on the lids from getting into the food.

☐ **Clean the can opener blade** after each use.

☐ **Take apart and wash blenders, food grinders and processors** immediately after use.

☐ **Throw away dirty sponges.**

☐ **Wipe up refrigerator spills** immediately.

☐ **Remove food particles** from kitchen counters.

☐ **Don't thaw meat at room temperature.** Thaw in the refrigerator or in the microwave. You can also defrost frozen foods in cold water, changing the water every 30 minutes. It's OK to refreeze foods that have been thawed in the refrigerator, but it is not a good idea to refreeze foods thawed in the microwave. Microwaves defrost foods unevenly, which might mean that one section of food gets warm enough for bacteria to start to grow, but not hot enough to kill the bacteria.

☐ **Wash all fruits and vegetables before cooking or eating raw.** After cutting a melon, either eat or refrigerate it within four hours.

Cooking safety tips

Cook foods at their recommended temperature. You may want to use a food thermometer to test heat levels. Listed below are some recommendations for heating foods.

- ❑ **Chicken and turkey — 170° F to 180° F.** Chicken will be white when it is done and its juices will run clear. The bone and some of the meat next to the bone may remain red, but this is not harmful.

- ❑ **Ground beef — 165° F.** There should be no pink in the center and juices should be clear. Small children, elderly people and people with lowered immunity should make an effort to steer clear of beef.

- ❑ **Veal, lamb and pork — 160° F.**

- ❑ **Roasts and steaks — 145° F.**

- ❑ **Shrimp — Cook three to five minutes or until the shells turn red.** You don't have to remove the vein in cooked shrimp. As long as it is refrigerated, shrimp is safe to eat for up to two days after you purchase it.

- ❑ **Oysters, mussels and clams — Steam an extra three to five minutes after they open.** When working with live shellfish, cook only those that have tightly closed shells or shells that close when you touch them. After cooking, discard any shells that do not open.

- ❑ **Flounder, swordfish, etc. — Cook at 450° F, 10 minutes for each inch of thickness.** The fish is done when the thickest part turns white and flakes easily with a fork.

- ❑ **Eggs — Cook until the white is firm and the yolk begins to harden.**

- ❑ **Maintain foods kept out of the refrigerator for more than two hours at a temperature of at least 140° F.** Otherwise, bacteria levels will skyrocket dangerously high. This is especially important for picnics and other outdoor eating events.

How to handle leftovers

Leftovers can mean a reprieve from cooking for a few days. Here are a few tips to keep your leftovers fresh and safe.

- ❏ **Refrigerate leftovers within two hours** of the meal.

- ❏ **Don't store large leftovers in one large container.** The food in the center of the container might not cool fast enough to stop bacteria from multiplying. Divide the remaining food into several smaller airtight containers.

- ❏ **Cut leftover meats into slices of three inches or less.**

- ❏ **Remove all stuffing from roast turkey or chicken and store it separately.** Also store giblets separately.

- ❏ **Check leftovers daily for spoilage.** Immediately throw away anything that looks or smells spoiled.

- ❏ **Leftovers should be reheated to at least 165° F.**

- ❏ **Use leftovers within three days.**

Food poisoning is most dangerous for the very young and old and for people with faulty immune systems. For severe symptoms, see a doctor or get emergency help.

Medical Sources ———————————————
   FDA Consumer (25,1:18)
   Tufts University Diet & Nutrition Letter (11,8:3)

The best bacteria-fighting cutting board: wood or plastic?

If you've been using plastic cutting surfaces to slice your meats and veggies, you might be surprised by this piercing news.

Plastic cutting boards can actually harbor bacteria, allowing them to survive in crevices and multiply. If you have grown accustomed to your plastic cutting boards, you're not alone.

For approximately the past 20 years, sanitation officials have encouraged us to use plastic cutting boards instead of wood, believing that it was easier to remove bacteria from plastic than wood

Even the Department of Agriculture has recommended using plastic cutting boards.

But very little research was conducted to demonstrate plastic's superiority over wood. In fact, one study performed 25 years ago found that cleaning bacteria from wooden cutting boards was just as easy as cleaning them from plastic boards.

Current research indicates that wooden surfaces are actually better at preventing food contamination and illness compared with plastic.

In a study at the University of Wisconsin, researchers contaminated both plastic and wooden cutting boards with common bacteria that cause food poisoning. In just three minutes, 99.9 percent of the bacteria on the wooden board couldn't be found and were presumed dead.

None of the bacteria placed on the plastic cutting boards died. In fact, when the boards were left overnight at room temperature, the bacteria on the plastic board multiplied. No live bacteria were retrieved from the wooden boards.

Even if a wooden cutting board were contaminated with a million or more bacteria, it would probably only take about two hours before 99.9 percent of the bacteria disappeared.

But most of us would probably never be dealing with this many bacteria at once, considering that the number of bacteria that might wash off a chicken would be about 1,000.

While wooden cutting boards appear to kill bacteria, they don't yield the dead bodies, but, instead, apparently absorb them.

And cleaning your wooden cutting board may be as easy as giving it a good wipe.

However, bacteria that is lodged in knife-cut grooves of plastic cutting boards can survive a hot soap-and-water wash and later contaminate other foods.

All types and ages of wood seem to be effective in fighting off the bacteria, including hard maple, birch, beech, black cherry, basswood, butternut and American black walnut.

Quite often, however, wooden cutting boards come from the factory treated with mineral oil, intended to make the wooden boards more like plastic, which unfortunately it does.

Bacteria survive longer on these cutting boards than on untreated, wooden cutting boards.

Researchers aren't exactly sure why or how wood works so well against bacteria. But for now, it seems that any way you slice, dice, chop or carve it — wooden cutting boards are the easiest on your knives and your best barrier against bacteria.

Medical Source ————————————————
Science News (143,6:84)

The preventable 'pork' poisoning

Cooking pork thoroughly can prevent disease. For years mom told us to cook pork chops thoroughly, but some people still aren't getting the message that trichinosis is a preventable disease.

Trichinella spiralis is a parasitic worm that causes trichinosis as it travels through the body after a person eats raw or undercooked meat, especially pork. *T. spiralis* then travels through the body and produces larvae that become enclosed in muscle tissue.

Five to 45 days later, symptoms such as mild flu-like feeling, nausea, vomiting and fever may appear.

More common second-stage symptoms include an accumulation of fluid around the eyes, sensitivity to light and retinal bleeding. Diagnosis is usually made from blood tests and muscle biopsies.

Sporadic outbreaks of trichinosis occur where people eat wild animals or home-butchered pork. However, recent cases in the Mid-Atlantic states region were linked to undercooked, commercially prepared bulk pork sausage.

Irradiation of pork with low doses of gamma rays to kill larvae, as well as meat inspection, can prevent the disease-infected meat from reaching our markets. Until these measures are set into effect, thorough cooking of pork is the best protection for your family's health.

Medical Source ─────────────────────
Southern Medical Journal (85,4:428)

Botulism: The fatal food poisoning

While most food poisoning is only uncomfortable and irritating, botulism can kill you.

Botulism is usually caused by eating improperly canned or preserved foods. Home-preserved foods, such as canned vegetables, cured pork and ham and smoked and raw fish, are often responsible for the illness.

These bacteria thrive in an oxygenless atmosphere with little acidity. Common canned foods that may harbor the bacteria include:

➤ Corn	➤ Green beans	➤ Soups
➤ Mushrooms	➤ Tuna	➤ Liver pâté

Some foods not packaged in cans may bring on a bout of botulism although poisoning associated with these items is rare. Keeping these foods in the refrigerator will significantly reduce any possible risk.

➤ Peppers	➤ Tomatoes	➤ Asparagus
➤ Eggs	➤ Salmon	➤ Stuffed eggplant
➤ Pickles	➤ Garlic	➤ Cooked potatoes
➤ Onions	➤ Beets	➤ Luncheon meats
➤ Lobster	➤ Smoked and salted fish	

Two simple steps will help you avoid botulism:

- ❑ Never eat food from bulging cans.
- ❑ Sterilize home-preserved food by pressure cooking it at 250° F. for 30 minutes.

Symptoms of botulism normally appear from eight to 48 hours after you've eaten the contaminated food. Nausea and vomiting commonly signal food poisoning and may also be indicators of botulism.

If you have any of the following symptoms, see a doctor immediately.

> Blurred or double vision
> Difficulty speaking, breathing or swallowing
> Paralysis

Eventually paralysis will shut down the respiratory system and the victim will suffocate. Death occurs in 70 percent of the people with botulism who don't receive medical treatment.

Medical Sources —————————————————

The American Medical Association Encyclopedia of Medicine, Random House, New York, 1989
Tufts University Diet & Nutrition Letter (11,8:3)

E. coli strikes again: Case of the 'natural' apple cider

E. coli O157:H7 is on the loose. If it catches up with you, you could be on the run.

The O157:H7 strain of E. coli bacteria has been linked to bloody diarrhea and hemolytic uremic syndrome, a disorder that can cause kidney failure and even death.

The E. coli bacteria is commonly present in intestines and feces of humans and animals. Most of the time this bacteria does not cause any problems. Some digestive bacteria is actually beneficial, helping to break down food. However, E. coli O157:H7 produces a poison that can cause serious problems.

Most illnesses occur when food and water become contaminated with E. coli as a result of unsanitary conditions, such as not washing hands after a bathroom visit or drinking water that has been contaminated by a sewage spill.

Unpasteurized milk and unwashed produce fertilized with manure contaminated with E. coli may cause illness. Usually one million or more bacteria need to be present to cause sickness.

When the bacteria gets into food or water, it multiplies rapidly. If you eat food or drink water that has accumulated substantial amounts of bacteria, you may experience cramping, diarrhea, vomiting and fever.

E. coli O157:H7 was responsible for one of the worst food poisoning outbreaks to ever occur in the United States. At a Pacific Midwest Jack-in-the-Box fast-food restaurant, contaminated hamburger meat made 400 people sick and resulted in the death of at least one child.

Investigation into the incident revealed that "the contaminated hamburger was improperly handled at the slaughterhouse, as well as being insufficiently cooked at the restaurant."

While any meat or poultry that is not properly handled could be a source of E. coli, most cases have been traced to fast food restaurants, not supermarkets.

However, a little common sense will protect you when you're eating out:

- ❏ Wash your hands with soap and hot water after bathroom visits.
- ❏ Tell pink beef to m-o-o-ve over. Well done is in. Steaks and other meat that is not ground is much less likely to harbor E. coli if it's undercooked. Still, health officials advise you not to eat steak tartare or other dishes containing raw meat.
- ❏ Don't depend on your nose to sniff out contamination. Meat infected with E. coli has no odor.

You should also avoid that amber, sweet smelling cider on sale at roadside stands in the fall. Investigators have linked apple cider to at least three outbreaks of E. coli. Unpasteurized apple cider appears to be an excellent growth medium for E. coli, which can survive in the cider for up to 20 days even when refrigerated.

Commonly, apple cider is made from "drops," apples collected from the ground. The infection is probably spread through rotten apples and fallen apples that become contaminated with animal droppings harboring the E. coli bacteria.

Both healthy and rotten apples are collected and pressed to make the cider. Only a small percentage, 33 percent in one study, of small apple cider producers brush and wash their apples before pressing them to make cider. Typically, these producers don't pasteurize or add preservatives to the cider.

If you just can't pass up that roadside apple cider, there are ways to reduce your risk of an E. coli infection.

☐ Ask if the apples used to make the cider were brushed and washed.
☐ Ask whether the cider is made from "drops," or from picked apples. Picked apples are preferable.
☐ Ask if the cider has been pasteurized or contains preservatives. The preservative sodium benzoate .1% reduced E. coli survival time from 20 to less than 7 days.
☐ Don't rely on your senses to tell you if the cider is contaminated. Cider tainted with E. coli has no strange odor, taste or appearance.

Despite this problem with homemade apple cider, most other apple products are safe. Commercial cider makers include several washing steps as well as pasteurization in their production process. Any E. coli in applesauce is eliminated in the cooking process.

With these tips in hand, you can prevent E. coli from cramping your style.

Medical Sources ————————————————————
University of California at Berkeley Wellness Letter (9,9:1)
Nutrition Action Health Letter (20,3:13)
The Journal of the American Medical Association (269,17:2217)
Medical Tribune (34,10:10)

New food packaging process may cause problems

Sometimes the last thing you want to do after a long day at work is to come home and make dinner, right? You might feel yourself choosing more and more microwave dinners and pre-packaged foods at the grocery store than you used to.

The increase in working women and senior citizens, and the changing family has challenged the food industry to create a new generation of quick and easy foods.

And now there's a new kid on the block in the food-processing industry known as "sous vide." Sous vide is French for vacuum-packed. But is this newcomer a friend or foe?

Sous vide isn't actually a new food, it's a new way to process and package foods that began in France. Fresh foods are vacuum sealed in heavy-duty plastic.

The package is then circulated in hot water for several hours. This process not only cooks the food, but pasteurizes it as well. Immediately after cooking, the packaged food is cooled in cold water.

The final product? Foods that have very little shrinkage, lots of flavor and freshness compared to other pre-packaged foods, very few preservatives, and a refrigerated shelf life of up to three weeks.

So, if the foods are great tasting and fresh, easy to prepare, and have an extended shelf life, what else do we need to know?

One serious concern is the safety of the food. Sous vide processing does not expose the food to extreme temperatures, (boiling or freezing), nor does it use preservatives — methods used in traditional processing to control spoilage by killing bacteria.

And sometimes food that is contaminated or bad might not always have an odor. What this means is that some sous vide food may have spoiled, but there might not be an odor signaling you not to eat it.

Sous vide may actually be a breeding ground for botulism and listeriosis. Both grow in conditions where there is almost no oxygen. Sous vide processing produces an almost oxygen-free environment which sets the stage for these two bacteria.

People most susceptible to botulism and listeriosis include pregnant women, babies and small children, the elderly and people who use antacids on a regular basis.

Another concern is the temperature fluctuations in the handling of sous vide food. Once the food is processed, it must be stored at 38° F. or less.

Handling and restocking of the items often means that the food is not kept at this temperature. This can lead to the growth of bacteria in the food which means a contaminated product.

According to one report, elderly people might be confused by how similar the packaging of sous vide foods, requiring refrigeration, looks like shelf-stable products that do not need to be refrigerated. In error, food could be stored in the cabinet instead of in the refrigerator, and the food would spoil.

Tips for making healthy choices in pre-packaged foods:

☐ Choose foods that are rich in vitamins and minerals. Try to get your nutrition from the food you eat rather than from supplements and pills.

☐ Check the expiration date on the package. If it is past the expiration date on the package, throw it out. It doesn't have to smell bad for it to be spoiled — you can't always smell poisonous bacteria.

☐ Store foods properly. Double check every label on a pre-packaged item. Often items that need to be refrigerated are packaged much like items that can be stored in the cabinet.

☐ Read preparation instructions carefully. The way you should prepare prepackaged foods will often vary depending on whether you are using a regular oven or a microwave oven.

☐ Check labels for fat, sodium and preservatives. This is particularly important if you are on a salt- or fat-restricted diet.

Medical Source ———————————————————
The Journal of Nutrition for the Elderly (11,3:45)

Trains, boats and planes: Travel cuisine to avoid

No one wants to think negative thoughts when taking a trip. You look forward to seeing the sights, buying souvenirs and getting a break from your everyday routine.

But one of the things you should remember is — food poisoning is a real possibility no matter what mode of transportation you use — airplane, train or ship.

Airplane food is usually prepared by caterers who are regulated by the

FDA (Food and Drug Administration), but sometimes food poisoning can occur.

For example, in 1988, 21 players of the Minnesota Vikings football team experienced cramps, fever, chills and diarrhea after eating an airplane meal. After an intense investigation, the contamination was traced to submarine sandwiches. The sandwiches had been prepared by infected food handlers employed by the airline caterer.

Train meals usually aren't catered. They are prepared on the trains in kitchen cars.

Two constant problems faced by these trains are space limitations involving refrigeration and mice infestation. The mice usually stow away while the trains are idle at freight yards.

Cruise ship food handlers experience some of the same problems that train food handlers encounter (storage and rodent problems). However, two additional problems can occur aboard ships.

One is the possibility of bacterial infection in food that often is served buffet-style. In other words, constant exposure and improper handling can increase the risk of food poisoning.

Another problem is the constant challenge of purifying sea water through plumbing systems that can experience drainage and back flow problems, possibly contaminating water used for preparing food, drinking water, bathing or showering and dish washing.

The FDA has provided guidelines to planes, trains and cruise ships to regulate equipment that could cause health hazards. They also make periodic inspections of equipment, food preparation and procedures. Travelers are also advised to call their FDA district office with any safety or sanitation complaint they may have after traveling.

While the FDA does not have the authority to monitor planes and ships from foreign countries, the United States Department of Agriculture, the Centers for Disease Control (CDC), and the United States Coast Guard have various jurisdiction, and they work with the FDA if a health crisis arises.

Such a problem occurred in February 1992, when 96 people aboard an airplane arriving in Los Angeles from Buenos Aires, Argentina, including passengers and crew members, became ill and were later diagnosed with cholera (infection involving severe diarrhea and vomiting). One passenger died in Los Angeles.

Health officials traced the poisonings to a cold seafood salad served aboard the plane.

Travelers — help reduce the number of food poisoning incidents — if you see or experience problems with food safety or sanitation, call the nearest FDA district office in your local phone book. Complaints will be investigated.

Medical Source ————————————————————
FDA Consumer (27,2:6)

Fact or fiction? Important food safety checklist

Most of us have grown up hearing "words of wisdom" from friends and relatives about food safety. You may be surprised to learn that some of these beliefs are fallacies. Here are a few:

Belief: Mayonnaise is a top bacteria carrier.

Fact: The high acid and salt content of mayonnaise may actually prevent bacterial growth. However, you should still keep any salads or sandwiches containing mayonnaise refrigerated.

Belief: Salmonella is found only in chicken, eggs and other animal foods.

Fact: Salmonella may grow on cantaloupe, watermelon and honeydew. To prevent contamination, wash all your fruits and vegetables and make sure all foods are refrigerated within two hours of heating or in the case of melons, within four hours of cutting.

Belief: Freezing kills disease-causing bacteria.

Fact: Freezing stops bacteria from growing. Heating food to the appropriate temperature is the only way to kill bacteria.

Belief: You can't refreeze thawed foods.

Fact: If the item has been thawed in the refrigerator, it's OK to refreeze it.

Belief: Food left out of the refrigerator for more than two hours is safe to eat as long as you warm it to the appropriate temperature.

Fact: Heating the food will probably kill the bacteria, but it won't eliminate the illness-causing poisons that some bacteria leave behind.

Belief: If the area near the chicken bone remains red after adequate cooking time at the appropriate temperature, the chicken is still not done.

Fact: If the chicken meat is white and its juices run clear, it's done. Most chickens sold these day are marketed very young, at about seven to nine weeks of age. In young chickens, the bones are still porous and when they are cooked, red pigment is drawn up to the bones from the bone marrow.

For more information:

For spur-of-the-moment food or nutrition questions you just can't find the answers to, try these sources.

- ❑ U.S. Department of Agriculture's Meat & Poultry Hotline 1-800-535-4555 from 10 a.m. to 4 p.m. EST. The number in the Washington, D.C., area is 447-3333. Monday — Friday.

- ❑ Seafood Hotline 1-800-332-4010 from noon to 4 p.m. EST. For Washington, D.C., residents, the number is 205-4314. Monday — Friday.

- ❑ Consumer Nutrition Hot Line 1-800-366-1655 from 10 a.m. to 5 p.m. EST. Monday — Friday.

Medical Source ————————————————

Tufts University Diet & Nutrition Letter (11,8:3)

CHEMICAL POISONING

Lead-poisoning: Arm yourself against an invisible danger

Lead poisoning continues to be a problem. It can have serious, long-lasting and life-threatening effects on children and adults.

In children, lead poisoning can cause long-term learning disorders and behavior problems, slowed growth, hearing loss, lowered IQ, colic, anemia, kidney damage, brain damage and death. Adults with lead poisoning may suffer from high blood pressure, hearing loss, anemia, shortened life span and brain damage.

Men with lead poisoning may also become infertile.

Children, however, are more at risk than adults. Since children tend to put everything (food or otherwise) into their mouths, they have a particularly high risk of absorbing lead in paint by eating or tasting the paint chips.

Lead builds up quickly in children because of their small size. Also, their incomplete development allows lead to enter the central nervous system more easily.

Recent studies indicate a strong connection between levels of lead exposure and IQ. Apparently, the more lead a child is exposed to during the crucial period of 15 months to 4 years, the greater the IQ decline.

The Centers for Disease Control and Prevention recommend that lead levels for children be less than 10 micrograms per deciliter of blood.

Researchers studied children with lead levels ranging from 0 to 15 micrograms and found that every time lead levels increased 10 micrograms, IQ scores dropped six points, and math, spelling and other academic subject scores dropped nine points.

Girls may be more sensitive to lead exposure than boys. The same amount of lead exposure resulted in a 7.8 point IQ decrease in girls compared to a 2.6 point decrease for boys.

Lead poisoning is a risk for almost all American children. It is reported that one in six children in the United States has ingested dangerous levels of lead in the blood.

You can lower your child's risk of lead poisoning by avoiding or reducing exposure to potential sources of lead. Also, have your child's doctor check at least once a year for lead poisoning.

If your child is at high risk for lead poisoning, you may want to have him checked more often. High-risk children include those who:

- ☐ Live in houses built before 1960, or in houses that are run down or are being remodeled.
- ☐ Have brothers or sisters with lead poisoning.
- ☐ Live near factories or smelters that release lead into the air.
- ☐ Live with someone who is exposed to lead on the job. Job-related lead exposure can be dangerous for the worker, and it can harm family members when brought home on clothes. Lead exposure can occur in a variety of jobs including:

➤ Auto mechanics	➤ Plastic makers
➤ Battery makers	➤ Steel welders, cutters
➤ Bridge repair crews	➤ Plumbers, pipe fitters
➤ Construction workers	➤ Lead smelters, refiners
➤ Gas station attendants	➤ Rubber product makers
➤ Glass makers	➤ Lead miners

Children often do not show definite signs of lead poisoning. Possible symptoms include:

➤ Headache	➤ Feelings of numbness or tingling
➤ Tiredness	➤ Trembling
➤ Weight loss	➤ Muscle or joint pain
➤ Stomach pain	➤ Vomiting

More severe lead poisoning may cause seizures and intense stomach cramps. A child or adult who has been exposed to lead and is suffering from these symptoms should see a doctor immediately.

The best treatment for lead poisoning is a healthy dose of prevention. Try to limit lead exposure as much as possible and have children ages one to six tested for lead poisoning at least once a year.

Ways you can help avoid lead poisoning include:

☐ **Test the paint in your house.** Exterior and interior lead-based paint accounts for half the cases of lead poisoning in children. Lead poisoning occurs when children eat lead-containing paint chips or breathe lead-contaminated air.

To reduce the risk of contaminating the air with lead, minimize sanding, scraping or other activities that create a lot of lead-containing dust or keep your children out of the house when you're renovating.

Remember, a new coat of paint or wallpaper isn't good enough to cover up the lead on walls — it can also peel or chip.

☐ **Test your tap water.** Tap water that travels through lead pipes, joints or faucets can sometimes absorb lead.

The hotter the water coming from the tap, the more lead it tends to absorb from the pipes. You may want to use only cold tap water for cooking and drinking.

If your water tests positive for lead, a lead-removing device may decrease lead concentrations. These units vary in effectiveness. Carbon, sand and cartridge filters will not eliminate lead in water.

☐ **Wash your vegetables in lead-free water.** Soil can cause lead poisoning in produce if the soil has become contaminated by lead paint, gasoline, smelting or industrial waste. If you suspect that your vegetables may have been grown in contaminated soil, you may also want to peel them.

Wash your hands after exposure to soil or dust you think may be contaminated.

☐ **Don't store food in containers made with lead compounds.** Food and Drug Administration Deputy Commissioner Michael Taylor attributes the majority of lead in food to storage problems. Foods or liquids stored in lead crystal or lead-glazed ceramics can absorb the lead from these dishes.

Imported foods may sometimes contain lead or absorb lead from cans that have been soldered with lead. Dishes from Latin America, Mexico and Spain are more likely to contain high levels of lead than American-made dishware. You can use a home-test kit to check your ceramics for lead glaze.

Medical Sources ————————————————————
American Family Physician (47,1:113)
Medical Tribune (34,1:25 and 34,3:6)
The Atlanta Journal/Constitution (April 7, 1993, B12)
The New England Journal of Medicine (327,18:1279)

Methanol: Good for the environment but toxic for you

We've all heard the news about gasohol: Use of this blend of gasoline and methyl alcohol (methanol or wood alcohol) may significantly reduce ozone and other kinds of air pollution. But the down side of increased methanol use is that methyl alcohol carries its own dangers.

The U.S. Department of Health and Human Services warns that poisoning by methanol can be difficult to recognize and very dangerous.

In the United States, we produce and use methyl alcohol abundantly. You probably don't realize it, but methanol is a key ingredient of all these products:

> ➤ Paint remover ➤ Windshield washing fluid
> ➤ Windshield de-icer ➤ Duplicating fluids
> ➤ Solid canned fuel ➤ Model airplane fuel
> ➤ Embalming fluid

Unfortunately, you can get a toxic dose of methanol by absorbing methyl alcohol through your skin or inhaling its fumes. If your skin comes in contact with methanol from one of these sources, be sure to wash it off quickly. Also, remove any clothing that becomes soaked with methanol and put the clothing outside to dry.

When you use a product containing methyl alcohol, be on the lookout for any or all of these symptoms:

> ➤ Eye and respiratory irritation   ➤ Headache
> ➤ Light-headedness   ➤ Nausea
> ➤ Sleepiness   ➤ Dizziness
> ➤ Ringing in your ears   ➤ Blurred vision

However, the most dangerous exposure to methanol comes from drinking it. Illegally made liquor sometimes contains methyl alcohol, and some people have accidentally swallowed methanol when siphoning gasohol from a gas tank.

If a person survives drinking methanol, exposure will likely blind the person or leave them brain damaged.

Take special care when you use any products containing methanol. In addition to being highly toxic, methyl alcohol is highly flammable and will burst into flames when exposed to sparks or fire.

If you believe that you have developed methanol poisoning, contact your doctor immediately.

Medical Source ────────────────────────
American Family Physician (47,1:163)

Aluminum poisoning at the workplace

Lack of coordination. Loss of balance. Memory loss. These are some of the symptoms of aluminum poisoning exhibited by 25 workers employed for over 10 years in an aluminum smelting plant.

The workers also suffered from joint pain, hearing loss and decreased abstract reasoning and concentration.

The aluminum smelting industry isn't the only one that exposes its workers to hazardous levels of aluminum. Studies have shown that aluminum exposure occurs in other industries, such as the mining industry, with equally harmful results.

A study comparing 631 miners exposed to aluminum to an unexposed group of 722 miners found the exposed workers ranked much lower than the unexposed when tested for perceptual accuracy, information processing and abstract reasoning.

While every person is different as far as how susceptible they are to the toxicity of aluminum, there is an extremely narrow margin between normal and lethally toxic levels of aluminum in the human brain, with the elderly being more susceptible.

More studies are needed to determine the "hows" and "whys" of the toxicity of aluminum. In the meantime, be aware of the symptoms characterizing aluminum disorders: incoordination, poor memory, difficulty in abstract reasoning and depression.

Medical Source ———————————————————
Archives of Internal Medicine (152,7:1443)

Focusing on family health

Children's health
Women's health
Men's health
Senior's health

CHILDREN'S HEALTH

Treating your infant's cold

It's 3 a.m. and your 5-month-old child has such a bad cold she can't sleep. So you give her some of her older brother's cough medicine, hoping you can all get some rest, right?

Wrong, says Dr. Anne Gadomski, a pediatric professor at the University of Maryland School of Medicine.

Both cough and cold medicines can be toxic to young children. Poison Control Centers in the United States get over 75,000 calls each year about reactions to cough and cold medicines, and most of these calls involve children under the age of 6.

One of the problems is that these drugs often have more than one ingredient. Only one product may contain an antihistamine, a decongestant, alcohol, an antitussive for coughs and an expectorant to promote productive coughing.

You may not know which ingredient or combination of ingredients is toxic to your child.

Some symptoms of a reaction to cough and cold medicine are:

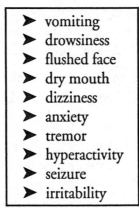

> vomiting
> drowsiness
> flushed face
> dry mouth
> dizziness
> anxiety
> tremor
> hyperactivity
> seizure
> irritability

If your baby has these symptoms after taking cold medicine, call your doctor or local Poison Control Center immediately.

Dr. Gadomski advises that you never give a cold or cough medicine to a child less than 1 year old except at the advice of your doctor. You should give cough medicine to children from 12 months to 2 years only if they are unable to sleep because of a cough.

Two medical studies have shown that children 5 years old and younger don't get any relief from over-the-counter cold medicines anyway. Cold medicines help a little to relieve symptoms in children age 6 and up, but adolescents and adults get by far the most relief from cold medicines.

If you must give a young child a cough or cold medicine, follow these safety tips:

❑ Follow label instructions carefully — never exceed the recommended dosage.

❑ Don't confuse tablespoon (Tbsp.) with teaspoon (Tsp.) abbreviations.

❑ Use child-resistant caps on all your medications.

❑ Never leave the caps off medications.

❑ Store your medicines out of the reach of children.

❑ Check your dosage cups carefully making sure you are giving your child the correct dosage. Never give an extra dose of any medicine hoping to help your child rest.

❑ Check with your doctor or pharmacist about drug interactions if your child is taking more than one medication at a time.

❑ Check with your doctor before you give your child aspirin.

❑ Choose a medicine with only one ingredient.

Since there is no cure for the common cold, all you can really do for your child is try to relieve the symptoms. Dr. Gadomski recommends these natural, nontoxic aids:

❑ Give your child plenty of decaffeinated liquids to drink.

❑ Use children's or infant's nose drops for nasal congestion. (Only use for a few days or you can get a "rebound effect.")

❑ Clear a stuffy nose with a child's nasal syringe.

❑ Use a vaporizer in the bedroom.

❑ Have your child sleep on her stomach or side.

□ Don't smoke around your child (children of smokers suffer more colds and respiratory infections than children of nonsmokers).

□ Encourage the hand-washing habit to prevent the spread of colds.

Contact your doctor or pharmacist if you have any questions at all about the dose or safety of a medicine for your child.

Medical Sources ————————————————————

Emergency Medicine (24,14:201)

The Journal of the American Medical Association (269,17:2258)

FDA Consumer (26,10:5)

Coping with children's croup

If your child's cold turns into a barking cough, hoarseness, wheezing, fever and a whistling when she breathes, she probably has croup. Croup is usually caused by an infection that causes swelling around the windpipe and the larynx (the voice box).

Some children under age 5 can get mild cases of croup again and again. When croup isn't accompanied by fever or other signs of a cold or infection, you can treat it at home if you keep a close watch on your child.

The first step you should take is to turn on the bathroom shower and sit in the steamy room with your child on your lap. You must be there to keep an eye on your child and to keep him very calm.

Some doctors think that "mist therapy" only works because children feel safer and can breathe easier when they know their parent is taking care of them.

Other at-home methods that seem to ease croup symptoms are:

□ A cool-mist vaporizer or humidifier

□ Plenty of liquids, especially when your child is coughing

□ Rest

□ A short walk outside or a drive in the car

□ No cough medicines unless your doctor recommends otherwise

Severe croup can cause respiratory failure, so call your doctor or go to the emergency room immediately if:

❑ Your child doesn't begin to breathe easier soon
after sitting in the steamy bathroom.

❑ He gets a high fever.

❑ He begins to drool or has trouble swallowing.

❑ He seems agitated, cranky or very uncomfortable.

❑ His lips and skin turn bluish.

Don't worry that your child will suddenly stop breathing, though. Respiratory failure occurs gradually. In cases of severe croup, your child will need to receive oxygen and treatment in the hospital.

Medical Source ―――――――――――――――――
American Family Physician (46,3:747)

Taking the heat out of childhood fevers

Most childhood fevers are not dangerous, but they always seem to strike a bit of fear and panic in the hearts of anxious parents.

Researchers from the Children's Hospital of Philadelphia questioned a group of parents on how to handle a child's fever and were astonished to discover that more than half of the parents answered incorrectly.

Listed below is standard information that no parent should be without:

❑ Most childhood fevers are due to harmless viral illnesses and will go away in a day or two without causing any damage or putting the child in any danger.

❑ Pay as much, or even more, attention to your child's behavior than to the numbers on the thermometer. If your child is playful, even if a bit subdued, then he is probably not in any danger.

❑ Always shake the mercury in the thermometer down below 96° F before taking your child's temperature. Forgetting this important step could give you a false reading.

❑ A child does not have a "fever" until his oral temperature is at least 100° F or his rectal temperature is at least 101° F.

❑ Don't use an oral thermometer on children under 5 years of age.

Lubricate a rectal thermometer with petroleum jelly, and insert it gently into the child's rectum about one inch. Hold it in place for two to three minutes before removing to read.

☐ For children over 5, use an oral thermometer. Remind your child not to bite down and hold the thermometer between his teeth. Instruct him to hold it gently under his tongue for two to three minutes.

☐ Don't get in a hurry to read the thermometer, thinking the mercury will go down while you are trying to read it. Take your time to make sure you read it correctly.

☐ Give your child acetaminophen (Tylenol, etc.) every four hours if his temperature is 103° F or less. Use the appropriate strength and dose for the child's age.

Give your child plenty of fluids (water and fruit juices — stay away from sodas). Don't wrap him up too much in pajamas and blankets — he doesn't need to get more overheated. Continue to take his temperature every four hours.

☐ If your child's temperature rises above 103° F, give him acetaminophen, just as above. Then, one hour later, sit him in a tub of lukewarm water and sponge-bathe him for about half an hour. He may shiver, complain of being cold or cry, but don't stop the bath.

If he still has a fever four hours after giving him the acetaminophen, give him another dose, and continue to give it every four hours as needed.

☐ You should call your child's doctor right away when your child has a fever and one or more of the following:

➤ He is three months old or younger.
➤ His temperature exceeds 102° F for more than 24 hours.
➤ His face, arms or legs are twitching.
➤ He is irritable or drowsy, even without medication.
➤ The fever (even a mild one) lasts for more than three days.

> He complains of bellyache, earache or pain on
  urination.
> He is vomiting, having diarrhea, wheezing or
  having any difficulty breathing.

☐ Always trust your "gut feeling" — if you think your child needs to
  see the doctor, forget the normal guidelines and don't hesitate to
  call. You know your child best of all.

Medical Source ───────────────────────
  Emergency Medicine (25,2:125)

Are you causing your baby's fever?

Naturally, you want to keep your baby warm and comfortable while he's
sleeping, so you turn up the heat in the house, perhaps put a space heater in
the baby's bedroom and cover your child with an extra blanket or two.

You're probably overdoing it. California researchers have discovered that
many parents are actually making their babies feverish when they bundle
them up for a nap.

Babies have an internal thermostat just like we do, but bundling and a
hot bedroom will override it. If you take a feverish baby to the doctor, he may
perform useless tests and start the baby on antibiotics, not realizing that
outside sources caused the high temperature.

Researchers don't know if getting babies too warm is a direct cause of
Sudden Infant Death Syndrome, but several studies seem to be pointing in
that direction. SIDS is more common in the winter months when babies are
wrapped in blankets, placed on hot sheepskins and put in overheated
bedrooms.

Only put slightly more covers on your baby than you would be
comfortable under and don't turn up the heat in the nursery. Thirty minutes
or an hour into the nap, put your hand under the covers to make sure your
baby is cool and comfortable instead of hot and sweaty.

Medical Sources ───────────────────────
  Pediatrics (92,2:238)
  The New England Journal of Medicine (329,6:377)

Febrile seizures: Don't panic

You've been on edge all night because your child is sick with a high fever.

Suddenly, you gasp in horror as you watch your child go into a seizure. It only lasts a few minutes, or even a few seconds, but you feel yourself beginning to panic.

What is happening to your child?

It is known as a "febrile seizure," and they look more dangerous than they are. They can occur in any child who is suffering from a fever — even a mild one. Your child will look as if he is suffering from epilepsy. The seizure may cause shaking, convulsions and even unconsciousness.

The seizures are generally brief and harmless, and cause no lasting damage, even if a child has them often.

Although most children will never experience a febrile seizure again, some children seem to have a genetic predisposition to febrile seizures and experience them more often than usual.

Also, children have different "fever thresholds" for seizures. This means that some children will experience a febrile seizure with a low fever while others must have a high fever before suffering from a febrile seizure.

Research suggests that anti-seizure medications don't help prevent future febrile seizures. Also, many doctors argue against using anti-seizure drugs after a febrile seizure because of the drug's negative side effects.

Talk to your pediatrician about what steps to take to avoid febrile seizures and what to do if one occurs.

Medical Source ————————————————
The New England Journal of Medicine (327,16:1122)

How to recognize a headache in your child

We think of headaches as a feature of stressful adult life, but the problem of headaches belongs to children, too. By age 15, three out of every four children have headaches.

Sometimes these headaches are severe enough to cause trouble at home and absences from school. If you discover the cause of the headache, you've taken the first step toward the cure:

❏ A sinus infection can cause a headache that hurts just over the sinuses, and a whole-body infection can cause a headache that hurts all over the head. Antibiotics may be the cure your child needs.

❏ Extreme physical exertion can cause a throbbing all-over-the-head headache in some children.

❏ Depression, especially in the teen-age years, or problems at school or home can cause headaches that never go away and never change in intensity. A depressed child will probably need professional counseling.

❏ A brain tumor, fluid on the brain or any other serious condition that creates pressure on the skull can cause headaches that get worse and last longer as time goes by. These headaches are present when your child wakes up in the morning and gradually get better during the day. Later, your child may have nausea and vomiting which bring relief from the pain.

❏ Certain foods and beverages, exercising too hard, lack of sleep, hunger, a blow to the head or changes in the weather can cause migraines.

Some migraine-triggering foods are hot dogs and luncheon meats (they contain nitrates), Chinese food that contains monosodium glutamate (MSG), and tyramine-containing chocolate, nuts and aged cheeses.

Before a common migraine headache, your child may become pale and experience a change in activity level and appetite. He will probably have at least three of these six symptoms:

> Stomach pain
> Nausea or vomiting
> Throbbing head pain
> A brief rest brings relief from pain
> Family member with migraines
> Pain on one side of the head

The good news is that half of children with migraines quit having them completely within a few years. If the headaches do continue into adulthood, they're usually less frequent and less intense.

If your child's headaches persist or are interfering with life or schoolwork, you should definitely consult your doctor.

Medical Source ————————————————
Emergency Medicine (24,15:69)

Smoking causes ear infections in children

More than a third of middle ear infections in young children are due to cigarette smoke exposure, one study estimates. Children with parents who smoke have more ear infections and longer-lasting infections than children who aren't exposed to smoke.

Why would smoking around kids have such an impact on their ears?

One theory is that smoke causes the respiratory tract to produce more mucus than usual. As a result, your child's eustachian tubes, which lead from the back of the throat to the middle ear, may become blocked.

Another possibility is that cigarette smoke reduces the defenses of the respiratory tract against bacteria. With defenses weakened, your child may experience more bacterial growth, which means more ear infections.

So, what's the bottom line? If you or someone you know is a smoker, don't smoke around small children. If you have to smoke, keep the room well-ventilated.

Medical Source ————————————————
Pediatrics (90,2:228)

Ear pulling not necessarily a sign of infection

The sight of your child pulling his ear is always upsetting. The first thought that may run through your mind is — "Oh no, another ear infection."

However, ear pulling isn't always a sure sign of infection.

Dr. Robert B. Baker reports that of 100 children brought into his office because they were pulling their ears, only 12 had ear infections.

None of the children who had only ear pulling as a possible symptom had infections. Only four out of 17 children who both pulled their ears and had a fever actually had an ear infection.

Dr. Baker advises that concerned parents whose children have this symptom by itself call their doctors before making an unnecessary trip.

Medical Source ———————————————————
Pediatrics (90,6:1006)

Easy ways to ease diaper rash

Cloth and disposable are still duking it out in the diaper wars. As far as diaper rash goes, the disposable variety with the super-absorbant gelling material in the center is winning, say New Jersey Medical School Drs. Janniger and Thomas.

These disposable diapers are also more resistant to leaks, which helps keep diseases from being passed around in daycare centers.

Below are a few guidelines to help prevent diaper rash:

❒ Never let your baby stay in a wet diaper. Change him frequently, clean the area with lukewarm water and pat dry. If your baby has a rash, don't use soap or store-bought baby wipes that contain irritants.

❒ Smooth on a small amount of zinc oxide ointment like Desitin two or three times a day to prevent diaper rash and to treat it. You can use a little cornstarch to dry your baby's bottom, but be careful. Some babies develop breathing difficulties when you use too much.

❒ Half of all diaper rashes quickly develop into a yeast infection or are part of a rash that has spread all over your baby's body. For the general rash, you can buy a nonfluorinated topical steroid, such as a cream that contains less than one percent hydrocortisone.

For the yeast infection, you might want to try an antifungal such as clotrimazole (brand names are Gyne-Lotrimin, Mycelex G and Lotrimin) available at your drug store or pharmacy.

Some doctors recommend a triple-punch treatment at the first sign of diaper rash: Combine equal parts of an antibiotic ointment such as Neosporin, an antifungal cream and a hydrocortisone cream, and rub the mixture on your baby's rash.

For pregnant women debating breast-feeding vs. the bottle: You may want to know that breast-fed babies have fewer diaper rashes because their urine is more acidic.

Very rarely, diaper rash can signal a more serious health problem. See your doctor if you can't cure the problem in a week, if your baby has a fever along with the rash and if any new symptoms develop while you're treating the rash.

Medical Source ———————————————————
  Cutis (52,3:153)

The dangers of diarrhea

Diarrhea in infants and young children can be dangerous because it can so easily lead to dehydration.

It's very important to give your child plenty to eat and drink when she has diarrhea. Eating and drinking won't make the diarrhea worse, and it will help prevent dehydration.

If your child does become dehydrated, The American Association of Pediatrics recommends that you "rehydrate" her within four to six hours and then restart her regular diet.

Some signs of dehydration are:

> ➤ A decrease in the usual number of wet diapers or bathroom trips
> ➤ An increased heart rate
> ➤ Weak pulse
> ➤ Dry mouth
> ➤ Loose skin
> ➤ Sunken eyes

To rehydrate your child, feed her small doses of a liquid salt and sugar mixture every 10 to 20 minutes. You can make your own rehydration fluid:

☐ Add one-quarter teaspoon of salt to a liter of Gatorade.
☐ Cut the Gatorade/salt solution in half with water.

You must use utmost care when making this solution because giving your child too much salt is dangerous.

If you can afford it, you may want to buy pre-packaged oral rehydration solution at the drugstore.

After four to six hours on this solution, your child should be able to resume her regular diet. The regular diet seems to shorten the course of diarrhea and help your child regain lost weight and nutrients faster.

Even infants less than six months old should be returned to their regular-strength formula or milk and not diluted milk.

A child should only be taken off milk if the infection that caused the diarrhea has made your child temporarily unable to digest lactose, a sugar found in milk. In that case, you may replace milk with yogurt or feed your child with a lactose-free formula.

Children who were already eating solid foods should eat carbohydrate-rich foods such as bananas, cereal, rice or potatoes once they have been rehydrated.

If the diarrhea continues, give your child one-half cup of the rehydration liquid for each cup of diarrhea passed. Call your pediatrician if your child's diarrhea doesn't get better or if she seems to be dehydrated again.

Medical Source —————————————————
Emergency Medicine (24,16:123)
The Lancet (341,8839:194)
American Family Physician (48,8:1381)

Deadly daycare diarrhea

Have a child in daycare? Watch out for diarrhea. It can be deadly.

Diarrhea, especially bloody diarrhea, is a common symptom of infection with a type of bacteria known as E. coli.

E. coli infection can lead to kidney failure and even death. Because of incomplete immune development, infants and young children have the greatest risk of becoming infected.

A large number of cases of E. coli infection may go undetected because there is no routine testing of preschool age children with diarrhea. In an 18-month study in Minnesota, 29 cases of E. coli were diagnosed at nine daycare centers.

Since the state of Minnesota constitutes only 2 percent of the total U.S. population, these findings seem to indicate that the problem is more widespread than it appears.

E. coli is normally spread through unsanitary conditions. You can help protect your child from this bacteria by teaching her to always wash her hands before eating or drinking and after visiting the bathroom. If your child is planning a trip to a local farm, warn her not to drink raw milk.

It is common for children who visit dairy farms to have an opportunity to taste fresh milk. However, studies have shown that as many as half the kids who drink unpasteurized milk develop symptoms of food poisoning three or four days later.

Diarrhea from E. coli normally resolves itself. However, since the bacteria can be so dangerous for children, it's a good idea to have your child tested for this bacteria before returning her to daycare and risk passing the infection on to other children.

If your child has diarrhea, be on the lookout for these symptoms:

> ➤ Headache
> ➤ Tiredness
> ➤ Shortness of breath
> ➤ Jaundice
> ➤ Very little urine is passed and
>   what is passed may be bloody

If you or your child has several of these symptoms, consult a doctor immediately.

Medical Sources

Medical Tribune (34,5:7)
Medical Update (16,10:4)

Microwaving baby's formula: Is it safe?

Store-bought formula and a microwave oven seem to be your best friends in the wee hours of the morning. Microwaves destroy many of the disease-fighting antibodies in breast milk, but is it safe for formula?

Fortunately, research has shown that the microwaving process does not cause a loss of heat-sensitive nutrients in the formula and seems perfectly safe if you follow these important safety tips:

- ☐ Always heat at least four ounces of formula. Heating smaller amounts can result in high temperatures that can scald your baby's mouth and esophagus as well as possibly destroy heat-sensitive nutrients such as vitamin C and riboflavin.
- ☐ Heat only refrigerated formula.
- ☐ Always place the bottle in the microwave standing upright. Do not place the bottle on its side in the microwave. If your bottles are too tall to fit in your microwave, try smaller bottles (no smaller than four-ounce bottles).
- ☐ Never leave the top on the bottle while heating it. Always leave the bottle uncovered to allow heat and steam to escape.
- ☐ Never heat a four-ounce bottle of formula for longer than 30 seconds.
- ☐ Never heat an eight-ounce bottle for longer than 45 seconds.
- ☐ After heating the bottle, replace the top and screw securely into place. Then invert the bottle 10 times to make sure all the heat is evenly distributed and to avoid dangerous hot spots in the formula. You do not need to shake the bottle vigorously.
- ☐ Never give your baby a bottle without testing the temperature of the liquid first. If the formula is warm to the touch, it may be too hot for your baby's mouth.
- ☐ When testing the temperature of the formula, place several drops on your tongue or the top of your hand, not on the inside of your wrist. Your tongue and the back of your hand are more sensitive to heat and can assess temperature more accurately.

Medical Source ———————————————
American Family Physician (47,4:902)

Breast milk — a perfect balance of nutrients

Breast milk. This nectar of infancy provides a perfect balance of nutrients for babies and protects them against infection.

Breast milk beats formula hands down for protecting babies against ear infections and viruses that cause stomach upset. Researchers have found that breast-fed babies have fewer and less severe bouts of diarrhea than formula-fed babies. Diarrhea can be a serious problem for infants because it can so quickly lead to dehydration.

Exactly what accounts for the infection-fighting power of breast milk? For years, researchers have attributed it to antibodies in the mother's milk. Now they think the protein mucin is responsible for at least half of breast milk's infection-fighting power.

In adults, mucins are found in the stomach and intestines where they work to fight off viruses. Dr. Robert Yolken, chief physician at Johns Hopkins Children's Center in Baltimore, who discovered the virus-fighting ability of mucin, speculates that newborns have not yet developed intestinal mucins. He believes the only protection babies get from mucin proteins comes from breast milk.

If researchers can find a way to artificially produce mucin, they may be able to use the protein as a supplement to give baby formulas the infection-fighting qualities of breast milk.

Until then, breast-feeding provides the best possible nutritional beginning for your child. To help your body produce the best milk possible, drink plenty of fluids and eat a healthy, well-balanced diet. Most of what you eat, drink and even do will affect your breast milk.

Keep reading to find out what your breast-feeding baby thinks about exercise, beer and smoking.

Exercise turns breast milk sour

If your newborn bundle of joy could speak in complete sentences, she might come out with a heart-felt groan: "Oh no — she's putting on her running shoes — well, there goes dinner."

Why such a groan? Because your breast milk tastes sour after you exercise, pediatric experts report. The sour taste comes from excess lactic acid produced by exercise.

Lactic acid is a natural by-product of vigorous or extended exercise. Your body uses sugars and carbohydrates as energy sources. Lactic acid is produced as your body breaks down the sugars and carbohydrates for energy.

The more you exercise, the more energy you need from sugars and carbohydrates. The more energy you use, the higher the level of lactic acid in your blood.

Shortly after exercise, your body breaks down the lactic acid, and the level of lactic acid in the blood returns to the pre-exercise level. However, immediately after exercise, the levels of lactic acid in the blood are high, and it spills over into the breast milk.

Fortunately, the lactic acid is not harmful to your baby. But it does make the milk taste sour. The level of lactic acid in the milk usually stays high for about 90 minutes — which means sour-tasting milk for at least an hour and a half after exercising.

So should I stop exercising? you ask. The answer is, no. Exercising is a healthy activity that you should try to continue as regularly as possible. To keep your baby from fussing or refusing to nurse after exercising, nurse your baby before you exercise or express your milk before exercising and save it for a feeding after your workout.

Beer and breast-feeding don't mix

Despite old wives' tales to the contrary, beer and breast-feeding don't mix. Beer actually does stimulate your flow of breast milk. Even so, babies apparently don't like the taste of alcohol.

Researchers observed 11 nursing mothers and their babies. In one testing session, the mothers were instructed to drink one regular beer and then feed their babies on demand for the next four hours. At the next testing session, the mothers drank one nonalcoholic beer and then breast-fed on demand as before.

On average, the babies drank 23 percent less milk when their mothers drank regular beer before breast-feeding than they did when the mothers drank nonalcoholic beer.

Interestingly enough, the mothers could tell no difference between the two breast-feeding sessions.

Stay away from beer or other alcoholic beverages while breast-feeding.

Babies don't like the taste, and alcohol ingested through breast milk can actually slow their motor development.

No smoking, please

Cigarette smoking spoils dinner for your breast-fed newborn, too. Smoking reduces the amount and quality of your breast milk.

Researchers found smoking mothers produced 21 percent less breast milk than nonsmoking mothers. After six weeks of breast-feeding, smoking mothers produced 46 percent less breast milk. The smokers' milk also had 19 percent less fat content than nonsmokers' milk. Less fat means babies get less calories, which they need to develop properly.

If you stop smoking before pregnancy or even just before giving birth, studies indicate that your milk production will go up and that you will be able to nurse as long as nonsmokers.

Medical Sources ————————————————
Science News (142,23:390)
Pediatrics (89,6:1245)
The Journal of the American Medical Association (269,13:1637)
Medical Tribune (34,1:21)

Soothing baby's teething pains

Teething is a natural process that starts four to eight months after birth, and something that parents and babies must endure. But take heart! At-home remedies and over-the-counter teething medications can lessen your baby's discomfort.

You may first want to try these simple at-home remedies before resorting to medicine.

❐ Let your baby chew on a wet washcloth that has been cooled in the freezer, a frozen teething ring or a cold apple slice wrapped in a wet washcloth.

If these home remedies don't relieve your baby's pain, an over-the-counter teething medicine will probably do the trick. These include Babee Teething Lotion, Baby Anbesol Gel, Baby Orajel, Baby Orajel Nighttime Formula and Dr. Hands Teething.

❒ Follow all directions for teething medications carefully.

❒ Apply the medicine to the painful area four to six times daily or as your dentist or doctor recommends.

❒ Do not use for babies less than four months old unless supervised by a dentist or doctor.

❒ If your baby develops fever, nasal congestion or seems listless, see a doctor immediately. These are not normal signs of teething and could indicate an infection.

Medical Source ——————————————————
U.S. Pharmacist (17,11:31)

Give your children the gift of healthy teeth

Preventing your children's tooth decay or damage can be a real challenge. The average child has one decayed permanent tooth by age 9, three by age 12 and eight by the age of 17. More than 60 percent of the teen-agers nationwide suffer from gingivitis, characterized by swollen, discolored gums.

However, there are steps you can take to lower your child's risk of tooth decay.

Before that first trip to the dentist, your child's doctor can be the key in identifying tooth decay, especially baby-bottle tooth decay. Baby-bottle tooth decay can already have done its most serious damage by the time the child first sees a dentist, normally around age 2.

If the doctor notices any signs of decay when he looks at your child's teeth during a routine exam, take your child to a dentist immediately.

Good bottle habits can help prevent baby-bottle tooth decay.

❒ Don't let your child carry around or feed for hours at a time on a bottle filled with sweetened liquids such as formula, milk, juice or soft drinks.

❒ Don't let your child take a bottle to bed.

❒ Don't take your baby to bed with you at night and let him breast feed at will.

❒ Take your child off the bottle by his first birthday.

❒ As your child grows older, watch for indications of tooth and gum disease, such as brownish teeth or red, irritated gums. Ask your child's physician to continue to mention any teeth or gum irregularities he notices.

Signs of tooth or gum damage:

> ➤ Swollen, discolored gums
> ➤ Misaligned top and bottom teeth
> ➤ Crowded or crooked teeth
> ➤ Bad breath
> ➤ Unusually quick loss of rear baby molars
> ➤ Injury to mouth
> ➤ Mouth breathing

Encourage your child to develop habits to help prevent tooth decay.

- ☐ Limit sugary, between-meal snacks.
- ☐ Brush and floss teeth every day.
- ☐ Use fluoride toothpaste and fluoridated water if possible. Fluorides strengthen tooth enamel and make it less susceptible to decay. You don't want to get too much fluoride, though (see story below).

For children between the ages of 5 and 13, you may want to have your dentist check to see if they need dental sealants. Children who seem to develop a lot of cavities are good candidates for sealants. Sealants are plastic coverings applied to the chewing surfaces of new molars before they have a chance to decay.

Another potential problem area you may want to be on the lookout for is mouth and facial injuries. During the past decade, 75 percent of mouth injuries occurred in people age 15 or younger. Sports and play were the most common causes of these injuries. Other causes include car crashes, falls and fights.

If your child plays competitive sports, encourage wearing mouthguards, helmets and other protective gear during practice as well as during actual competition.

Protective gear should also be used in recreational activities such as skateboarding and bicycling. Make sure the standard mouthguard provides enough protection. Otherwise you may want to have your dentist make a customized one.

Teen-age years are a popular time to take up smoking or chewing tobacco. Besides other risks associated with these activities, they can damage the teeth and gums. These products can cause swollen, irritated, receded gums and stained teeth.

Teens may be less likely to use tobacco products if they understand the unsightly effects they can have on physical appearance.

Your child's dental care doesn't have to make you grit your teeth in despair. Following a few simple tips and knowing what danger signs to look for can make the whole process a lot less painful.

Medical Source ———————————————
Journal of Family Practice (35,4:459)

Fluoride for kids: How much is enough?

Fluoride is flourishing these days — and the increase in fluoridated water and toothpaste has sent most tooth decay out to lunch. However, too much fluoride can cause fluorosis, in which the teeth turn a mottled brown color.

To be sure that children get adequate fluoride protection against cavities, most dentists and pediatricians prescribe fluoride supplements, which may come in the form of fluoride gels, rinses, drops, pills or vitamins.

Fluoride supplements are especially helpful if taken while the teeth are forming. The American Academy of Pediatrics recommends beginning fluoride supplements within two weeks of birth and continuing them up to age 16.

The only problem is, supplements can lead to a fluoride overdose and possible teeth discoloration if you live in an area where local water supplies are heavily fluoridated.

Your dentist or doctor can test a water sample to check fluoride levels in your water supply or may request this information from the local water treatment plant, health department or dental school. Since fluoride levels may vary from year to year, your dentist should check them often and adjust your child's prescription accordingly.

Only about half of all dentists and pediatricians check fluoride levels in the local water, so you should ask your dentist if he has done so.

To keep your child from getting too much fluoride, you should also report to your dentist or pediatrician what toothpaste your baby uses, what you feed him and any changes you make in his diet.

For instance, instant baby foods mixed with fluoridated water contain almost as much fluoride as the water itself. Meat-based baby foods have high levels of fluoride due to ground bone particles. Soy-based formulas contain higher levels of fluoride than milk-based formulas.

Breast-fed babies may need more supplements because they get very little fluoride compared with formula-fed babies.

If fluoride supplements are recommended for your child, don't give them with milk or baby formulas. These can reduce fluoride absorption by 60 to 70 percent. You certainly don't want your child to get too little fluoride, either.

Medical Source ⎯⎯⎯⎯⎯⎯⎯⎯⎯⎯⎯⎯⎯⎯⎯⎯⎯⎯
American Journal of Diseases of Children (146,12:1488)

What causes Sudden Infant Death Syndrome?

Why do 7,000 perfectly healthy American babies die in their sleep every year for no apparent reason?

Sudden Infant Death Syndrome (SIDS) remains a mystery, but researchers have found that the gasp reflex, the ability to revive yourself when your blood-oxygen supply is too low, is just not strong in infants from a few weeks to 1 year old.

Researchers noticed in laboratory tests that the same thing happens to mice. The gasp reflex is strong in newborn mice and in adult animals, but the mice seem to pass through a gap in their development during which they have trouble breathing quickly and deeply when they need oxygen.

Reducing the risk of SIDS

The American Academy of Pediatrics says you can slash the risk of SIDS if you put your baby to sleep on his back or his side. Researchers in study after study have found that babies who sleep on their stomachs are at a higher risk of SIDS.

Parents have traditionally preferred the tummy-down, or prone, position for their babies. They worry about babies choking when they vomit, and they've probably noticed that most babies sleep more soundly on their stomachs.

If you have a specific medical reason to put your baby to sleep on her stomach or if your baby absolutely won't fall asleep any other way, you can still reduce the risk of SIDS:

☐ Do not wrap your baby in a blanket or sheet and lay him on his stomach. Place covers over him loosely. Tight covers prevent your baby from moving freely, and when she gets into a position where it's hard to breathe, she tends to stay there.

Wrapping your baby in covers, also called "swaddling," is not dangerous for babies sleeping on their backs. In fact, it may give your baby a feeling of security and help her rest better.

☐ Don't put your baby to sleep on his stomach if he's been sick that day or the day before with nasal congestion, cough, chest noises, fever or diarrhea.

☐ Do not overheat your baby's bedroom during the winter.

☐ Place your baby on a firm mattress. You should avoid soft, fluffy pillows and mattresses made of sheepskin or natural fibers such as ti-tree bark or kapok. These surfaces increase SIDS risk in infants sleeping on their stomachs 20-fold.

Soft surfaces allow your baby's head to sink in too far, especially if he tends to turn his face down. Babies simply suffocate when they "rebreathe" too much carbon dioxide and not enough oxygen.

If you put a 2-pound bag of sugar on a mattress and there's still a dent five minutes after you move the bag, the mattress is too soft.

In the United States, we have a much lower rate of SIDS than New Zealand and Tasmania, Australia, even though twice as many babies are put to sleep on their stomachs here. Americans tend to use harder mattresses while Tasmanians and New Zealanders use soft, natural-fiber mattresses and sheepskins.

If you follow these recommendations, it's possible that placing your baby on his stomach to sleep won't increase SIDS risk at all.

However, until scientists are more certain about what causes SIDS, placing your baby on her side or back at bedtime is a smart move.

Medical Sources ———————————————————

The New England Journal of Medicine (329,6:337 and 425)
Canadian Medical Association Journal (149,5:629)
Pediatrics (91,6:1112)
Journal of Pediatrics (122,6:874)
American Journal of Diseases of Children (147,6:642)
The Journal of the American Medical Association (267,17:2359)

Childproofing your home

More infants die each year from injury than children in any other age group. Most infant injuries occur in the home, and most could have been avoided with a few simple precautions.

☐ Make sure your baby's sleeping area is safe. Unsafe sleeping conditions are the most common cause of accidental death among infants. Check for loose or missing crib slats or any spaces in which your baby's head could get caught, such as between the mattress and crib rails. Make sure all parts of the crib are secure.

Do not let your baby sleep on a couch or any place where he could slip between the cushions and suffocate.

Exercise caution in letting infants sleep with children or adults. Six infants in a child injury study suffocated when the person they were sleeping with rolled on top of them.

☐ Do not leave infants unattended in or near bathtubs, toilets or buckets filled with water. Drowning or scald burns may result.

Also, don't bathe infants in the kitchen sink while the dishwasher is running. Two infants were severely burned when scalding water from the dishwasher backed up into the sink.

For safety purposes, water heaters should be set at approximately 125° F or lower. Even when water heaters are set at safe levels, dishwashers often produce much hotter water. Infants can sustain severe burns when exposed to scalding water for as little as one second.

☐ Keep all plastic dry-cleaning and grocery bags well out of children's reach. One child suffocated after he crawled into a closet and pulled down a plastic bag hanging from a rack.

☐ Install smoke detectors in your home and periodically check them to make sure they work. The younger the child, the higher his risk of dying from smoke inhalation.

☐ Buckle your child properly and securely into a car seat when traveling. Even in minor collisions, infants who aren't in car seats are vulnerable to serious injury. One nine-month-old girl was being nursed when she was killed.

☐ Do not leave your infant where he can fall or hit his head on sharp or hard objects.

☐ Keep all items on which a baby might choke out of reach. One infant choked to death on skin cream that had been left in her crib.

☐ Make sure your baby stays warm. Two infant boys died after being left unattended one winter night in unheated homes.

☐ Do not leave infants with other children without adult supervision. One baby died after a young sibling gave him a bottle filled with alcohol.

If you are preparing your home for a new baby or have children already, be sure to follow these tips to ensure that your family stays safe and happy.

Medical Sources ————————————————
American Journal of Diseases of Children (146,8:968)
Pediatrics (91,1:142)

Breath-holding may be a reaction to stress

Breathe easy, parents. If your child holds his breath, even to the point of turning blue and passing out, it probably doesn't mean that he has behavior disorders, psychological problems or is even extremely difficult or willful.

Breath-holding may simply be an involuntary response to stress caused by anger, frustration, pain or surprise. These attacks are usually harmless although they may seem quite alarming at the time. Even if your child passes out, breathing quickly resumes as a natural reflex.

The attacks may begin at six months or less and last up to age 11. Breath-holding incidents normally decrease and eventually disappear with age, often stopping around age 5.

Don't avoid correcting your child for fear of causing a breath-holding attack. Be patient, firm and consistent in your treatment of the child. A lack of discipline could lead to real behavior problems.

Medical Source ————————————————
The Journal of Pediatrics (122,3:488)

When your child comes home with lice

Head lice infestation is no longer solely the problem of the poor and unwashed.

These human, blood-sucking parasites infiltrate the homes and heads of 10 to 40 percent of America's schoolchildren every year, regardless of socio-economic status or personal hygiene habits. However, head lice do seem to prefer elementary-school-age, Caucasian females.

The way head lice spread is to blame for this bias. Since head lice don't jump or fly, they hitch rides from head to head to head.

Shared combs, brushes, clothes (like in a children's game of "dress-up"), earphones and bed pillows are all favorite modes of transportation for lice.

While lice pose no real health threat, they are an inconvenience and an embarrassment.

How can you tell if you're infested? An itchy scalp is often the first sign of a lice problem. When lice feed on blood they cause an allergic reaction, similar to that from a mosquito bite.

If you suspect your child may have lice, carefully examine her scalp for light-brown insects, about one-eighth of an inch long (adult lice). Since adult lice scurry and hide from any light, it might be easier to check for lice eggs, or nits.

Nits are yellowish, oval eggs that the mother louse cements to the hair shaft, usually near the root. The eggs need the body heat to hatch. Nits are usually laid on the hair on the back of the neck, behind the ears, and on the crown of the head.

During your lice inspection, don't be tricked by nit impostors, such as dandruff or hair spray residue that might look like nits but are not. These nit look-alikes can be flicked freely from the hair. Real nits are much more difficult to remove.

If you do find lice, steer clear of old wives' tales and traditional family remedies for head lice.

More often than not, these home treatment recipes don't kill the little critters and may even end up harming the person seeking relief.

The following treatments are dangerous and they don't work:

> Gasoline
> Kerosene
> Sulfur
> Larkspur lotion
> Garden insecticides
> Dog lice/flea shampoos

There are plenty of over-the-counter (OTC) head-lice shampoos, creme rinses and gels that can be safer and more effective than prescription remedies. Some of these are:

> A-200 Pyrinate
> Barc
> Licetrol 400
> Nix
> Pronto
> R&C
> RID
> Tisit Blue
> Triple X Kit

Most commercial treatments are a mix of natural insecticides made from the chrysanthemum flower and petroleum products.

One OTC treatment is a little different from the other head-lice preparations on the market and perhaps the best of the lot. Nix Creme Rinse contains an artificial form of the natural insecticide used in its commercial "cousins." Nix is quick and easy to use, and usually only requires one application. The downside is it may cause some itching.

One warning: If you or the person you're treating is allergic to chrysanthemums, ragweed, kerosene or petroleum products, do not use any over-the-counter lice treatments. Ask your doctor what kind of remedy might work best for you.

Also, if the lice-infested area is red or hot to the touch, or if a rash or skin irritation appears during treatment, stop and call your doctor immediately.

Once you've completed your treatment, it's tedious but very important to remove all the nits.

You can do this by either combing or picking out every egg on every strand of hair. Sometimes, it may be necessary to cut affected hairs below the nit. However, there is no need to shave your child's head.

When you're sure every household member has been inspected (treated, if necessary) and declared lice-free, then it's time to clean out lice hideouts.

- ☐ First, wash and dry everything that is washable (clothes, sheets, towels, etc.) for at least 20 minutes on the hottest cycle.
- ☐ Stuffed toys, furniture, mattresses and other things that won't fit in the washing machine can be dry-cleaned or vacuumed thoroughly.
- ☐ All combs and brushes need to be soaked in very hot water for five to 10 minutes.
- ☐ While it may be a tempting shortcut, don't douse your home with household lice sprays. They aren't very effective and may not be safe.
- ☐ Finally, don't worry about treating the family pets. Head lice don't survive long once they're off humans, and they can't live on cats, dogs and other common household animals.

Medical Source ——————————————————————
U.S. Pharmacist (17,9:18)

Health tip for your high-school sports star

If your teen-age daughter is involved in high-school or junior high-school athletics, you need to be more involved than watching her sporting events or manning the concession stand. In fact, your involvement could have a huge impact on her athletic performance.

Adolescent athletes frequently suffer from anemia. Anemia is defined as a low level of hemoglobin or red blood cells in the body.

The most common cause of anemia in adolescents is not getting enough iron in the diet. Iron is one of the central components of the red blood cell.

Many female teen-age athletes suffer from mild anemia caused by iron deficiency or menstrual blood loss, and the anemia is sometimes slightly exaggerated by the athletic activity.

Although this condition is not dangerous, it can interfere with the athlete's performance.

The anemia can cause increased fatigue, diminished endurance (especially evident in endurance events, such as long-distance running), shortness of breath and a scary sensation of a racing or pounding heart. The athlete will tire more easily during the sporting events and not perform as well throughout the events.

Parents of adolescent athletes (both male and female) should take the teen-ager to the local health department from time to time to check for anemia.

The screening test for anemia is quick and simple and usually involves just a finger-prick to analyze the blood. The results are available within a few minutes.

Teen-agers who have trouble with iron-deficiency anemia should:

☐ Increase their intakes of iron-rich foods, such as red meat, beans, grapes, raisins, and tomato and apple juice.
☐ Eat citrus fruits or drink citrus fruit juices with the iron-rich foods to increase the body's absorption of the iron.
☐ Avoid tea and coffee when eating iron-rich foods because they decrease iron absorption.

Teen-agers with severe anemia should visit their doctors to evaluate the situation. Occasionally, more aggressive measures need to be used to fix the underlying problem.

Medical Sources —————————————————
American Journal of Diseases in Children (146,10:1201)
American Family Physician (47,5:1266)

Buy a helmet when you buy a bike

Remember your first bike? It probably took you a couple of days (and a few spills) to get used to riding it.

Back then we didn't worry about getting hurt and certainly not about losing our lives in bicycling accidents. But doctors say, even if we didn't, our parents should have.

Each year in the United States 400 children are killed and nearly 400,000 are seriously injured in bicycling accidents. Though studies indicate that using safety helmets could significantly reduce the incidence of head injury and death, fewer than 10 percent of cyclists wear them on a regular basis.

Most kids will admit that wearing a helmet is smart, but don't because of outside influences. Apparently, kids don't want to wear helmets because they are afraid their friends will make fun of them.

Some states have laws requiring the use of helmets while bike riding. Even if your state doesn't, consider making bike helmets a family law in your house.

Medical Sources —————————————————
Pediatrics (91,4:772)
The Atlanta Journal/Constitution (July 15, 1993, D5 and May 13, 1993, E4)

WOMEN'S HEALTH

Natural ways to avoid PMS

If your friends and family try to avoid you once a month and you feel miserable just before your menstrual period, you may suffer from a serious case of PMS, or premenstrual syndrome.

There's no medical cure for the emotional and physical symptoms that beset most women seven to 10 days before their period. The best therapy is exercise, stress management and a well-planned diet.

Although almost all women experience some symptoms of PMS, only 5 to 10 percent of women have symptoms so severe that their lives are disrupted with missed business meetings and even suicide attempts.

Over 100 physical, emotional and behavioral symptoms have been linked to PMS. Here are a few of the more common ones:

➤ Breast swelling and tenderness	➤ Fatigue
➤ Nausea and vomiting	➤ Stomach or pelvic pain
➤ Sinus infection, hay fever	➤ Abdominal bloating
➤ Diarrhea or constipation	➤ Change in sex drive
➤ Decreased concentration	➤ Fluid retention, swelling
➤ Increased thirst or appetite	➤ Anxiety
➤ Mood swings, crying spells	➤ Joint and muscle pain
➤ Insomnia or too much sleep	➤ Backache
➤ Decreased efficiency, clumsiness	➤ Acne, hives
➤ Food cravings, compulsive eating	➤ Depression
➤ Tension or migraine headaches	➤ Cramps
➤ Tension, irritability, anger	➤ Irregular heartbeat

Women who suffer from PMS often complain that they feel out of control. Making a few changes in your lifestyle and nutritional habits can improve symptoms and help you regain the feeling of being in charge.

❒ Get regular exercise. This helps the majority of women suffering from PMS. Studies have linked regular exercise to less breast tenderness, fluid retention and stress. Exercise also stimulates production of the brain's natural substances that make us feel better and help us feel less pain. Forty-minute aerobic sessions three to four times a week could do wonders, but walking briskly 20 minutes a day will give you healthful effects, too.

❑ Practice stress management. Be good to yourself during that critical week or two before your period.

➤ Plan to reduce or eliminate stressful activities or big projects during the time you expect your symptoms to appear.

➤ Plan an activity that is strictly for relaxation.

➤ Join a PMS group, take time out for a hobby or practice yoga.

➤ Let your family know what to expect from you during this time so they can provide emotional support.

➤ Get plenty of rest.

❑ Watch your diet. This is especially important during the two weeks before your period.

➤ Eat low-fat, balanced meals that supply plenty of protein (meat, fish, poultry, dairy products and eggs).

➤ Limit salt. This will help decrease swelling of hands and feet, reduce bloating and breast tenderness.

➤ Eliminate foods and drinks that contain caffeine such as coffee, tea, soft drinks and chocolate.

➤ Stay away from alcohol and tobacco, which worsen symptoms and increase your feeling of being out of control.

➤ Eat less refined sugar, such as pure table sugar. Carbohydrate-rich meals can reduce your craving for sweets.

➤ Eat plenty of complex carbohydrates (cereals, vegetables) and fibers (root vegetables, fruits and whole-grain breads and cereals).

➤ You may want to take magnesium and calcium supplements. Both seem to help prevent moodiness and reduce pain and water retention.

Researchers have found the nonsteroidal anti-inflammatory drug naproxen sodium to be safe and effective in treating some of the symptoms of PMS. This is especially useful in people whose complaints include pain.

Pyridoxine, one of the B6 group of vitamins, is often recommended to treat PMS, but the evidence for its effectiveness is slim. Many women who take B6 for PMS suffer side effects from an overdose of the vitamin.

If your PMS symptoms are severe, talk to your doctor. He may prescribe medicine for some of your symptoms. He also needs to rule out other health problems that could fluctuate with the menstrual cycle and can be treated, like migraine headaches or depression.

Medical Sources ─────────────────────────────

Drug Therapy (23,3:67)

U.S. Pharmacist (16,12:29)

American Journal of Obstetrics and Gynecology (168,5:1417)

Magnesium prevents menstrual migraines

Women who suffer from migraine headaches are more prone to have headaches along with their periods than any other time. These headaches are called menstrual migraine attacks and they usually coincide with other symptoms of PMS.

Studies indicate that some people who suffer from migraine, menstrual migraine or premenstrual syndrome are deficient in the mineral magnesium.

The migraine headache seems to start when magnesium in the body dips to a low level. Then the migraine sufferer seems to lose even more magnesium during the headache attack.

In one scientific study, menstrual migraine sufferers who took magnesium supplements experienced less pain, fewer migraines and improved PMS symptoms compared with the volunteers who were given a placebo.

Overprocessing of foods can destroy magnesium, and it also can be washed out of the body through the use of diuretics.

Some foods rich in magnesium are:

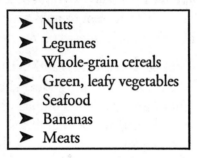

> ➤ Nuts
> ➤ Legumes
> ➤ Whole-grain cereals
> ➤ Green, leafy vegetables
> ➤ Seafood
> ➤ Bananas
> ➤ Meats

Magnesium is found in most multi-vitamin supplements. If you take vitamins, check the label to make sure that you are getting the right amount of magnesium. The recommended dietary allowance for females ages 11 to 14 is 280 milligrams, 300 milligrams for females ages 15 to 18, and 280 milligrams for females ages 19 and over.

Medical Source ———————————————————
Headache (32,3:132)

Nitrous oxide: no laughing matter if you're trying to get pregnant

Having trouble getting pregnant? If you work in a dentist office and are exposed to nitrous oxide, the side effects might not leave you laughing.

Up to half of the dentists in the United States sometimes give nitrous oxide (laughing gas) to their patients as a relaxing anesthetic. For some time researchers have suspected that prolonged exposure to laughing gas can cause liver disease and miscarriages.

New data indicates that dental assistants who regularly work around nitrous oxide in the office are less fertile than normal.

Women who are not exposed to laughing gas usually take an average of six menstrual cycles to get pregnant. Women exposed to nitrous oxide for five or more hours weekly take an average of 32 cycles to conceive. Although research has not focused on male dental workers, lowered fertility could also be a consequence of exposure for them.

There is some equipment available to protect dental workers from exposure. However, if you are trying to get pregnant, avoiding exposure to nitrous oxide could be your key to success.

Medical Sources —————————————————
The New England Journal of Medicine (327,14:993)
The Wall Street Journal (Oct. 10, 1992, B11)

Fetal hearing — a womb full of noise

Be careful what you say. Your unborn baby is listening.

Can he recognize your voice? He certainly can.

In a study done on eight mothers in the early stages of labor, researchers inserted special microphones into the mothers' uteruses.

They found that babies in the uterus are not surrounded by a protective blanket of silence. Their world is full of sound.

The voice that your fetus hears most clearly is yours. This explains why he will so quickly recognize and respond to your voice after he is born.

He hears low-frequency sounds better than high-frequency sounds. With the exception of his mother, he can hear male voices, such as his father's, better than he can hear female voices.

Researchers caution that loud noises may be just as damaging to fetal ears as they are to our own.

Studies indicate that children born to mothers exposed to high levels of industrial noise are more likely to have hearing loss than children who are not exposed to loud noises.

If you work in a loud environment and are pregnant or planning to conceive, you may want to consider a quieter job for the next several months.

Tell your unborn baby a story or sing him your favorite lullaby. You're guaranteed a captive audience.

Medical Source —————————————————
Obstetrics and Gynecology (80,2:186)

At last: a good reason for morning sickness

You wake up in the morning and run to the bathroom. Every time you smell food, you feel sick. Even the smell of soap in the shower can make you want to throw up.

If this seems all too familiar to you, you might feel comfort in knowing that the sickness you feel happens for a very good reason. It protects your unborn child from potentially damaging toxins.

According to biologist Margie Profet of the University of California, Berkeley, women have a more sensitive sense of taste and smell during pregnancy so that their bodies will reject foods that contain naturally occurring toxins.

A bitter taste or strong odor might be the cue for pregnant women to feel "morning sickness" and then avoid a potentially dangerous food. Coffee, tea, bitter or pungent vegetables, and meat that is less than fresh are all loaded with chemicals that could harm your baby. In other words, your body is protecting you and your baby, naturally, from dangerous foods.

There's more reassuring news for morning sickness sufferers. Several studies have indicated that women who are nauseated during early pregnancy have lower rates of miscarriage.

If you are pregnant, consult your doctor about an appropriate diet for you and your baby.

Medical Source ――――――――――――――――――――
Science (257,5071:743)

Exercise your morning sickness away

Don't stop exercising when you find out you're pregnant. Moderate exercise is perfectly safe for your unborn child, and it may even ease your symptoms of morning sickness.

Women who exercise three times a week report fewer morning sickness symptoms (nausea and bloating) than women who don't exercise. Exercise doesn't seem to have any effect on birth weight, length of labor or type of delivery.

The American College of Obstetrics and Gynecologists recommends that you exercise frequently but not strenuously. Strenuous exercise can sometimes slow down the growth of the unborn baby by interfering with your body's breakdown of carbohydrates into sugar. The baby might not get enough fuel for normal growth.

You should also eat right before you exercise to prevent your blood sugar from dropping too far. Exercise normally makes your blood sugar levels drop, especially during the last stage of pregnancy. Drastic drops in the blood sugar level can negatively affect your baby, even causing brain damage if the blood sugar level stays too low for too long.

If you don't normally exercise, talk with your doctor before beginning an exercise program when you're pregnant.

Medical Source ————————————————————

> *Medical Tribune* (33,12:33)
> *The Physician and Sportsmedicine* (20,12:26)

Pregnancy and your sex life

Concerned that having sex during the last trimester of your pregnancy may bring on a premature delivery? You may have heard that sex could rupture membranes or that orgasm or nipple stimulation could cause uterine contractions.

For most women, that's not true at all. Sexual intercourse one or more times a week in late pregnancy is perfectly healthy, unless you have certain types of vaginal infections.

Pregnant women who have a vaginal infection called *Trichomonas vaginalis* or *Mycoplasma hominis* are more likely to have a preterm delivery when they engage in frequent sex. Having sex frequently seems to push the harmful bacteria from the vagina into the cervix, the neck of the uterus. The lining of the uterus may become dangerously inflamed.

Other bacterial infections, such as the common yeast infection, don't have this same effect.

If you're interested in having sex one to three times a week in late pregnancy, ask your doctor to screen you for the *T. vaginalis* and *M. hominis* infections. If you don't have the infections, frequent sex should not increase your risk for preterm delivery.

In fact, your desire to have sex in late pregnancy probably indicates that you feel well and you're having a very healthy pregnancy. Women without infections who have sex one or more times a week actually seem to have fewer preterm deliveries than women who don't have sex.

Warning: You can have too much sex when you're pregnant even when you're infection-free. Engaging in sexual intercourse five or more times a week in the last trimester will increase your risk of early delivery.

Medical Source ————————————————————
   American Journal of Obstetrics and Gynecology (168,2:514)

Birth defect from common decongestant?

Just because a medicine is available over-the-counter doesn't mean you shouldn't check with your physician before taking it, if you are pregnant, that is. If you are pregnant, you should be especially cautious because any medicine you take also affects your unborn child.

Studies show that women in their first trimester of pregnancy who take over-the-counter drugs containing pseudoephedrine, a common decongestant, for hay fever, colds or the flu have given birth to babies with gastroschisis.

Gastroschisis is a hole in the baby's abdominal wall that allows the baby's intestine to protrude outside the body. Surgery is required immediately to close the hole. Babies who were exposed to pseudoephedrine while in the womb seem to have a three times greater risk of developing gastroschisis.

Further research is being done to prove the link between this over-the-counter drug and the abdominal defect.

In the mean time, if you need to use a nasal decongestant while you're pregnant or if you are trying to become pregnant, try using saline nasal drops, or ask your doctor about a safe alternative.

Medical Source ————————————————————
   Science News (141,17:262)

Buckle up for baby and you

Strapping on a seat belt may just save two lives, instead of one.

In car accidents, moms-to-be who buckle up with a lap belt and diagonal shoulder strap significantly reduce injury to themselves and their unborn baby. Yet, researchers say only one in seven pregnant women use seat belts. Most expectant moms say they're afraid buckling up will harm their baby.

The truth is, buckling up the wrong way can be dangerous. But a seat belt placed properly can be a lifesaver.

Pregnant women need to make sure the diagonal strap goes over the shoulder, between the breasts and around the side of the pregnancy swelling or "bump." The lap belt needs to rest on the upper thighs. This way the energy from the crash impact is distributed in a less harmful way.

So, if baby's on the way, play it smart! Always buckle up and remember to keep it above and below the "bump."

Medical Source ————————————————————
British Medical Journal (6827,304:586)

How many extra pounds are safe?

Unfortunately, "eating for two" doesn't mean you can eat everything in sight.

Pregnancy is one of the few times in your life when it's easier to hide a few extra pounds, but if you gain too much weight or if you are overweight to begin with, you're more likely to have complications during pregnancy.

The more overweight you are and the more weight you gain during pregnancy, the more likely you are to deliver an unusually large baby.

The larger the baby, the greater your chances of needing a Caesarean section or developing other complications such as pregnancy-induced diabetes or toxemia.

So, exactly how much weight should you gain when you're pregnant? The National Academy of Sciences recommends the following guidelines:

> ➤ Thin women — 28 to 40 pounds
> ➤ Average-weight women — 25 to 35 pounds
> ➤ Heavier than average women — 15 to 25 pounds
> ➤ Obese women — at least 15 pounds

Be sure to consult your doctor or nutritionist to make sure that you're getting the proper nutrition for you and your baby while maintaining sensible weight limits.

Medical Source ———————————————
Medical Tribune (33,18:22)

Hot tubs out cold for pregnant women

A dip in the hot tub at the end of a long day can be relaxing for you, but it can actually cause birth defects in your unborn baby.

For some years, researchers have known that too much heat causes birth defects in other mammals. And now doctors are taking this concern one step further and analyzing whether exposure to heat from a fever, hot tub or sauna might be responsible for neural tube defects in humans.

Neural tube defects occur when the baby's neural tube fails to close normally during the first six weeks of development in the womb. The neural tube develops into a baby's brain and spinal cord.

When researchers interviewed 23,000 New England women who had recently had babies, they concluded that exposure to heat from a hot tub, sauna or fever in early pregnancy more than doubled their risk of neural tube defects compared to those women without heat exposure.

Can you still take a shower? Apparently warm showers and baths are fine for you and your baby. A bath is too hot if it leaves your skin red for several minutes after you get out of the bathtub.

Medical Sources ———————————————
The Journal of the American Medical Association (268,7:882)
Developmental Medicine and Child Neurology (34,8:661)

Lead mugs not practical for pregnant women

Too much lead can tumble an entire kingdom. Historians suspect this is what happened to some ancient empires whose leaders became deranged or died from lead poisoning.

Back then, the risk of lead poisoning was very high since lead was used to sweeten wine, line aqueducts and form the base of clays and paints used to decorate utensils.

In the United States, lead levels are the lowest they've been in recorded history. Even at these levels there is still a risk of lead poisoning, especially for children and pregnant women.

Normally, adults absorb 10 to 15 percent of the lead they ingest. Children and pregnant women can absorb up to 50 percent of the lead they consume. The greater absorption rate is due to their increased need for calcium. The body absorbs lead just as it does calcium because it cannot distinguish between the two.

Large quantities of lead can damage an unborn baby's nervous system, cause premature birth and low birth weight.

Although government agencies and manufacturers carefully monitor lead levels in food, small amounts still manage to creep in from lead crystal and pewter and silver-plated hollow ware, and from the glazes and paints used on ceramic dinner ware. Lead also gets into food through soil and water.

Ceramic cups and mugs that have been improperly fired seem to pose the biggest problem. FDA researchers estimate that about 80 percent of the lead adults are exposed to is leached from cups and mugs that are used regularly to hold hot acidic drinks.

Your local FDA office or FDA headquarters (301/443-4667) can provide you with information about kits consumers can use at home to test ceramic ware for lead. Most ceramic manufacturers in the United States also have toll-free product information numbers.

Occasional use of lead-glazed dishware is not a problem, even for pregnant women.

Here are some tips to help you keep lead levels low.

- ❐ If you are pregnant, do not drink hot acidic liquids, such as coffee, tea or tomato soup, from ceramic cups or mugs. Use plain glass or plastic mugs instead. Avoid using lead crystal ware on a daily basis.
- ❐ Do not use lead crystal bottles to feed your baby.
- ❐ Do not store fruit juice or other acidic foods in ceramic containers.
- ❐ Do not store liquid in lead crystal containers.
- ❐ Do not use antique or other collectible dishware on a daily basis.

❑ Do not serve food or drinks in products that warn "Not for Food Use — May Poison Food. For Decorative Purposes Only."

❑ Do not use ceramic items in which the glaze turns a dusty or chalky gray color after washing.

Medical Source ————————————————————

FDA Consumer (27,3:19)

Fishy eating habits during pregnancy

"There's something fishy about your eating habits," should be the claim of husbands of pregnant women.

But "something fishy" doesn't mean ice cream and pickles.

It means fish.

Eating fish throughout the pregnancy seems to improve the health of the baby, suggests medical research. Women who eat a lot of fish rich in omega-3 oils tend to have fewer premature births, and the babies tend to weigh more at birth.

Full-term deliveries and higher birth weights usually indicate stronger, healthier babies.

Researchers do recommend eating fish to increase your omega-3-oil intake instead of taking fish-oil supplements. Apparently, the supplements have the same beneficial effects for the baby, but the mother might suffer negative effects.

One of the actions of fish-oil supplements is to reduce the amount of "sticky" clotting factors in the blood. In nonpregnant women, this can reduce the risk of strokes due to blood clots.

However, the reduction in clotting factors can be dangerous in pregnant women, because the women tend to bleed more during delivery than they should. Too much blood loss during delivery can be dangerous, and even life-threatening.

To avoid side effects, stay away from fish-oil supplements. Instead, eat more fresh fish, and enjoy a long and healthy pregnancy.

Medical Source ————————————————————

The Lancet (340,8811:118)

Vitamin guidelines for pregnant women

"Remember, you're not just eating for one anymore."

It's the admonishment every newly pregnant woman hears when she sits down to eat.

Wanting to make sure she provides all the proper nutrients and vitamins for the new baby, a pregnant woman will often go overboard and eat far too much. She might even take handfuls of vitamins at a time.

All these excesses could do the baby more harm than good.

A pregnant woman often does need an increased amount of many nutrients and vitamins, but getting too much of some vitamins can cause tragic results, such as mental retardation.

Some vitamins cross over the placenta more easily than others. The danger occurs when too much of the vitamin accumulates in the placenta and developing baby. The baby's kidneys and liver are not mature enough to process the vitamins, and poisonous levels build up and endanger the baby's health.

Listed below are some guidelines on a few vitamins expectant mothers should know:

❑ **Vitamin A:** Too much vitamin A before or during pregnancy increases the risk of birth defects. You should get no more than 8000 IU (or 2400 micrograms) per day. This includes any form of vitamin A, from supplements to retinol or cod liver oils. Avoid eating liver because of its high vitamin A content.

❑ **Vitamin D:** Most pregnant women get enough vitamin D from the sunlight and from a healthy, well-balanced diet, so extra supplements are not necessary. Getting too much vitamin D during pregnancy can cause abnormal facial features in the baby, as well as mental retardation in some babies. The recommended daily allowance (RDA) for vitamin D in pregnant women is 10 micrograms per day.

❑ **Folic acid:** Taking folic acid supplements before and during pregnancy reduces the risk of having a baby with spina bifida, which can cause disorders ranging from slight walking problems to severe crippling and mental retardation.

Many American women don't get enough folic acid. The RDA for folate in pregnant women is 400 micrograms per day. Liver, yeast, leafy vegetables, legumes and some fruits are good dietary sources of folate.

☐ **Vitamin K:** Taking vitamin K during the last one to two weeks of pregnancy can help lower the risk of the baby's hemorrhaging from the umbilical cord, circumcision site, etc.

The RDA for vitamin K in pregnant women is 65 micrograms per day. Green, leafy vegetables are the best source of dietary vitamin K. Milk, dairy products, meats, eggs, cereals, fruits and vegetables are also good sources.

☐ **Vitamin B12:** The body stores B12 very efficiently. In fact, the vitamin stores will often last for three to five years, even when you don't get any B12 in the diet.

So, you don't need B12 supplements unless you're a strict vegetarian who doesn't eat meat, eggs or dairy products. The RDA for vitamin B12 in pregnant women in 2.2 micrograms per day.

☐ **Calcium:** The developing baby needs lots of this extremely important mineral to form teeth, bones, healthy nerves and muscles. The body will actually "leach" calcium out of your bones to provide it for the fetus.

This leaves your bones weak and breakable. Most pregnant women do not get enough calcium, and they often suffer up to 10 grams of bone loss during pregnancy.

Lots of dairy products and other calcium-rich foods (broccoli, kale, collards, lime-processed tortillas, tofu) will provide enough calcium for the mother and baby. The RDA for calcium in pregnant women is 1,200 milligrams per day.

Women who cannot tolerate dairy products (due to lactose intolerance) should take at least a one-gram calcium supplement daily. During the last trimester, they should take two grams daily.

☐ **Iron:** Iron deficiency is very common in pregnant women. The fetus takes up about 360 milligrams of iron, and a pregnant woman's total blood volume goes up more than her red blood cell volume.

Many women don't like to take iron supplements because they can cause nausea and constipation. Eating iron-rich foods such as red meat, eggs and dark poultry meat is very important. Many breads and cereals are iron-fortified.

Drink citrus fruit juices when you eat iron-rich foods to increase the absorption of iron. The RDA for iron in pregnant women is 30 milligrams per day.

❒ **Zinc:** Zinc deficiency is rare because the body stores zinc efficiently. Alcoholics, cigarette smokers and older women who have already had several children may need extra zinc. Zinc-rich foods are meat, poultry, eggs and seafood (especially oysters). The RDA for zinc in pregnant women is 15 milligrams per day.

If you eat a well-balanced diet with a good mix of meats, cereals, dairy products, fruits and vegetables, you can take care of most of your vitamin and mineral needs.

Do not take vitamin or mineral supplements unless you are under the close supervision of your doctor. Remember that you can have too much of a good thing.

Medical Source ————————————————————
U.S. Pharmacist (18,2:34)

Snacking during labor

Probably the last thing you want to do while you're in labor is eat, right? But that's just what a new study suggests you do — if you want to shorten the time you're in labor, that is.

Although many doctors still advise women in labor to drink clear liquids and not to eat, a new study may change that advice.

Angela Flanagan, a midwife at Jubilee Hospital in Belfast, Ireland, conducted a study of 90 women in labor at the hospital. Half the women followed the traditional recommendation of fasting (going without food), and the other half were allowed to eat until they went into the advanced stages of labor.

The women who were allowed to choose from foods such as scrambled eggs, toast, jelly and ice cream not only reduced labor time by one-and-a-half hours, but they also required fewer labor-inducing drugs and painkillers than those who fasted.

Dr. Kieran Fitzpatrick, who participated in the study, said that the infants born to the "snacking" mothers also had stronger heartbeats and better muscle tone than those born to the fasting mothers. One possible reason for the increased heartbeats of the babies could be that they were less sleepy because the mothers used fewer painkillers.

Of course, any woman who is a candidate for surgery requiring general anesthesia, such as a Caesarean section, should not eat while in labor. But, where there are no complications, a little snack may strengthen both mother and child.

Medical Sources ————————————————
Medical Tribune (33,18:22)
Medical World News (33,8:14)

Beating the baby blues

You expected to be happy and carefree, enjoying all the daily wonders of a newborn child.

Instead, you sit and stare out the window, if you're not crying your eyes out instead. You feel tired, lonely and hopelessly inadequate in your new role as "mother."

You're not alone. As many as 50 to 80 percent of new mothers experience the mild postpartum depression known as the "baby blues." And as many as 15 percent of new mothers experience a deeper postpartum depression.

Women with the baby blues find themselves feeling moody, weepy and anxious. Often, they have difficulty concentrating, which can make it harder to carry out simple day-to-day activities like cooking and cleaning.

Symptoms usually begin a day or two after delivery and last several weeks.

Full-scale postpartum depression is a little more serious. It typically begins about two weeks after childbirth and may last for more than a year.

Some of the warning signs of postpartum depression include:

☐ Poor appetite or excessive weight gain.
☐ Difficulty sleeping well or disturbances in sleep patterns (beyond the baby's feeding schedule).
☐ Feelings of guilt, lack of interest in life and mood swings.
☐ Excessive worry, irrational fears (phobias) or extreme fatigue.
☐ Thoughts focus obsessively on the care and health of your baby.
☐ Fear of being criticized for poor mothering skills.
☐ Inability to concentrate or make decisions.
☐ Physical symptoms, such as headaches and breast tenderness.

The mild form of postpartum depression usually represents a new mother's adjustment from her previous lifestyle to one that includes a new person. Some of the depression arises from feeling ill-equipped to care for a new baby.

Most women begin to feel confident in their mothering skills after a few weeks. The baby blues start to slip away as the joy of the new baby fills your life.

Unfortunately, some new mothers have additional factors to deal with that can turn a simple case of the baby blues into serious postpartum depression.

A few of the risk factors for developing postpartum blues are:

☐ Additional sources of tension, such as moving, changing jobs, divorce, death in the family, financial difficulties, marital conflict, etc.
☐ Unplanned pregnancy, especially among unmarried teenagers.
☐ Irritable, sick or temperamental infant that doesn't always enjoy cuddling, making you feel inadequate or unloved.
☐ Poor relationship with your own mother, or lack of maternal role model.
☐ Lack of support system from husband, parents, family and friends.

Although postpartum depression feels as if it will never end, most new mothers simply need a lot of reassurance and support.

"New mother support groups" provide you with the opportunity to discuss your feelings of depression, inadequacy and worry with other mothers in the same boat.

Counseling from the pediatrician, family doctor, a therapist or a social worker often helps soothe your anxieties and fears.

Grandparents and the child's father can help relieve postpartum depression by getting involved in the care of the infant. Everyone "pitching in" lets you rest and helps you feel a family support system of encouragement and assistance.

Make arrangements with grandparents or a baby-sitter to keep the baby for short periods of time every now and then to allow you time away from the baby.

Spending this time alone, with your husband or with friends will help you get back into the swing of things and feel as though some things are still the way they used to be before the baby came.

Time away from the baby can also make you eager to see the baby again and makes your time together more enjoyable instead of tiring.

New mothers who feel tense should practice some stress-relief or relaxation exercises. Some simple ways to help reduce stress are:

- ❐ Physical exercise — taking daily walks, attending low-impact aerobics classes or doing simple exercises at home.
- ❐ Sitting quietly and listening to soothing music.
- ❐ Reading a favorite book or watching a favorite old movie.
- ❐ Taking short mid-day naps to ease tension and increase energy for the rest of the day.
- ❐ Taking slow, deliberate breaths to calm down in moments of anger, frustration or irritation with the new baby or other daily aggravations.
- ❐ Prayer and meditation.

And, finally, you should feel free to pursue outside interests and hobbies that you enjoyed before the baby came, even though your free time may be more limited now.

If you still have difficulty dealing with postpartum depression, you should seek help from your family doctor.

He can offer medical help that will help relieve the symptoms and allow you to enjoy your new bundle of joy.

Medical Source ———————————————————
  Postgraduate Medicine (93,3:103)

Hormone replacement therapy and cancer: balancing your risk

When your body stops producing the hormone estrogen at menopause, you usually begin to experience hot flashes, night sweats, vaginal dryness which causes pain during intercourse, and other aggravating symptoms. Your risk of heart disease and osteoporosis also dramatically increase.

Hot flashes, heart disease and osteoporosis weren't always a problem, but now women live more than a third of their lives after the age of menopause. That's why doctors so often recommend hormone replacement therapy.

Osteoporosis is a disorder in which the bones become thin and fragile and tend to fracture and break easily. Women past menopause are most commonly affected because your body needs estrogen to maintain bone mass.

Five years of estrogen replacement therapy has been shown to reduce hip, arm and vertebrae fractures by 50 to 75 percent. Once estrogen therapy stops, bone mass starts to deteriorate. Hip fractures aren't just annoying — if you fracture your hip when you're very old, you have a good chance of not surviving it.

Cardiovascular disease is another serious problem that women over 50 face. Heart attack is the most common cause of death in women past menopause. For every five American women who die, three die from heart disease and fewer than one each die from cancer and from all other causes put together.

Researchers estimate that estrogen therapy may reduce coronary disease by as much as 45 percent. Hormone replacement therapy could be especially important to you if you are at an increased risk of heart disease because of family history or other factors.

Other women who may greatly benefit from hormone replacement therapy include those who had early menopause, missed periods often, have a thin, slight frame, smoke, have a family history of osteoporosis, or have been recently treated with glucocorticoids.

Risks of hormone replacement therapy

Researchers have linked hormones such as estrogen and progestogen to more than 40 percent of cancers that develop in women. Normally, your risk for hormone-related cancers is greater before menopause than after because menopause decreases the production of estrogen and progestogen.

Hormone replacement therapy slightly increases your naturally lowered postmenopausal risk. Estrogen taken alone can increase your risk of uterine cancer three to six times after five years of use and up to 10 times after 10 years of use. However, this risk can be almost eliminated by taking progestogens along with estrogens for 12 days each month.

Women who undergo hormone replacement therapy have a slightly higher risk (about a 10 percent increased risk) of developing breast cancer than women who do not.

The effect that the combination therapy of estrogen and progestogen has on breast cancer has not been widely studied. A study done in Sweden suggests that combination therapy may present a greater risk than estrogen used alone.

Women already at increased risk for breast or uterine cancer (they have a family history of it, for instance) need to seriously consider the risks of hormone replace therapy. For other women, the benefits of the treatment may be equal to or greater than the risk of cancer.

If you decide that hormone replacement therapy is worthwhile for you, taking estrogen continuously instead of in 21-day cycles seems to be better. Any woman who still has her uterus should also take progestogen. It may be best to take estrogen orally since implanted estrogen may cause dependence.

Estrogen can cause breast tenderness and sometimes stomach upset. This may mean the dose is too high.

Progestogens can cause breast tenderness, bloated feelings, depression, anxiety and irritability. Taking the progestogen last thing at night or taking half the dose in the morning and the rest at night may help. If not, you may want to ask your doctor about trying a different progestogen.

You may want to ask your doctor about other factors that could increase your cancer risk before beginning hormone replacement therapy. By carefully weighing your risks for hormone-related cancer, osteoporosis and heart disease, you can make a decision about hormone replacement therapy that will be most beneficial for you.

Medical Sources —————————————————————
Science (259,5095:618 and 633)
British Medical Journal (305,6866:1403)

The best time to perform breast self-exams

Since hormone replacement therapy does increase the risk of developing breast cancer, monthly breast self-examinations become more important than ever. Early detection of questionable lumps in the breast is the key to treating breast cancer successfully.

For the best, most accurate results in the breast self-examination, women on hormone replacement therapy should perform the exam on the same day each month.

Hormone therapy can influence the levels of hormones in the body at different times of the month. The changing hormone levels can cause differences in the size, shape and feel of the breast from day to day.

Performing the self-examination on the same day of each month eliminates the confusion of normal daily changes and allows you to detect changes that are not related to hormone levels.

If you detect any changes in the shape, size, feel or look of your breasts, or if you develop any discharge from your nipples, call your doctor right way.

Medical Sources —————————————————————
Medical Tribune (34,1:7)
Health After 50 (4,12:8)

Slow, deep breathing leaves hot flashes out in the cold

Do hot flashes make you lose your cool? Try regulating your breathing.

Hot flashes, also known as hot flushes, are caused by varying hormone levels. In a process that is not well understood, changing hormone levels dilate the blood vessels in the skin. Blood rushes to the skin, generating heat and making you feel flushed.

Researchers studied 33 menopausal women who had not received any estrogen therapy (which controls hot flashes) and who were having an average of five hot flashes a day. They divided the women into three different groups. One group was taught regulated breathing; one was taught muscle relaxation and one biofeedback relaxation.

Only the women who were taught regulated breathing experienced a significant decrease in hot flashes. While the normal adult breathes 15 to 20 times a minute, the women in the regulated breathing group were trained to breathe only six to eight times per minute and to breathe much deeper than they normally would. This reduced their frequency of hot flashes by almost 39 percent.

Before you turn to medicine to control your hot flashes, ask your gynecologist for more information about regulated breathing techniques.

Medical Source ————————————————
American Journal of Obstetrics and Gynecology (167,2:436)

Vitamin D has negative impact on estrogen therapy

Many women on estrogen replacement therapy also take vitamin D to help protect their bones against osteoporosis, the brittle-bone disease.

However, if you have healthy bones and are taking estrogen to lower your risk of heart disease, you may want to reconsider that daily dose of vitamin D.

Hormone replacement therapy works to prevent heart disease because it lowers total blood cholesterol levels and raises the level of HDL cholesterol (the good kind). Vitamin D supplements seem to interfere with this positive effect on cholesterol.

Scientists gave 0.5 micrograms of cholecalciferol (a form of vitamin D) to women on estrogen replacement therapy. That's one-tenth the Recommended Dietary Allowance of vitamin D for women over 50.

The researchers found that the vitamin-D supplements negated the positive effect that estrogen has on the HDL cholesterol levels of postmeno-pausal women. In other words, hormone replacement therapy seems to be more effective against heart disease when you don't take vitamin-D supplements.

Talk to your doctor about the impact of vitamin D supplements on estrogen replacement therapy. Do not stop taking your vitamin supplements without consulting your doctor. You may need vitamin D to protect against osteoporosis more than you need the cholesterol-lowering effect of estrogen.

Medical Source ————————————————
Archives of Internal Medicine (152,11:2265)

Estrogen eases carpal tunnel syndrome

Do your hands tingle and go numb even when you're not excited or cold?

If they do, you may be suffering from a common condition known as carpal tunnel syndrome, which causes numbness, tingling and pain in your thumb, index and middle fingers.

Carpal tunnel syndrome is caused by pressure on the nerve that runs from the neck to the hands at the point it passes into the hand.

Interestingly, more women seem to suffer from the syndrome than men, especially pregnant women, women who have recently started taking birth control pills, and women who have had gynecological surgery. In one study, one out of three women who had had their ovaries removed had carpal tunnel syndrome.

Researchers believe that menopause may cause changes in forearm fat and fluid retention, which may lead to carpal tunnel syndrome. Women who begin estrogen replacement therapy seem to experience significant improvements in their carpal tunnel syndrome symptoms.

Low estrogen levels may also be connected to fibromyalgia (pain in fibrous tissue, such as tendons and cartilage). Two common signs of low estrogen levels are loss of rapid eye movement sleep and depression, which are also symptoms of fibromyalgia.

Researchers believe that estrogen replacement therapy can be helpful in relieving carpal tunnel syndrome as well as fibromyalgia.

Consult your doctor for more information about estrogen replacement therapy if you think it could be beneficial for you.

Medical Source —————————————————————
   British Medical Journal (304,6823:382)

How to build stronger bones

Osteoporosis is the crippling, painful disease that causes fragile, breakable bones and disfigurement in millions of women past the age of menopause.

It's responsible for countless numbers of hip fractures, broken bones, rounded shoulders, aching backs and the need for wheelchairs.

Fortunately, it's a disease that in many cases can be avoided, even if you have a family history of it.

Although everyone — men and women alike — is going to experience some degree of bone loss when they get older, the effects of bone loss are less severe if you have more bone mass to begin with.

Young women need to take simple measures to increase their bone mass while they are still able to do so.

Scientists recently conducted a study on 156 women in their 20s and found that exercise, calcium intake and the use of oral contraceptives all had positive effects on bone mass.

Taking calcium daily seemed to have the greatest positive effect on the rate of bone-mass increase in the spine. Regular exercise had the second-greatest influence, and the use of oral contraceptives also had a notable, positive influence on bone mass.

None of the women in the study exercised too heavily (none were marathon runners, etc.), and none of them took megadoses of calcium. Women can increase their bone mass simply by exercising for 30 minutes three times a week and getting the recommended daily allowance of calcium.

Scientists warn that increases in bone mass usually stop around age 30. Beyond age 30, calcium and regular exercise can certainly help prevent bone loss, but it will no longer contribute to increases in bone mass.

This news should not discourage women past age 30 from taking calcium. A recent study of over 3,000 women aged 69 to 106 suggests that taking calcium and vitamin D supplements reduces the risk of bone fractures at any age.

Women who took extra calcium and vitamin D for 18 months experienced almost half the hip fractures and about a third fewer fractures of other bones compared with the women who had received a placebo.

If an elderly person does break a bone because of osteoporosis, they may need protein supplements as well as vitamins if they don't eat a proper diet. An older person who doesn't get enough protein will suffer through a longer-than-normal healing process after breaking a bone.

Researchers gave daily protein supplements to a group of people over age 60 who were admitted to the hospital with a broken thigh bone. These people had fewer complications and greater bone mass once the bone healed than people who didn't receive protein.

Be careful, though — too much protein in your diet can also be dangerous.

The amount of protein in the supplements contained only enough to raise the volunteers' dietary intake to the recommended daily allowance.

It is important for young and elderly women to get a balanced diet with the recommended daily allowance of protein, vitamins, minerals and nutrients to help keep their bones as healthy as possible.

Medical Sources ————————————————
> *The Journal of the American Medical Association* (268,17:2403)
> *The New England Journal of Medicine* (327,23:1637)
> *The Journal of the American College of Nutrition* (11,5:519)

Steps to build and preserve bone mass

- ☐ Be sure you get the recommended dietary allowance of calcium every day. The RDA for calcium in females ages 11 to 24 is 1,200 milligrams, 800 milligrams for women ages 25 and over and 1,200 milligrams for pregnant women.
- ☐ Milk, cheese, yogurt and other dairy products are great sources of calcium. Since these can be fatty, try to use the low-fat versions.

❏ Wheat bread is a good source of calcium. Although it doesn't contain a large amount of calcium, the calcium in wheat bread is easily absorbed and used in the body.

❏ Yeast helps increase the availability of calcium in the body. So eating breads with yeast ensures that the calcium present in the bread will be easily digested and used in the body.

❏ Several different types of beans (such as soybeans, navy beans, pinto beans and red beans) are good sources of calcium.

❏ Green, leafy vegetables like broccoli, kale and collards are good, natural sources of calcium.

❏ Begin exercising regularly to increase your bone mass. Try to lean toward smooth, nonjarring exercises such as walking, bicycling, swimming and low-impact aerobics instead of high-stress, high-impact sports such as basketball, long-distance running and high-impact aerobics.

❏ Moderate social drinking of alcohol may help prevent bone loss. People who drink moderate amounts of alcohol seem to have thicker and stronger bones than nondrinkers and heavy alcohol drinkers. Drinking large amounts of alcohol can actually lead to increased bone loss and an increased risk of osteoporosis.
Medical researchers don't recommend drinking as a way to prevent osteoporosis. They were just encouraged that this popular American habit has a positive side effect.

Talk to your doctor about a proper diet and a healthy exercise plan that will help you build healthy bones.

Medical Sources ───────────────────────

The Journal of the American Medical Association (268,17:2357)
British Medical Journal (306,6891:1506)
The Atlanta Journal/Constitution (Oct. 16, 1992, D4)

MEN'S HEALTH

Pelvic exercises may cure impotence

It can strike any man, at anytime, at any age — impotence. But, now, instead of worrying, waiting or going under the surgical knife, some men may be able to exercise their way back up to full sexual capacity.

Impotence — a taboo topic for most men — is more common than you may realize. In the United States, it is estimated that 10 to 15 million males are impotent at one time or another.

The older a man gets, the more likely it is that he will have to deal with impotence. As many as one in three men over the age of 60 has difficulty with erections.

While experts disagree on the exact mechanics of an erection, they do know that an increased blood flow to the penis is needed to enlarge the organ, and muscle contractions are necessary to sustain the erection. Although being unable to get and maintain an erection is often caused by stress or other mental pressures, sometimes the culprit is physical, not mental.

In some cases, the blood flow to the penis becomes disrupted or drains from the area prematurely. Usually, when this occurs, doctors prescribe medication or surgery to correct the dysfunction.

The cure can be as bad as the problem. The operation can leave the penis sore, swollen and numb for anywhere from one week to six months.

But, now, there may be a more appealing alternative. A team of Belgium urologists treated 150 men who suffered from a disruption in penile blood flow. Some men had operations and others did special pelvic muscle exercises, called Kegels. Kegels are contractions of the pelvic floor muscles — an exercise pregnant women have been doing for years to help with childbirth.

One year after treatment, 58 percent of the men who performed the Kegels were completely cured or were so satisfied with their improvement that they did not opt for surgery. While the short-term results for those in the surgical group were better than the exercise group, more of those who had surgery had trouble with impotence returning over the long run.

Some skeptical doctors say that the pelvic muscles don't have any influence on the mechanism for trapping blood in the penis and that the men in the study may have improved because of the beneficial psychological effects of the therapy.

At any rate, if you are suffering from impotence, please see your doctor and advise him of these studies. If your case is mild, then Kegels just might do the trick.

Kegel exercises:
1) Identify the pelvic muscles that need exercising. You can do this by stopping and starting the flow of urine several times when using the bathroom.
2) Tighten the muscles a little at the time. Contract muscles slowly, hold for a count of 10 and relax the muscles slowly.
3) Repeat these exercises for the anal pelvic muscles. To find these muscles, imagine you're trying to hold back a bowel movement, without tensing your leg, stomach or buttock muscles.
4) Then practice tightening all pelvic muscles together, moving from back to front.
5) Start by repeating each exercise five times three to five times a day. Gradually work up to 20 or 30 repetitions at once.

Ask your doctor for more information about how to do the exercises. Performing the Kegels incorrectly can cause hemorrhoids.

You will find that you can perform your Kegels just about anywhere or anytime. Chances are good that "pumping it up" with these pelvic exercises will have you back in top shape in no time.

Medical Sources ———————————————

Medical Tribune (34,5:19)
British Journal of Urology (71,1:52)
Obstetrics and Gynecology (81,2:283)

Prevent impotence with low-fat diet

Men! Watching your fat and cholesterol intake now might prevent impotence years down the road.

Researchers in New Zealand discovered that rabbits fed a high-fat, high-cholesterol diet developed impotence from plaque buildup in the arteries of the penis.

The same conditions have been found in men with similar diets, especially in men whose arteries are already damaged by smoking and high blood pressure.

Since erections depend on blood flow to the penis, cholesterol blocking the arteries is one of the chief causes of impotence.

Changing your diet after you've found out about the problem may not reverse it. You can reduce your chances of ever developing this problem if you start a low-fat, low-cholesterol diet now — before it's too late.

Medical Source ———————————————
Medical Tribune (33,12:14)

Older men: Exercise improves sex life

Want to maintain an active sex life into your senior years? Then you'll be glad to hear that there is a definite link between sexuality and physical activity.

Apparently, a moderate 60-minute workout three times a week can be your ticket to better sex. To prove this, researchers in California tested 95 middle-aged couch potatoes for nine months.

Seventeen of the men walked regularly, while the rest worked out at 75 to 80 percent of their aerobic capacity over three times a week.

The results: The men who exercised more vigorously reported better sex and more of it!

The improvement probably stems from increased levels of the male hormone, testosterone, and improved circulation and breathing.

Another reason? Regular workouts can improve sex because you look better and feel better about yourself when you exercise regularly — you have less fat, better muscle tone and a higher self-esteem.

Medical Source ———————————————
The Physician and Sportsmedicine (21,3:199)

Vasectomy link to prostate cancer is unclear

Vasectomies prevent unwanted pregnancies, but do they also cause prostate cancer? A few recent studies have suggested this possibility.

Men who've had a vasectomy often have higher levels of testosterone than other men. Too much testosterone may contribute to the development of prostate cancer.

One study reported that men with vasectomies have about a 60 percent increase in risk for prostate cancer. However, increases in risk below 200 percent are generally considered small.

Some researchers suspect that vasectomized men don't have a higher risk of prostate cancer at all. They believe that doctors simply found more prostate cancers in these men because they were examined more closely than other men usually are.

In any case, there is not sufficient evidence to indicate a strong link between vasectomies and prostate cancer. Neither is there any evidence that a vasectomy increases a man's risk of developing an enlarged prostate.

Researchers continue to search for causes of prostate cancer. In the meantime, don't avoid vasectomies or have your vasectomy reversed in an attempt to avoid prostate cancer.

If you're considering a vasectomy, talk with your doctor about the risks and benefits. If you do decide in favor of this operation, you should still have regular screenings for prostate cancer after you turn 40.

Medical Sources ───────────────────────

Journal of the National Cancer Institute (85,7:527)

Annals of Internal Medicine (118,10:793)

How to cope with common prostate problems

Most men will suffer from prostate troubles sometime in their lives. Prostate problems can be uncomfortable, but most are minor and can be easily treated.

The prostate is a small, doughnut-shaped gland that encircles the urethra, the tube that carries urine to the penis. The prostate is responsible for producing most of the whitish-colored fluid that transports sperm.

Prostatitis

Prostatitis, an inflammation of the prostate, is the first prostate problem most men experience. This disorder generally affects men in their 20s and 30s, although older men can also develop prostatitis.

The inflammation is often caused by a bacterial infection that spreads from the urethra. The infection may or may not be sexually transmitted. Symptoms include:

> ➤ Low back pain
> ➤ Difficult urination
> ➤ Painful or burning sensation when urinating
> ➤ Chills
> ➤ High fever

Getting plenty of rest, drinking lots of fluids and medicine will relieve prostatitis. If you have the nonbacterial form of prostatitis (which is more difficult to treat than the bacterial type), hot baths, pain medicine and periodic prostate massages can be helpful. Abstain from sex until the pain lessens.

Prostate enlargement

More than half of all men over fifty have symptoms caused by an enlarged prostate gland. As most men age and their hormone levels change, the prostate begins to grow.

As the prostate enlarges, it squeezes the urethra, making it difficult for men to urinate, which is often the first sign of an enlarged prostate. Other symptoms include:

> ➤ Dribbling following urination
> ➤ A feeling that the bladder is not completely empty
> ➤ An urgent need to urinate
> ➤ Having to get up in the middle of the night to urinate
> ➤ Straining to urinate
> ➤ Painful or burning sensation when urinating
> ➤ Less forceful or interrupted stream of urine
> ➤ Frequent urinating

In most men, symptoms only worsen with time. Symptoms may also become worse during stressful situations or during very cold weather. Occasionally symptoms may disappear without any type of treatment.

Considering the types of complications that can result from prostate enlargement, it's best to see a doctor as soon as you have any problems. Conditions caused by an enlarged prostate may include:

> ➤ Constipation
> ➤ Infection
> ➤ Bladder stones
> ➤ Kidney disease or failure

Sometimes prostate problems can be caused by an underlying disorder that has not been diagnosed. Problems that can affect your prostate include:

> ➤ Diabetes
> ➤ Urinary tract infections
> ➤ Kidney disease
> ➤ Nerve disorders

How to cope with an enlarged prostate

☐ Stay away from spicy foods, alcohol, coffee and other caffeinated drinks. These will irritate your prostate gland. You can still have decaffeinated colas, of course.

Many pain relievers for colds, headaches and hay fever also contain caffeine. Whenever possible, replace these medications with ibuprofen or another pain reliever that does not contain caffeine.

☐ Don't drink coffee, tea or cola right after dinner.

☐ Allow yourself several uninterrupted minutes to urinate. This will help you empty your bladder more completely.

☐ Avoid anticholinergic or sympatholytic drugs. Over-the-counter medicines that can worsen symptoms include many cough and cold remedies, hay fever products, bronchodilators and appetite suppressants.

☐ Avoid diuretics if at all possible, or at least take the smallest dose allowed. Taking the diuretic early in the day may also help.

Treatment options: What to do

If your prostate symptoms are only mild and do not present a danger to your overall health, your best bet would probably be to put up with them and avoid any type of therapy, surgical or otherwise. If you and your doctor do decide that treatment beyond what you can do at home is necessary, you have quite a few options to consider.

Medicine

Medication effectively relieves symptoms of prostate enlargement in some men. It is certainly worth giving this option a try before turning to surgery.

Terazosin, doxazosin and prazosin are all anti-hypertensives, drugs used to lower blood pressure. They also seem to work quite well in relieving prostate problems. Side effects from these drugs include dizziness, headache and fainting.

Taking acetaminophen a half hour before taking terazosin can make headaches less severe. Headaches normally subside after taking the medication for several weeks. Prazosin is associated with more sexual problems than terazosin or doxazosin.

The drug flutamide modestly reduces symptoms of prostate enlargement. While it does not cause impotence, it may cause stomach upsets or cause some men to develop unusually large breasts.

Finasteride relieves moderate symptoms of prostate enlargement without causing sexual problems in most men.

Hormone therapy

Hormone therapy has also been used to successfully treat enlarged prostates. However, the treatment must be continuous or the gland will return to its former size. Although this procedure is effective, many men don't choose this route because it often causes sexual dysfunction.

Hyperthermia

Recently, high heat levels have been used to destroy excess prostate tissue. This technique reduces bladder blockage and has very few complications. It does not affect sexual function. This procedure can be performed on an outpatient basis and requires only a mild painkiller. Long-term effects from this procedure are not known.

Laser destruction

In this procedure, a laser beam is used to destroy excess prostate tissue. This treatment has a shorter recovery period and fewer complications than surgery.

Balloon dilation

During this procedure, a deflated balloon is inserted into the prostate, inflated and then withdrawn. This treatment relieves the symptoms of an enlarged prostate for at least a year in three out of four men who undergo the procedure. Balloon therapy is most effective in men with mild symptoms.

Surgery

If you have any of the following conditions, your doctor may recommend surgery.

☐ Previous urinary retention that required catheterization
☐ Low urinary flow rate
☐ Increased urine in your bladder or urine trapped in your kidneys
☐ Blood in your urine
☐ Severe urinary tract infection

There are three types of surgery used to treat an enlarged prostate.

Prostatectomy — All or part of the prostate gland is removed. This type of surgery is recommended for men with glands too large for other types of surgery or who need to have another disorder corrected, such as bladder stones.

TURP — Transurethral resection of the prostate. Most men choose TURP instead of prostatectomy because it is associated with a shorter hospital stay, is safer (no actual incision), requires less catheterization time after surgery and is less stressful on the body.

Infection occurs in 15 to 30 percent of the men who undergo this operation. Temporary incontinence is common for a short while after surgery, but total incontinence occurs less than 1 percent of the time.

Impotence affects 5 to 35 percent of the men who undergo this process. Half or more of these men experience retrograde ejaculation, in which semen is forced backward into the bladder. These men still experience the sensation of orgasm although they may note that it "feels different."

TUIP — Transurethral incision of the prostate. This surgical procedure is often recommended for men with small prostate glands who are having problems. TUIP will not cause retrograde ejaculation. This method offers the same relief of symptoms as TURP, but it's not known how long TUIP is effective.

If you are diagnosed with prostate enlargement, discuss your treatment options with your doctor. He will be able to help you decide what will work best for you.

Medical Sources ——————————————————
> *U.S. Pharmacist* (18,4:41)
> *FDA Consumer* (26,3:29)
> *Geriatrics* (47,12:39)
> *American Family Physician* (48,6:1144)

How to take your prostate medicine

- ❒ Take medicine exactly as prescribed.
- ❒ Don't miss doses.
- ❒ Don't take aspirin for pain relief if you've recently undergone prostate surgery. Take acetaminophen or ibuprofen instead.
- ❒ Talk with your doctor or pharmacist if you notice your symptoms getting worse, if you have any questions about your medicine and before taking any over-the-counter medication. Some of these drugs can actually worsen your symptoms.
- ❒ Keep medicine in a child-proof container and well out of the reach of children.

Medical Sources ——————————————————
> *U.S. Pharmacist* (18,4:41)

Nutrition and your prostate

Mom was right! You are what you eat. The more problem foods you eat, especially fatty foods, the more health problems you have, even when it comes to your prostate.

Men who eat a high-fiber diet that includes plenty of fruits, raw vegetables, cereals and grains seem to lower their risk of prostate cancer. A high-fiber diet may decrease the amount of testosterone in the body, thus slowing prostate growth.

Fats, on the other hand, seem to raise the levels of testosterone and other male hormones, stimulating the prostate to grow. Any cancer cells within the prostate grow as well.

The fat in red meat seems to be especially dangerous. After studying the health records of more than 47,000 men, researchers found that men who eat large amounts of red meat are 2 1/2 times more likely to develop advanced prostate cancer than men who eat very little red meat. Nutritionists recommend that you eat red meat only once or twice a week.

Eating a lot of fat doesn't appear to cause you to develop cancerous cells in the prostate. Cancerous cells develop in 60 to 70 percent of all men who live to the age of 80.

A large fat intake seems to activate any cancer cells you may have in your prostate, making them deadly where they lay dormant before. The more fat you eat, the faster prostate cancer seems to progress.

Adopting a low-fat lifestyle

For maximum health, you should consume no more than 30 percent of your daily calories from fat. On average, the normal man only needs 30 to 60 grams of fat per day. Adults need a minimum of 15 to 25 grams of fat per day to keep their bodies functioning normally. Your body needs fat, just not in excess!

If figuring the specific amount of fat in your diet gets to be a real chore, just remember this rule: Most of your food should have no more than 3 grams of fat per 100 calories. Look for fat grams per serving on food labels.

For foods without labels, consult a book such as *Controlling Your Fat Tooth* by Joseph C. Piscatella or *The Complete Up-To-Date Fat Book* by Avery Publishing Group.

If you eat less fat, you'll not only lower your risk of prostate cancer, you'll have more energy, sleep better, have lower grocery bills and more control over your weight.

The zinc link

Zinc prevents prostate problems, claim recent advertisements. Doctors, however, are not so certain. While the prostate contains more zinc than any other part of the body, how it is used or what its exact function is remains unknown.

Whether or not zinc will prevent prostate cancer is debatable, but higher zinc levels do appear to help urination. Men with prostate cancer or other prostate problems often find it difficult to urinate.

Zinc in combination with the vitamins B12 and E may provide relief of prostate problems. This combination of vitamins and minerals appears to shrink the enlarged prostate, making it easier to urinate.

Men with an enlarged prostate who take this vitamin/mineral combination also report that they have less dribbling following urination and don't make as many trips to the bathroom during the night.

Does this mean you should take a zinc supplement to make sure you get enough zinc each day? Opinions differ on whether it is better to get zinc through a supplement or through a well-balanced diet.

Unfortunately, many zinc-rich foods are high in cholesterol. Too much cholesterol in the diet is often a problem for men in the 40 to 90 age range, when prostate problems tend to flare up. You don't want to create a new problem, such as heart disease or stroke, by trying to solve your prostate problem.

If you're interested in changing your diet or in using zinc and vitamin supplements, talk with your doctor. Having the right amount of zinc in your body is critical. What might be right for one man will not necessarily be right for you.

Some foods high in zinc are nuts, sunflower seeds, wheat germ and bran, milk, eggs, onions, brewer's yeast, many seafoods, beef liver, meat, lentils, molasses, peas, beans and poultry. Cooking or other processing methods can lower the amount of zinc a food contains naturally.

The following vitamins may also be beneficial for the prostate. We've listed the most common foods that contain these vitamins:

Vitamin B12 — Liver, kidney, chicken, beef, pork, fish, eggs and dairy products

Vitamin C — Orange juice, citrus fruits, tomatoes, broccoli, brussels sprouts, cabbage, strawberries and green peppers

Vitamin D — Milk, tuna, sardines, egg yolks, margarine, fish liver oil and salmon

Vitamin E — Peanuts, cabbage, spinach, asparagus, wheat germ, whole-grain bread, vegetable oils and rice

Will pumpkin seeds do the trick?

Some advertisements claim that pumpkin seeds, saw palmetto, golden rod and flaxseed oil help the prostate function normally. There is no evidence to prove that these claims are true.

However, men who take such compounds may experience relief from their prostate symptoms simply because they believe the products are working.

Researchers agree that the best thing you can do for your prostate is to eat a well-balanced diet. Make sure you get plenty of the basic foods, while being careful not to eat or drink too much.

Talk with your doctor before you make a major change in your diet to control your prostate problems.

Medical Sources ————————————————

Annals of Internal Medicine (118,10:793)
Journal of the National Cancer Institute (89,19:1571)
Medical Tribune (34,21:8)
Nutrition Action (20,2:5)
Nutrition Research Newsletter (12,11/12:117)
The Complete & Up-To-Date Fat Book, Avery Publishing Group, Garden City Park, New York, 1993
Controlling Your Fat Tooth, Workman Publishing Company, Inc., New York, 1991
The Atlanta Journal/Constitution (Oct. 6, 1993, B4)

Healthy sperm need vitamin C

Attention, all future fathers.

The health and well-being of your future children could be in danger, and you might hold the key to their safety in your hands — if you're holding an orange, that is.

Yes, an orange.

Scientists now suspect that a single orange a day can provide enough vitamin C to help prevent the possibility of birth defects in your children.

Numerous studies show that men who have low levels of vitamin C in their bodies seem to have an increased number of genetically damaged sperm.

How can low vitamin C levels damage the sperm? you ask.

During the everyday processes of metabolism, the body produces waste products known as radicals, or oxidants. Radicals can cause genetic damage to all the cells in the body, including sperm cells. In fact, these oxidants are more harmful to cells than many manmade chemicals that everyone worries about.

Vitamin C is known as an "antioxidant," which means that it breaks down the dangerous oxidants into harmless forms that can be removed from the body.

Not getting enough vitamin C means that the body can't get rid of all the oxidants quickly enough, so they can get into cells and damage the DNA.

Scientists think that most of the genetic damage caused by low vitamin C levels is repaired by "self-repair mechanisms" soon after the egg is fertilized.

However, the greater the damage to the sperm, the less likely that those self-repair mechanisms can fix everything, and the greater the chances of birth defects in the fetus.

The solution to the problem is simple: Eat more fruits and vegetables.

The minimum recommended daily allowance (RDA) for vitamin C is 60 milligrams per day, which is about the amount contained in one orange.

Men who smoke need to take in more vitamin C every day than other men. Some of the chemicals in cigarette smoke destroy vitamin C in the body.

Fruits and vegetables rich in vitamin C include green and red peppers, collard greens, broccoli, spinach, tomatoes, potatoes, strawberries, oranges and other citrus fruits. Meat, fish, poultry, eggs and most dairy products also contain small amounts of vitamin C.

Medical Source ————————————————
Proceedings of the National Academy of Sciences (88,11003)

Chemical imbalance linked to male aggressiveness

If heavy traffic or a cranky cashier makes you fighting mad, you could have a chemical imbalance. Recent studies have found that some men who tend to become aggressive and violent in stressful situations do not have the enzyme that helps people cope with stress.

During stressful situations, chemicals in your body stimulate changes in your heart rate and blood pressure. Unfortunately, your body's natural response to stress can make it harder for you to cope. (In caveman days, when a "stressful situation" meant you were about to be eaten by a wild boar, you would have been glad of the extra burst of energy and adrenaline your body provided.)

Normally, enzymes present in the body regulate your chemical reactions to stress, slowing down or speeding up these processes as needed.

Men who become unusually aggressive or violent under stressful conditions do not have the enzyme that should slow down their body's reaction to stress. This means that they experience stress for longer periods of time than most people, increasing their tendency to react with aggression or violence.

Medical Source ——————————————————
Medical Tribune (34,22:7)

Stress leads to early death in men

Middle-aged men who get divorced, fired or charged with a crime have a high risk of dying early, report Swedish researchers.

However, it may not always be the stressful events themselves that lead to an early death. Alcohol abuse causes many cases of stressful life events and early death.

Cancer and heart disease may also be linked to stress and early death. Men who had experienced many stressful events tended to develop these disorders.

Dangerous stressors include worry, divorce, financial problems and prosecution for a crime. Men who worried about a family member doubled the risk of premature death.

Divorce, separation or a forced move to a new location before the age of fifty tripled a man's risk of early death. Men prosecuted for a crime had the greatest risk of premature death — 25 percent of the men in this study prosecuted before their 50th birthday died earlier than expected.

You can control the quality and length of your life. Don't let stress send you to an early grave.

Medical Source ─────────────────────────
Medical Tribune (34,22:7)

Senior's health

Alzheimer's disease: the aluminum link

Everyone dreads Alzheimer's disease, or senile dementia, and for good reason. It affects about one out of every three people by the time they reach their 80s.

The mind-robbing disease usually strikes between the ages of 40 and 60, progressing over a few months to five years to the point where you can't recall the names of your children or how to brush your teeth.

If you knew anything you could do to prevent it from happening to you, you would try it. That's one reason everyone jumped on the bandwagon when researchers discovered large amounts of aluminum in the brain tissues of Alzheimer's victims.

Does the slow accumulation of aluminum in the brain cause Alzheimer's disease? Should we avoid aluminum soft-drink cans, aluminum cookware and even our tap water if its aluminum content is higher than it should be?

After 30 years of research, the jury is still out. While some researchers found excessive aluminum in the brain tissues of Alzheimer's sufferers, other scientists said the aluminum came from chemical agents the researchers used to analyze the brain tissue.

Other studies do seem to point to a weak link between Alzheimer's and aluminum:

❏ Population studies have shown that people were more likely to have Alzheimer's if they had been drinking from public water supplies treated with aluminum sulfates to make them clearer.

❏ Animal studies seem to show an Alzheimer's/aluminum link. When researchers injected aluminum into the brains of rabbits and cats, changes in their behavior and their brain mimicked changes in Alzheimer's victims.

❏ People with kidney failure who have undergone dialysis have shown a loss of intellectual function similar to Alzheimer's when the dialysis fluid is made from water containing large amounts of aluminum. This condition is called dialysis dementia.

☐ An experimental drug that draws aluminum out of the body seems to slow down the progression of Alzheimer's disease.

Researchers seem to agree that there's no doubt that aluminum is poisonous to our bodies and our brains if it gets into our nervous system. It's just that aluminum is present everywhere on the earth, and our bodies are expert at keeping the harmful metal out.

We get rid of aluminum through our urine and feces, and our brains have a mechanism called the "blood-brain barrier" that is supposed to prevent certain substances like aluminum from entering.

Most scientists believe that our brains couldn't possibly absorb enough aluminum to cause Alzheimer's, but some scientists are still holding on to the aluminum/Alzheimer's link.

If you want to be on the safe side and avoid taking in large amounts of aluminum, the best thing to do is worry only about the big sources of aluminum:

☐ Some antacids contain 200 times more aluminum than we would normally take in in one day. Watch out for these.

☐ Washing down buffered aspirin with orange juice isn't a good idea. The mixture gives you a substance called aluminum citrate. This form of aluminum is absorbed by your body at five times the rate of normal aluminum.

☐ You may want to avoid aerosol antiperspirants. The aluminum in aerosol form may be more readily absorbed into the brain through the nose.

Other, smaller sources of aluminum:

☐ Canned, noncola soft drinks contain almost six times the aluminum as bottled, noncola soft drinks. Canned cola drinks contain three times the aluminum of bottled cola drinks. Canned beer doesn't have a high aluminum content.

☐ Aluminum pots and pans can leach a good deal of aluminum into acidic foods. When boiling water or baking fish or a cake, little aluminum travels from the pan to the food. Acidic foods such as rhubarb and black currants take in a lot more aluminum from the cookware.

☐ Some public water sources contain more than the recommended amount of aluminum. The World Health Organization and the European Economic Community recommend a maximum aluminum concentration of 7.4 mcM/L in drinking water. You can take care of this aluminum source by drinking pure well or bottled spring water.

☐ Small amounts of aluminum can be found in scores of other products: cosmetics, paper products, foil and prepackaged foods, to name a few. You may lose your mind more quickly by trying to avoid all these products than by ingesting the aluminum they contain.

Medical Sources ─────────────────────

Taber's Cyclopedic Medical Dictionary (Philadelphia, F.A. Davis Co., 1989)
Canadian Journal of Public Health (83,2:97)
The Johns Hopkins Medical Letter (5,1:8)
University of California at Berkeley Wellness Letter (9,7:1)
Medical Tribune (33,22:6 and 33,14,17)
Food Safety Notebook (3,12:111)
Medical World News (33,12:12)

Vitamins A and E and Alzheimer's

In one recent study, researchers found low levels of the "antioxidant vitamins" in Alzheimer's victims. Low levels of vitamins A and E may expose brain cells to damage by "free radicals."

Antioxidant vitamins absorb loose, oxygen-carrying free radicals before they can damage cells and tissues in the body.

Researchers aren't sure whether the low levels of vitamins A and E are a cause or an effect of Alzheimer's disease. Nevertheless, it certainly won't hurt to take a vitamin supplement or to make sure your diet provides these nutrients.

Good sources of vitamin A are egg yolks, spinach, liver, milk, carrots, squash, sweet potatoes and peaches. Vitamin E is found in vegetable oils, wheat germ, whole grains, nuts, margarine, soybeans and dark-green, leafy vegetables.

Medical Source ─────────────────────

Stay Healthy (6,7:27)

How to avoid falling accidents

The fear of falling is a familiar sensation for many elderly people, and for good reason. Nearly one-third of people over 60 fall every year.

One out of every 20 people who fall suffers serious injury. Some people don't even survive the extremely common hip injury.

Many elderly people who have experienced one fall will begin avoiding all risks of falling again, so they become stationary and immobile — a condition that can sap your strength and will to live. Many accidents can be avoided by making a few simple changes in daily routines:

❑ Install better lighting systems in your house. Often people fall over books, shoes and articles of clothing because they didn't see them on the floor in a dark room or hallway.

❑ Tape down all loose throw rugs or area rugs with double-sided tape. The loose edges often stick up just enough to catch a toe. Make sure the rugs don't slide around on the floor.

❑ Install handrails on staircases in your house. (And remember to make sure the stairs are properly lighted.)

❑ Make regular visits to the eye doctor. Make sure your prescription glasses are the correct strength. You don't want to fall over objects or uneven pavement because you can't see.

❑ Many older people fall simply because they don't get enough exercise and they lack muscle strength and coordination. Exercise and balance training can help you reduce your chances of falling by as much as 50 percent.

Even when elderly people who exercise do fall, the stronger muscles and quicker reflexes prevent the fall from causing as much damage as it would normally.

Before beginning an exercise program, get a full checkup and physical exam from your doctor. He can help you choose an exercise program that's right for you. For example, a person with asthma or other lung problems might need to exercise indoors instead of outside with dust and pollen in the air.

❑ Walking is an excellent exercise because it strengthens your calf and ankle muscles, which are particularly important in maintaining balance and avoiding falls. Begin slowly, walking for just a few minutes at a time at first. Many doctors encourage older people to eventually walk up to six miles a week — two miles on three different days.

☐ Weight-stack machines at the local gym or YMCA help strengthen the thighs, buttocks, stomach, lower back and arm muscles. Increased tone in arm muscles helps quicken coordination and helps you catch yourself (with railings, tabletops, etc.) when you lose your balance.

☐ A simple, at-home exercise for people who can't get out of the house will help develop strength and tone in the lower legs:

➤ Place a book on the floor next to a tabletop or railing you can hold onto for balance.

➤ Then stand on the edge of the book, lower your heels to the floor, and then raise your heels as high as you can.

➤ Do 10 "leg-lifts" at a time, and then rest. Build up to three sets of 10 at least three days each week.

➤ After building up to that point, try holding a book or a half-gallon of milk to add a little extra weight and improve muscle strength.

☐ Be sure to warm up and cool down slowly when you exercise. Simple stretches will help warm up your muscles and prevent cramps while you exercise. Taking a few minutes to stretch and cool down after the exercise routine will help avoid sore muscles and stiff joints that could increase your risk of falling.

☐ Make sure you wear the proper shoes. You can trip over the toes of shoes that are too big. Shoes that are too tight can decrease blood flow and feeling in the feet and increase the likelihood of falls. Also wear good socks to help avoid rubbing hard-to-heal blisters on your feet.

☐ If you exercise outside, you should make an appointment with your family doctor to get your hearing checked. Many people are involved in accidents because they didn't hear someone come up behind them on a bike, or they didn't hear a dog barking, etc.

Reducing the risk factors for falling will help you enjoy a more active and happy day-to-day routine and avoid the agony of broken bones.

Medical Source ───────────────────────

The Physician and Sportsmedicine (20,11:147)
Medical Tribune (33,24:2)

Incontinence: Beat the bladder blues

Over 12 million older Americans find that uncontrolled urine loss really puts a damper on their social activities.

The pelvic muscles that control urine flow do weaken with age, but incontinence is usually a symptom of some underlying medical problem.

Two-thirds of all the people who suffer from incontinence are women. The more babies a women has delivered naturally the more likely she is to be incontinent, especially when exercising, coughing, sneezing or laughing.

Low estrogen levels after menopause are a common cause of incontinence in women, and an enlarged prostate is the most common cause of incontinence in men.

Some medicines that may produce temporary urinary incontinence include:

> ➤ Muscle relaxants
> ➤ Diuretics, including alcohol and caffeine
> ➤ Hallucinogens, sedatives, sleeping pills, tranquilizers, hypnotics
> ➤ Alpha-blockers
> ➤ Sympatholytics
> ➤ Narcotic painkillers, such as codeine and morphine
> ➤ Alpha-agonists
> ➤ Anticholinergics
> ➤ Calcium channel blockers
> ➤ Beta blockers

There are several different types of persistent incontinence. You can just lose urine during physical activities (stress incontinence), or you can get an intense desire to urinate and not be able to hold it long enough to reach the toilet (urge incontinence).

Arthritis, bladder infections, stroke or fecal impactions (a large mass of hard feces that cannot be evacuated from the rectum) can make you unaware that you need to urinate. This is called functional or behavioral incontinence, and it can cause you to lose large amounts of urine at once.

An enlarged prostate gland, an injury or a nerve or muscle disorder can cause dribbling, an almost continual loss of urine (overflow incontinence).

One effective method that teaches you to be continent is gradually increasing the amount of time between bathroom trips, called bladder training.

Scientists recently studied the effects of bladder training on 123 women over the age of 55 who suffered from urinary incontinence.

Each volunteer determined their maximum dry period (how long they could go without urine leakage), and they urinated just inside that period of time.

For example, if a woman's maximum dry period was 60 minutes, she urinated after 50 minutes. The volunteers used wristwatches with alarms set to tell them when to urinate.

After doing that for a week, they added 30 minutes to their time periods. If someone had been going to the bathroom every hour, then they had to start going every hour and a half instead.

The interval was increased by 30 minutes every week until everyone had a two- to three-hour period of dryness in between planned trips to the bathroom.

At the end of the six-week training period, 12 percent of the women in the study were cured from their urinary incontinence. And 75 percent of them experienced at least a 50-percent improvement in their symptoms.

Talk to your doctor about beginning a bladder control training program. Many researchers consider it the treatment of choice for incontinence.

Medical Sources ————————————————

Emergency Medicine (24,14:26)
U.S. Pharmacist (18,4:65)

Tips for taking control of bladder problems

- ☐ Avoid alcohol and caffeine. These are diuretics, drugs which help remove excess water from the body by increasing the amount lost in the urine. They cause you to need more frequent bathroom breaks.
- ☐ Check with your doctor or pharmacist before starting new over-the-counter medications. Cold remedies that contain antihistamines can cause men with enlarged prostates to retain urine.
- ☐ Limit use of sedatives and tranquilizers.
- ☐ Lose excess weight.
- ☐ Stop smoking. The prolonged and violent coughing of many smokers weakens the pelvic muscles responsible for bladder control.
- ☐ Take advantage of support measures, such as protective undergarments, adult diapers and bedside commodes. Many people do not use these items because of embarrassment or cost. However, the price of such products is decreasing.
- ☐ Improve access to the bathroom. Install adequate lighting to, from and in the bathroom. Secure rugs and electrical cords. Install grab bars. Adjust the height of the toilet seat.
- ☐ Contact organizations dealing with incontinence.

Help for Incontinent People Inc. at 1-800-Bladder publishes a newsletter, *The HIP Report*, every three months, which contains articles by doctors, nurses and other members on treating incontinence. The publication advertises the most recent products for dealing with incontinence and includes discount coupons.

The Simon Foundation at 1-800-23SIMON offers help and education to people with incontinence. They can provide referrals to a nationwide network of health care professionals and to "I WILL Manage" support groups. They offer a free information packet and a copy of the *Informer*, their quarterly newsletter.

The Agency for Health Care Policy and Research at 1-800-358-9295 provides information on urinary incontinence in adults.

See your doctor if you suffer from incontinence. Untreated incontinence can cause unnecessary social isolation, depression, anxiety and skin problems. For the elderly, it may mean entering a nursing home before you really need to.

If self-help measures provide no relief, medicines are available which improve storage and emptying of the bladder. You may decide to periodically drain your bladder with a catheter or to have surgery.

Take control. You don't have to let incontinence limit your lifestyle.

Medical Sources ———————————————————
Postgraduate Medicine (93,2:083)
The Johns Hopkins Medical Letter (5,3:8)
Medical Abstracts Newsletter (13,2:4)

Pelvic exercises improve bladder control

If you're stressed by incontinence after menopause, Kegel pelvic exercises may provide relief.

These exercises are especially beneficial for women with mild or moderate stress incontinence, such as occurs with severe coughing or strenuous activities. But no matter how severe your incontinence, give Kegel exercises a try before turning to treatments that require extensive recovery time, such as surgery.

Kegel exercises are designed to strengthen the muscles and ligaments at the bottom of the stomach, which form the pelvic floor. They support the uterus, vagina, bladder, urethra and rectum and control urine flow. These muscles and ligaments commonly stretch and weaken with childbirth and age.

1) First, identify the pelvic muscles that need exercising. You can do this by stopping and starting the flow of urine several times when using the bathroom. Or place a finger just inside the opening of the vagina and then squeeze the finger by contracting the muscles surrounding it.

2) Contract the muscles slowly, hold for a count of 10 and relax the muscles slowly. Imagine the contraction of these muscles as an

elevator rising to the top of a building. Tighten and release the muscles slowly, one floor at a time.

3) Repeat these exercises for the anal pelvic muscles. To find these muscles, imagine you're trying to hold back a bowel movement, without tensing your leg, stomach or buttock muscles.

4) Then practice tightening all pelvic muscles together, moving from back to front.

Practice tightening your pelvic muscles four times each day. These exercises are easy to perform when you're sitting, standing, walking, driving, watching TV, listening to music or cooking. Start by repeating each exercise five times. Gradually work up to 20 or 30 repetitions.

Your doctor may be able to offer some suggestions that would increase the effectiveness of your pelvic exercises or get you enrolled in a class that gives detailed instructions on how to perform Kegel exercises for maximum benefit.

You might also want to try vaginal weights, which are inserted like tampons. You attempt to keep the weights in place by squeezing your pelvic muscles together for 15 to 30 minutes. Repeat the exercise twice a day. Ask your doctor for more information about vaginal weights.

Whatever method of exercising your pelvic muscles you choose, continue your workout for three to six months.

Medical Source _____
Obstetrics and Gynecology (81,2:283)

Bladder control up in smoke

Smoking can totally blow bladder control. Women smokers more than double their risk of developing urinary incontinence compared with women who've never smoked.

The risk of incontinence increases with the number of packs smoked per day and the number of years smoked. Smoking may also worsen existing incontinence.

The frequent and violent coughing typically associated with smoking may damage the nerves and muscles which control urine flow and prevent urine from escaping involuntarily. Some of this damage may be irreversible since women who have quit smoking also have an increased risk of incontinence.

The compounds that make up tobacco smoke may also affect proper bladder functioning. Smoking decreases estrogen levels, which can contribute to deterioration of urethral muscles.

However, if you do stop smoking, your estrogen levels won't drop as quickly and coughing won't continue to stress or damage pelvic or urethral muscles.

If you have surgery to correct your bladder problems yet continue to smoke, your urinary incontinence will probably recur.

Medical Source ————————————————————
American Journal of Obstetrics and Gynecology (167,5:1213)

Healthy eating puts sparkle in golden years

"Growing old gracefully" has become one of the most popular goals in the nation today. With the current life expectancy of 75 years (compared to 47 years at the turn of the century), people are living longer and wanting more out of life.

People over age 65 are no longer quietly waiting to die. They are pursuing hobbies, traveling with friends and family and even starting new careers.

The 65-and-over age group now makes up a huge 12 percent of the U.S. population, and experts expect the number to double to almost 65 million people over the next 40 years.

All of these facts lead to one message: Older people must make sure they are getting all the proper vitamins, minerals and nutrients they need to ensure the best quality of life for as long as possible.

A healthy diet can help you maintain a healthy mind and a high level of activity, plus reduce your risk of coronary heart disease, high blood pressure, cancer and diabetes.

As you age, it becomes increasingly important that you focus on "prevention" instead of "cure." Boosting your immune system and preventing diseases through good eating habits ensures good health with minimal effort instead of fighting out of the sick bed.

Unfortunately, some nutritional surveys indicate that many older people are malnourished and suffer from nutrient deficiencies. Older people do tend to eat fewer high-fat foods than younger people. They also eat less fast food and drink fewer soft drinks than their children and grandchildren.

But many older people haven't increased their intake of fruits, vegetables, high-fiber breads and cereals. These foods will help you fight something as serious as colon cancer and something as annoying as constipation.

Your nutritional needs change when you get older and your diet must change to meet those needs. You're probably less active than when you were younger, so you may eat less food because you're not hungry.

You may have slowly and unconsciously adopted a poorly balanced, nutrient-deficient diet that is having dangerous effects on your immune system and your organs.

Listed below is a chart of the Recommended Daily Allowances for essential vitamins and minerals for adults over age 50.

	Men	Women
Vitamin A (micrograms)	1,000	800
Vitamin D (micrograms)	5	5
Vitamin E (milligrams)	10	8
Vitamin K (micrograms)	80	65
Vitamin C (milligrams)	60	60
Thiamin (milligrams)	1.2	1.0
Riboflavin (milligrams)	1.4	1.2
Niacin (milligrams)	15	13
Vitamin B-6 (milligrams)	2.0	1.6
Folate (micrograms)	200	180
Vitamin B-12 (micrograms)	2.0	2.0
Calcium (milligrams)	800	800
Phosphorus (milligrams)	800	800
Magnesium (milligrams)	350	280
Iron (milligrams)	10	10
Zinc (milligrams)	15	12
Iodine (micrograms)	150	150
Selenium (micrograms)	70	55

Remember that RDA values for vitamin and minerals are intended as a general guideline. Some people may have additional requirements. Check with your doctor.

If your doctor tells you that you need a vitamin/mineral supplement, pick one that contains a broad spectrum of vitamins and minerals (at least 11 or 12) in doses of 100 to 200 percent of the RDA. Two good over-the-counter supplements that meet these standards are Centrum and One-a-Day Maximum Formula.

Many supplements contain healthy amounts of most vitamins and minerals except for calcium and magnesium. You may decide you need an extra calcium and magnesium supplement after reading the label on your multivitamin bottle.

Here are some good guidelines for creating a well-balanced diet that meets an older adult's needs:

- ❏ Eat at least four servings of grain products every day. (One serving is equal to one slice of bread, one ounce of cereal or 1/2 cup of rice or pasta — the "serving" sizes are pretty small.)
  Choose grain products that are also good sources of fiber, such as brown rice, whole-grain pasta, and whole-grain breads and cereals. If the cereal box says it contains less than six grams of fiber per ounce, buy some unprocessed bran to sprinkle on top.
- ❏ Eat six to seven servings of fruits and vegetables per day. (One serving is equal to one medium apple or banana, 1/2 cup of canned fruit, 1/2 cup of cooked vegetables or one cup of raw vegetables.) If possible, choose a variety of fruits and vegetables (at least seven different kinds each week, including dried fruits). Try to eat the peel or skin of vegetables (like potatoes) as often as possible: It's a good source of fiber.
- ❏ Drink three to four cups of low-fat milk every day. People who don't like milk should eat the same amount of yogurt each day. If you have lactose intolerance or other problems digesting dairy products, take calcium supplements or medication like Lactaid to make the digestion easier.

❑ Eat three to six ounces of fish, poultry and lean red meat each day. To minimize the amount of fat, remove skin from poultry, trim visible fat from all meats and avoid frying.

Basic daily menu for older adults

Breakfast

➤ High-fiber cereal, low-fat milk and fresh fruit (or juice and dried fruit)

Light lunch

➤ Vegetable or bean soup with whole-grain crackers or a bran muffin, fruit and low-fat milk or nonfat yogurt

➤ Pasta salad or potato salad with vegetables, fruit and low-fat milk or nonfat yogurt

➤ Sandwich on whole-wheat bread (chicken, turkey, tuna, salmon or low-fat cheese sandwich) with raw vegetables, fruit and low-fat milk or nonfat yogurt

➤ Fruit salad with cottage cheese and bran muffin or whole-wheat bread

Snacks

➤ Bran muffin
➤ Whole-grain crackers
➤ Graham crackers
➤ Oatmeal cookies with raisins
➤ Low-fat cheese
➤ Fig bars
➤ Nonfat yogurt
➤ Fresh or dried fruit
➤ Raw vegetables with low-fat salad dressing

Dinner

➤ 3 to 6 ounces of fish (2 to 3 times per week), low-fat poultry (2 to 3 times per week) or lean red meat (1 to 2 times per week), or non-meat meal, such as beans and rice (1 to 2 times per week); two or three servings of vegetables, and bran muffin or whole-wheat bread.

Older adults who have a regular exercise program will burn more calories and energy than the average, low-activity person. Exercisers will need to take in more food each day.

Most long-term diseases of aging can be prevented or delayed by good nutritional health. If you adopt healthy eating habits, growing old gracefully won't have to be a conscious effort — it will just happen naturally.

Medical Sources —————————————————
> *Geriatrics* (47,10:56)
> *Nutrition Today* (27,5:15)
> *FDA Consumer* (26,6:3)
> *Medical Tribune* (33,23:10)
> *The American Journal of Clinical Nutrition* (55,4:823)
> *Recommended Dietary Allowances, 10th Edition* (National Academy Press, Washington D.C., 1989)

High-protein diet puts bedsores to rest

A soft, cozy bed can turn into a torture chamber if you are stuck in it for a week or more. Your body begins to ache at all the points that "comfortable" mattress touches.

If you stay there long enough, the pressure will cut off your blood supply, your tissues will start to die and you will develop bedsores, or pressure ulcers.

Bedsores may at first be only red, flaky patches of skin, but a small area can quickly grow very deep as the tissues and muscles under the patch of skin die away.

You can help heal and prevent the painful and potentially dangerous bedsores simply by eating a diet high in protein. Many people who are bedridden lose their appetite and their interest in healthy foods. They become malnourished, and this leaves them at a high risk for developing bedsores.

In one study, nursing home residents with bedsores drank or were tube-fed an eight-ounce can of high-protein liquid supplement along with their regular meals. Their bedsores got much better.

The people who were able to eat the most protein and take in the most calories healed the best. Even though they took in extra calories, they gained very little weight.

People with pressure ulcers probably need more protein and calories than other bedridden people because nutrients actually drain out of the oozing ulcers. You also need more protein and calories if you have a fever or infection, which often accompany bedsores.

Eating more protein may make a bedridden person feel so much better that he's able to do gentle exercises or walk slowly. Any movement will help relieve pressure and do wonders for healing and preventing bedsores.

Battling bedsores

- ❏ Turn a bedridden person from side to side every two hours. Place him at 30-degree angles rather than completely on his side.
- ❏ Provide plenty of nourishment, especially foods containing iron and protein.
- ❏ Try not to pull a sick person across bed sheets or upholstery. The friction will lead to bedsores.
- ❏ Good skin care is important, but avoid harsh soaps and alcohol-based products.
- ❏ Keep incontinence problems under control. Wet skin breaks down easily.
- ❏ Some helpful devices are chair cushions made of foam, air, water or gel, heel protectors, splints and a 4-inch egg-crate mattress pad.
- ❏ Avoid the reclining-sitting position. Sliding down in bed will aggravate the skin. A padded footboard also helps prevent sliding.
- ❏ Antibiotic ointments will help stop infection in raw, draining bedsores. Deep pressure ulcers will need the care of a doctor or nurse.
- ❏ If possible, walk slowly or do gentle exercises to keep pressure from building up and creating bedsores.

Medical Sources ————————————————
Journal of the American Geriatrics Society (41,4:357)
American Family Physician (47,5:1207)

How to help someone else get a good night's sleep

Nursing home nurses seem to have missed the message about caffeine and insomnia.

If you know someone living in a nursing home who can't get to sleep at night, you may need to talk to the nurse.

In an attempt to be helpful, some nurses seem to be encouraging residents who are sleepy during the day to drink caffeine to stay alert and attentive.

The problem is, the residents are sleepy during the day because they can't get to sleep at night. The caffeine in coffee and tea only adds to the cycle of insomnia and daytime sleepiness.

In one study, the nursing home residents who slept poorly had, on average, more than twice as much caffeine in their blood in the evening than the ones who slept well. The many nursing home residents who take sleeping pills had even higher average levels of caffeine in their bodies at night.

If you have a relative in a nursing home, keep an eye on her diet, especially on how much coffee, tea and cola she drinks. You may hold the answer to someone else's sleepy days and sleepless nights.

Medical Source ─────────────────────
Age and Aging (22,1:41)

Understanding the mind/body connection

Depression
Chronic fatigue
  syndrome
Stress
Sleeping problems
Eating disorders

DEPRESSION

Depression — symptoms and risk factors

Are you depressed and you don't know why? More people are depressed these days than ever. The risk of depression seems to rise with each generation.

Possible causes could be the higher divorce rate, increased drug and alcohol abuse and increasing numbers of people living in cities.

About 11 million Americans suffer from depression each year — even children are affected. Research indicates that depression can occur in preadolescents and is common in teens.

Depressed people might experience some of the following symptoms:

> ➤ Sad or irritable mood
> ➤ Feelings of worthlessness, self-reproach, hopelessness or excessive guilt
> ➤ Difficulty thinking or concentrating
> ➤ Fatigue and loss of energy
> ➤ Loss of interest or pleasure in usual activities, including sex
> ➤ Changes in appetite, weight and sleep
> ➤ Constantly fidgeting, feeling restless or moving slowly and lethargically
> ➤ Suicidal thinking or attempts

If these symptoms are present but do not interfere with your daily activities, you may be mildly to moderately depressed.

Depression is caused by chemical changes that take place in the body. These changes can be triggered by a variety of causes including heredity, social and psychological factors and biologic factors, such as physical illness, hormonal imbalance and medication.

Identifying the cause of your depression will help you in treating it.

Below are some risk factors for depression:

- ☐ **Heredity** — If your family has a history of depression, you may be more likely to develop it yourself.
- ☐ **Light deficiency** — If your depression is worse in fall and winter, you may be suffering from Seasonal Affective Disorder (SAD) syndrome. Ask your doctor about light therapy.
- ☐ **Illness** — Any illness that causes a chemical change in your body, such as a stroke, can lead to depression.
- ☐ **Drugs** — Over-the-counter and prescription medications, as well as some illegal drugs such as cocaine and LSD, can cause depression. Sometimes a combination of medicines can cause depression. Symptoms include tiredness, problems waking up in the morning, early-morning waking or insomnia.
- ☐ **Advancing age** — Sometimes retirement, illness, pain or decreased mobility that may accompany aging can contribute to the development of depression.
- ☐ **Stressful events** — Death of a loved one, job loss or change in a close relationship can bring on depression.
- ☐ **Thought patterns** — Although depression is a physical illness, changing your thought patterns can help. Stressful events or other causes may trigger a bout of depression, but the meaning and importance you give stressful events determines whether or not you'll come out of the depression quickly.

When you are depressed, negative thought patterns tend to keep you from coping effectively with problems. If you have any of the following thought patterns, get rid of them immediately:

- ☐ You must be loved or approved of by everyone.
- ☐ You must be competent in every respect to be worthwhile.
- ☐ People must be severely blamed or punished when they are bad.
- ☐ Life is terrible when things are not the way you want them to be.
- ☐ People have no control over their own happiness.
- ☐ You should worry constantly about possibly dangerous situations occurring.

☐ Avoiding difficulties and responsibilities is easier than facing them.

☐ You should depend on others and rely on someone stronger than yourself.

☐ Your past history determines your present and future life.

☐ You should get upset over other people's problems.

☐ There is a perfect solution to every problem and you must always find it.

☐ You should never have pain or discomfort.

☐ The world is always good and fair.

Try these tips for beating depression:

☐ Learn about depression. Your family doctor can recommend self-help books on depression and answer any questions you have. Educate your family so they can provide support.

☐ Keep a journal about how you feel. Ask a close friend or relative to observe and comment on negative thought patterns or beliefs you seem to have. Note the progress you make.

☐ Think about family problems or other upsetting situations that may be contributing to your depression. If you've recently lost a loved one or you've undergone upheavals in your personal life, talking your feelings over with a friend or family member can be helpful.

☐ Get regular exercise. If you haven't exercised in a long time, start slowly. If you have trouble motivating yourself and following a regular schedule, exercise with a friend or join an exercise group.

☐ Do at least one thing you like to do every day whether you feel like it or not.

☐ Don't isolate yourself. If certain people make you feel worse, limit contact. You may want to determine what depresses you about that person. Building close relationships helps protect against future depression. Close friends and family can make coping with stressful life events easier. You may want to try volunteer work or simply go someplace where other people congregate, such as a library, mall or museum.

Consider joining a local support group. The National Foundation for Depressive Illness may be able to provide you with details about free support groups in your area. Call 1-800-248-4344 for information. Support groups such as Adult Children of Alcoholics or Overeaters Anonymous may help you cope with other problems that can contribute to your depression.

☐ Set practical goals for feeling better. If a job seems too large to accomplish, break it down into a series of smaller tasks. Make a list of daily duties to complete, such as cleaning the house or yard. Note in your journal the progress you make.

The amount of work you do may seem trivial compared to the work you did before you became depressed. However, it's important to remember that reversing depression consists of a number of small, seemingly unimportant steps before life seems to improve.

☐ Reward your progress with something special, like a new book or trip.

☐ Don't increase your consumption of nicotine or caffeine to make yourself more energetic. These stimulants only increase anxiety and contribute to a feeling of being out of control. Alcohol and sedatives also worsen depression.

☐ Be patient and go easy on yourself.

If these techniques do not improve your depression, see a doctor for counseling or medication. Doctors regard depression as much a medical illness as an ulcer or high blood pressure. And you may find comfort in knowing that 80 percent of all the people treated for depression improve.

Medical Sources ————————————————

Medical Tribune (34,1:14)
FDA Consumer (27,2:18)
Archives of Family Medicine (2,1:76)
American Family Physician (47,2:435)

For seniors only: coping with stress and depression

If you are suffering loss of memory and concentration, the cause of the confusion just might be stress or depression.

You can control stress and avoid depression by following these tips:

☐ Give yourself permission to admit when you are sad or worried. Older people often suffer losses that are upsetting.

☐ Establish a buddy system with a friend. Regular contact can foster friendship and boost your spirits. Living alone, giving up a job, losing a loved one or worrying about money can cause depression.

☐ Practice an exercise routine. The more a person rests, the less energy he has. Mall walking with others can be an easy, companionable way to get fit.

☐ Eat a sensible diet. Medical authorities stress seniors' need for fruits, fruit juices, vegetables, whole grains and milk products. Try freezing one-person portions of meat, poultry and fish in aluminum foil for ease in cooking and clean up.

☐ Enjoy companionship with your meals. Join a lunch club or other organized program. Share a meal with a neighbor. Listen to the radio or read a newspaper while you eat.

☐ Get regular checkups. Illnesses like diabetes or thyroid disorders, anemia, arthritis, ulcers or cardiovascular disease can make you feel bad.

☐ Ask your doctor if depression could be a side effect of a drug you are taking. A normal dose of medicine for a younger adult might actually be toxic for an older person.

☐ Practice relaxation. Learn to meditate or use music to help you relax.

☐ Find a new challenge. Change your routine by starting a new hobby, volunteering for community work or enrolling in a class.

☐ Seek out humor. Laughing exercises your cardiovascular system and makes you feel better.

☐ Treat yourself to something special. Whether your treat is eating a favorite food or using the fancy china, be good to yourself.

Medical Sources ——————————————————
Senior Patient (1,4:30 and 2,7:31)
Postgraduate Medicine (91,1:255)
Tufts University Diet and Nutrition Letter (7,2:7)

Light therapy helps sufferers of winter depression

Are you feeling sad? Craving starchy foods and sweets? Gaining weight and having a hard time getting up in the morning? You may be suffering from winter depression, also known as SAD (seasonal affective disorder).

Symptoms seem to appear late in November and disappear by the following April. Some of the symptoms include daytime drowsiness, fatigue and diminished concentration. SAD affects four times as many women as men.

Studies done over the years have found a treatment to help make the "blues" disappear. The treatment involves exposure to bright lights every morning or evening for a week or two during the winter. Morning exposure seems to produce the greatest relief.

The traditional light treatment requires you to sit in front of a large light box for several hours each day. However, a more convenient form of light therapy may be just as effective.

The new treatment, called simulated dawn, works while you sleep. A low-intensity light, gradually increasing in brightness from 4 a.m. to 6 a.m. to resemble dawn, seems to improve symptoms of SAD.

In two studies, 23 SAD-affected people spent a week in their bedrooms using a special light bulb that produced a gradual light similar to dawn.

The treatment of 18 other affected people consisted of 30-minute dawns peaking at a light level similar to moonlight, or two-hour dawns using light only slightly stronger than moonlight. Symptoms of depression greatly improved in those receiving the light simulating a natural dawn.

Apparently, some SAD sufferers have a delayed secretion of melatonin at night, a hormone that helps regulate sleep. Low-intensity lights simulating dawn might prompt melatonin secretion an hour or two earlier.

The eye's sensitivity to light may be a factor in winter depression. The retinas of people with SAD seem to have difficulty getting more light out of shorter days in winter.

People with SAD seem to spend less time outside than those who are not affected. SAD sufferers should take a walk every day for about an hour in the winter sunlight.

If you think winter depression is getting you down, talk to your doctor about simulated dawn therapy.

Medical Sources ─────────────────────

Science News (142,4:62)
Medical Tribune (33,12:2)

CHRONIC FATIGUE SYNDROME

How to cope with Chronic Fatigue Syndrome

Have you been totally well and active — then suddenly were hit by an acute infection and have since been sidelined with prolonged fatigue?

Chronic Fatigue Syndrome (CFS) is characterized by debilitating fatigue, headaches, sore throat, low-grade fever, weakness, muscle and joint pains, lymph node pains, gastrointestinal trouble, memory loss and difficulty in concentrating—basically, an overall impairment in your immune system. All of these symptoms must last for at least six months to be regarded as CFS.

Experts suspect that abnormal sleep patterns may be an important cause of CFS because many of the symptoms can be imitated in healthy people by disrupting their sleep.

While there is no cure yet, you may want to try some of these techniques to help reduce stress and anxiety:

- ☐ Avoid caffeine, tobacco and salt.
- ☐ Don't eat right before going to bed.
- ☐ Try to manage your time better so that you don't feel rushed all the time.
- ☐ Learn to relax. Sit down and let all of your muscles go limp. Take long, slow, deep breaths.
- ☐ Try keeping a "fatigue diary" of all your daily activities, including level of fatigue and the possible causes of your fatigue.
- ☐ Learn how to deal with stress by meditating, praying, talking to a friend or therapist, donating your time and energy to others or learning a new skill.
- ☐ Think of something that gives you a lift, rediscover an old friend, forgive yourself, go to the zoo or go for a walk.
- ☐ Ask your doctor if medications you are taking, such as antidepres-

sants, antihistamines and blood pressure drugs, could be causing your fatigue. Taking a pain reliever occasionally can help with the aches and pains that may make you feel tired.

☐ Buy all your prescriptions from the same place, so your pharmacist can watch out for fatigue-causing interactions between drugs.

☐ Eat properly — lots of carbohydrates and very little fat.

☐ Exercise regularly. You'll have more energy.

For more information and support, you can write to the National CFS Association at NCFSA, 3521 Broadway, Suite 222, Kansas City, MO 64111.

Medical Sources ────────────────────

Emergency Medicine (25,1:77)
Postgraduate Medicine (91,4:069)
Medical Update (16,9:2)
British Medical Journal (306,6886:1161)

Stress

Is stress harming your health?

Do you stress yourself out during the workweek — juggle several projects at once, swing through emotional highs and lows as you argue with a co-worker one minute then impress your boss the next, and come home so tired that you fight with your spouse over who should take the trash out?

You think you can handle the stress because you sleep in and chill out on the weekends. You need to think again.

The effect of long-term stress on your body is like running an engine in high gear on a nonstop trip from Virginia to California. Your hormones, blood pressure, heart rate and nerves are constantly changing to meet the mental and physical challenges you face every day.

Stressors such as exertion, trauma, infection, fear, anxiety, social defeat, humiliation, disappointment and even intense joy send your hormone levels soaring and put your nerves on edge.

Your body tries to counterbalance the systems working overtime in response to stress by kicking the other systems into high gear.

Have you ever noticed that you tend to come down with a cold or an infection not during a busy workweek, but on the following weekend? Your body works like a seesaw:

When stress weighs down one end of the board, your body tries to stay balanced by weighing down the other end. On the weekend, one of those weights is suddenly lifted, and your body goes crazy trying to get back in balance again.

Even ulcers and upset stomachs develop most quickly while you're resting and recovering after periods of prolonged stress.

So don't count on that relaxed weekend to rejuvenate your stressed-out body.

When your nerves and hormones are constantly elevated in response to stress, you are at increased risk of many serious diseases, including:

> ➤ Cancer
> ➤ Heart disease
> ➤ Rheumatoid arthritis
> ➤ Asthma
> ➤ Diabetes
> ➤ Ulcers, inflammatory bowel disease and other stomach disorders
> ➤ Depression
> ➤ Obesity
> ➤ Psoriasis and other skin diseases
> ➤ Common cold, mononucleosis and other viral infections

Some diseases are connected to the hormone changes stress seems to cause. Imbalances in certain hormones increase the risk of heart disease by speeding along hardening of the arteries and changing how body fat is made and distributed.

Other diseases are directly connected to stress's effect on the nervous system. Asthma automatically gets worse when you get anxious or upset.

Since nerve cells and immune cells often act together (the immune cells tell the nerve cells when you need to have a fever, for example), stress can weaken the immune system when it puts your nerves on edge.

The immune system is the headquarters for white blood cells, which fight off all things foreign to your body — cancer cells, cold viruses, bacteria, etc. The so-called "stress hormones," adrenaline and cortisol, depress the immune system, too.

Stressful events can cause instant and long-lasting drops in your white blood cell count and in other useful antibodies. That might explain why researchers consistently find that people under stress will get sick when infected with a cold virus while nonstressed people can fight the cold off.

Nerve cells can also give off substances that keep immune cells from doing their job of fighting diseases, as in the case of the red, itchy skin disease — psoriasis. A weakened immune system is only one explanation of why stress increases your risk of cancer. Stress causes the same changes in the genes of rats that known cancer-causing agents cause.

If you have a history of workplace problems over the past 10 years, you have 5.5 times the colorectal-cancer risk of someone with little on-the-job aggravation.

You simply don't have the option of skipping work when you're feeling stressed, so what can you do to bolster your body against disease? Try the following tips to help relieve stress:

☐ Take care of your body and you'll take life in stride. Exercise, a proper diet and adequate rest can make all the difference in your ability to handle stress. A balanced diet of vegetables, fruits, grains, dairy products and small amounts of meat will keep your immune system strong. Avoid caffeine because it is a stimulant and can worsen anxiety.

Exercise will relax you, help you rest better and help you feel good about yourself. However, high-intensity exercise on the level of a marathon runner can cause your body to put out too much of the stress hormones and depress your immune system. Too little exercise is a more common problem than too much.

☐ Be nice. Bolster your immune system and your marriage. A stressful argument with your spouse can instantly cause a drop in your white blood cell count and make you more susceptible to disease. Reduce your stress by discussing issues with your spouse calmly.

☐ Resist the call of alcohol. The numbing effect of alcohol may seem to decrease stress in the short term, but the social stigma of drinking, your own feelings of worry and guilt, and the harm it does to your body will actually increase your stress over the long haul.

☐ Get some of that old-time religion. Religion is a wonderful stress reliever because God and your church give you social networks and personal support to help you cope. Religious people also tend to avoid self-destructive behaviors like drinking and drugs. But, you have to attend church regularly for it to help.

❏ Seek out humor. Laughter really is the best medicine. It releases "feel-good" chemicals in your brain and enhances blood flow. Laughter increases your heart rate, blood pressure and muscle tension. When you stop laughing, these levels temporarily drop below normal, leaving you feeling very relaxed.
Find movies, comedians and books that make you laugh, put cartoons on your refrigerator and office bulletin board, and don't take yourself so seriously all the time.

❏ Make your home and office smell nice with flowers, spices, perfumes or fragrant sprays. Pleasant smells may trigger brain chemicals that work against stress. Your nose quickly adapts to your own body fragrance, so simply wearing your favorite perfume won't help.

❏ Control your time so it doesn't control you. A day with too much or too little to do can make you stressed and anxious. Plan to help others a few times a week. Your own worries will look smaller when you get involved with others.

❏ Avoid disastrous thinking. If you describe situations as "awful," "horrifying" and "terrible," you may not be seeing things realistically. How you perceive a threat to your happiness or well-being will determine your body's response. Overstating threats will only create unnecessary stress.

❏ Focus on a relaxing scene. Imagine yourself lying on a beach and feel the sun making you warmer and warmer, melting your stress away.

If your stress isn't relieved by these techniques, talk with your doctor.

Medical Sources ————————————————
Science News (144,10:153 and 13:196)
The Atlanta Journal/Constitution (May 14, 1993, B6)
Archives of Internal Medicine (153,18:2093)
Medical World News (34,5:23)
American Family Physician (47,3:575)
Health & Healing (3,2:1)
UC Berkeley Wellness Letter (10,1:4)

Take five: 5-minute stress relievers

These exercises are perfect for relieving stress during a hectic day at the office. After a tense meeting with the company president, a run-in with a co-worker or a rush to meet a deadline, take five:

Stress reliever No. 1:

☐ Sit in a comfortable position and close your eyes (unless it makes you nervous to close your eyes at work).

☐ Point your toes back towards your face and tighten your shins. Hold for five to 10 seconds. Release and relax for 20 to 30 seconds.

☐ Point your toes downward and tighten your calves, thighs and buttocks. Hold for five to 10 seconds, then release and relax for 20 to 30 seconds.

☐ Take a deep breath, arch your back slightly and push your stomach out. Hold for five to 10 seconds, then relax for 20 to 30 seconds.

☐ Hunch your shoulders forward and up to your ears. Wrinkle your face up like an old, dried apple. Hold for five to 10 seconds, then relax.

After each step, note the difference between body tension and relaxation. You should feel your muscles relaxing in waves throughout your body.

Stress reliever No. 2:

☐ Raise your right arm out to your side and over your head while breathing in. Breathe out. Breathe in and stretch your right arm up to the ceiling. Breathe out.

☐ Repeat with left arm.

☐ Let your arms come down slowly while you breathe out. Continue to breathe deeply for about 20 seconds.

☐ Place your feet shoulder-width apart. Slowly let your head hang forward until your chin touches your chest.

☐ Start to curl forward and bend over very slowly. Breathe deeply. Let your arms dangle and hang down as far as you can comfortably. Don't strain or bounce. Sway gently from side to side.

☐ Now, on each inhale, raise back up a little. On each exhale, relax. In this way, slowly roll your body up until your spine and head are straight.

Your body should feel looser and more relaxed.

Medical Source ───────────────────────
Less Stress in 30 Days, New American Library, New York, 1986

The benefits of thinking positive

The flip side to all this bad news about stress and disease is that happiness, contentment and good social vibes can increase your resistance to disease. Take a look at these encouraging studies:

☐ People with cancer who are relaxed and optimistic about their chances of survival live longer than anxious people trying to cope with cancer on their own, say researchers at the University of California at Los Angeles.

Thirty-four people with a deadly skin cancer went through a six-week program of relaxation techniques, coping strategies and cancer education. Another group the same age, sex and with the same seriousness of cancer didn't receive counseling.

Ten of 34 people in the uncounseled group died within six years, but only three of the group that received counseling died.

☐ Your chances of surviving a heart attack are better if you have emotional support. In one study of heart attack victims, those with supporting companions and family members had better survival rates and less severe heart problems than people without support.

☐ A group of 110 people aged 60 to 70 gave their immune system a boost by living in a resort facility for 11 days and learning about exercise, diet, stress management and changing their lifestyle. Blood samples were taken before and after the program. The people who reported feeling less stress after the program had increased levels of the disease-fighting white blood cells in their bodies.

Medical Sources ───────────────────────
American Journal of Cardiology (71,4:263)
American Family Physician (47,5:1253)
The Atlanta Journal/Constitution (Sept. 22, 1993, B4)

Is laughter really the best medicine?

Laughter seems to help people keep positive attitudes in sometimes bleak surroundings. And it also helps keep your body healthy.

Laughter is more than simply jovial activity. It is a complex and coordinated arrangement of 15 separate facial muscles and is accompanied by changes in the normal breathing pattern.

Laughter causes an increase in pulse rate and breathing rate, which increases the amount of oxygen in the blood. The muscles involved in laughter undergo a light physical workout during the laughter, which helps to improve and maintain muscle tone.

And, during hearty, boisterous laughter, a larger group of muscles undergoes a stronger workout. This is especially helpful for bedridden patients who don't get much exercise otherwise.

Following bouts of laughter, the involved muscles begin to relax, helping to ease muscle tension that builds during the day and helping to break the spasm-pain cycle that is often seen in many nerve problems and in rheumatism.

People who suffer from lung problems like emphysema also benefit from laughter. Doctors refer to this laughter therapy as "humor respiration." The laughing, chuckling and chortling involved in humor respiration help to increase air exchange in the lungs, increase blood oxygen levels, and clear mucous plugs out of the airways. And the laughter just seems to make the patients feel better.

Laughter also causes an increase in heart rate and blood pressure, which serves to exercise the heart muscle and increase circulation of blood, oxygen and nutrients from the heart to the whole body.

Increased blood circulation helps promote the movement of important immune system elements throughout the body, helping the body to fight infection and illness.

Increased circulation also reduces the risk of blood clots forming in vessels and, therefore, reduces the risk of some types of heart attacks and strokes.

Although scientists are still conducting studies on the effects of laughter on the nervous system and the brain, they suspect that laughter has beneficial effects on mental functions such as alertness and memory.

As scientists learn more about the benefits of laughter and mirth, they hope to use it as a complement to the natural healing process and possibly add "laughter therapy" to many medical treatment routines. Feelings and attitudes have always seemed to play an important role in achieving and maintaining good health — scientists are just trying to figure out why.

Medical Source ───────────────────────

The Journal of the American Medical Association (267,13:1857)

Man's best friend — a natural remedy for stress?

Dogs might offer more than the morning newspaper and your evening slippers. Sometimes a dog can be nature's best remedy for stress or illness.

The presence of a dog can act as a "natural drug" for its owner by helping to lower blood pressure and other bodily responses to stress. The dogs seem to help reduce the effects of stress because they provide unconditional love and support without criticizing the owner's actions.

Researchers studied 96 people with heart disease released after care in a heart unit at a hospital. They found that the people who owned pets had a higher survival rate one year after release from the hospital than the people who did not have pets, even after accounting for individual differences in the extent of heart damage and other medical problems.

In fact, owning a pet seemed to be a better indicator of a successful recovery than the presence of a spouse or extensive family support.

In another study, 345 elderly pet owners reported fewer doctor visits over one year than did 593 elderly people without pets. Some study evidence indicates that touching, stroking and cuddling pets reduce a person's heart rate and blood pressure.

Scientists state, however, that these benefits probably do not extend to those people who are afraid of animals or are uncomfortable around animals.

But for those who enjoy the company of a pet, the faithful companions might help you enjoy a longer, more stress-free life.

Medical Source ───────────────────────

Science News (140,18:285)

SLEEPING PROBLEMS

Trouble sleeping? Try these natural sleep aids

A lack of sleep can definitely interfere with your daily performance. So what can you do when it's 3 a.m. and you're staring at the ceiling wishing you could fall asleep? And who are the people most likely to develop sleeping problems?

Although up to 40 percent of us complain of insomnia from time to time, the people most likely to have problems sleeping are women; older adults; and people with diabetes, hypertension, anxiety, depression or diseases that obstruct breathing.

If you have trouble sleeping, try these natural sleep aids:

- ☐ Establish a good sleep routine (set a regular bedtime and a regular wake-up time and stick to it every day), and keep a diary of your sleep habits.
- ☐ Limit the amount of salt you eat. Researchers studying sleep disturbances in athletes have reported a link between insomnia and eating too much salt.
- ☐ Don't watch television, read or work in bed.
- ☐ Complete your exercise routine at least three to four hours before bedtime to increase slow-wave sleep, the most restful phase of sleep.
  Research shows that men over sixty who exercise regularly fall asleep in half the time it takes nonexercisers to get to sleep. The exercisers also wake up less during the night and enjoy a longer period of restorative slow-wave sleep.
- ☐ Avoid cigarettes and alcohol within three to four hours of bedtime, and do not drink caffeine for six hours before you go to bed.
- ☐ Try using earplugs if you have a noisy sleeping partner.
- ☐ Make sure the temperature in your bedroom is comfortable and keep your curtains or blinds closed to keep your bedroom dark.

❏ Learn relaxation techniques or try massage and hot baths.
❏ Take a short nap during the day if you've lost sleep. It can help your performance without reducing your need to sleep at night.
❏ Talk to a friend, relative or neighbor if troubles are keeping you awake.

Most of us tend to be overstimulated and underrested, trying to cram too much into our daily lives. This daily stress, the foods we eat, and drugs and alcohol just before going to bed can have adverse effects on the quality of our sleep.

Some people suffer from delayed sleep phase syndrome, a more severe case of insomnia. People who are affected by this sleep disorder tend to be classified as night owls who prefer to sleep between the hours of 4 a.m. and noon.

Although this type of sleep pattern could be useful to someone working the night shift, it is very frustrating to anyone trying to live a normal life.

The solution, in this case, might be to gradually push forward your sleep time until it is more in tune with a normal work/sleep cycle. Once the proper bedtime has been set, it should be reinforced — stick to the sleeping and rising times every day.

If your insomnia persists for long periods of time, talk to your doctor.

Medical Sources ————————————————————
Archives of Internal Medicine (152,8:1634)
Postgraduate Medicine (92,2:157)
Medical Tribune (33,12:40)
The Physician and Sportsmedicine (10,9:75)
Geriatrics (47,10:65)
The Lancet (340,8824:884)

Get plenty of sleep to avoid a heart attack

It's not the kind of advice you hear from your doctor, but perhaps it should be.

Why? Because getting plenty of sleep seems to cut down on the kind of sleep that could trigger heart attacks. The kind of sleep that might be related to heart attacks is REM sleep, named for the Rapid Eye Movements that occur when you're dreaming. What do dreams and REM sleep have to do with heart attacks? you ask.

Well, scientists know several things that connect REM sleep to heart attacks. First, they know that when REM sleep occurs, the sympathetic nervous system is activated.

The sympathetic nervous system is the branch of the nervous system that controls involuntary bodily functions, such as breathing, blood pressure and heart rate.

Second, scientists have observed that most heart attacks occur in the morning, just after a person wakes up.

Third, they know that REM sleep occurs more frequently in the hours just before dawn, right about the time when many people suffer from heart attacks.

The surge of sympathetic discharge might be the trigger that causes the high incidence of heart attacks in the early morning hours.

So, shouldn't I avoid lots of sleep to lower my risk of heart attack during REM sleep? you ask.

Just the opposite.

People who spend less time in bed suffer from sleep deprivation, and people suffering from sleep deprivation often experience a rebound effect. In other words, your body tries to make up for lost time by going through unusually heavy periods of REM sleep.

Instead, sleep specialists recommend getting plenty of sleep. This can help cut down on long periods of heavy REM sleep and perhaps reduce your risk of a heart attack.

Medical Source ────────────────────────
Science News (143,6:85)

Sleep apnea — what it is and what to do

If your spouse falls asleep while you're talking to him, it's not necessarily because you're boring him or because he didn't get his eight hours of sleep last night.

His daytime sleepiness might, in fact, be part of a larger, potentially dangerous health problem.

The Greeks called it "apnea" or want of breath. Sleep apnea is a sleeping disorder that can place stress on your heart and possibly increase the risk of stroke and heart attack.

Sleep apnea is an ailment in which the sleeper actually stops breathing for 10 to 20 second intervals repeatedly throughout the night. After each breathless pause, the sleeper gasps for air, then repeats the cycle.

Although snoring and snorting during sleep are common symptoms of sleep apnea, not all snorers suffer from apnea.

A recent report estimates that while one in 10 adults snores, only one in 10 snorers has sleep apnea.

Additional symptoms of apnea include:

> daytime sleepiness
> headache, irritableness, forgetfulness upon awakening
> loss of interest in sex
> depression

Sleep apnea can be dangerous for your health because it puts "stop and go" stress on your blood vessels and heart every night.

But daytime sleepiness also makes you dangerous to yourself and those around you, since drivers with sleep apnea are up to five times more likely to fall asleep at the wheel.

The typical victim of sleep apnea is a middle-aged, overweight man. But women also develop this disorder, especially after menopause when hormones no longer offer protection from the changes of aging.

Most cases of sleep apnea result from obstructed airways. A less common form of apnea can also develop when the diaphragm and chest muscles fail to work properly.

This second form of apnea happens more among older, less healthy people. However, you can have a combination of the two problems causing sleep apnea.

Most researchers agree that any or all of these factors can play a role in sleep apnea:

> obesity (20 percent above ideal weight)
> hypothyroidism (deficient activity of the thyroid gland)
> jaw abnormalities
> longer than normal tongue or soft palate
> alcohol or tranquilizers
> antihistamines

If you have sleep apnea, any of these influences can temporarily cut off air flow through your breathing passages while you sleep. And when you've stopped breathing, you won't inhale again until the amount of oxygen in your blood gets so low that your brain gets a signal to jump start your breathing again.

Here are some natural ways to help control your problem without surgery or mechanical devices:

> Don't sleep on your back.
> Lose excess weight.
> Avoid alcohol and tranquilizers.
> Don't take antihistamines at night.

If you have reason to believe that you or your spouse has sleep apnea, talk to your doctor.

Medical Sources ————————————————————
> *British Medical Journal* (300,6739:1557)
> *FDA Consumer* (26,5:33)
> *Emergency Medicine* (24,6:83)

Test your sleep knowledge

☐ Adults require at least eight hours of sleep.
False. Sleep needs vary from person to person.

☐ Most people get enough sleep.
False. Many people ignore their bodies' signals that tell them they

need more sleep.

☐ Sleep is a period of quiet inactivity — the brain "turns off." **False.** The brain uses as much energy during sleep as when you are awake.

☐ You turn over as many as 40 times a night while you are asleep. **True.** You can also awaken during the night as many as 15 times without remembering it.

☐ Eating chocolate too close to bedtime can ruin a good night's sleep. **True.** Chocolate, as well as alcohol and drugs, can interfere with sleep.

Medical Source ────────────────────
Geriatrics (47,10:65)

EATING DISORDERS

Recognizing and understanding eating disorders

Anorexia nervosa and bulimia nervosa are two of the most common eating disorders, but they often go unrecognized because friends and parents don't know the warning signs.

People suffering from anorexia nervosa refuse to eat for fear of becoming fat, and they continue to see themselves as fat even after losing massive amounts of weight.

Bulimia nervosa is an eating disorder characterized by binge eating cycles followed by self-induced vomiting.

Bulimics are often on starvation diets before their binge cycles, and they, too, are afraid of becoming fat.

Bulimia nervosa is the more common of the two eating disorders. It affects between four and 10 percent of adolescent and college-age women. Although both disorders are more common in women, men are sometimes affected.

Despite the fact that eating disorders are relatively common, many people suffer silently for months or even years without the help of family or friends largely because people don't know what the warning signs are.

Listed below are some of the most common characteristics of anorexia and bulimia.

Anorexia nervosa:
- ☐ People suffering from anorexia often hide their food (in napkins, pockets, school milk cartons, etc.) instead of eating it. Later, they throw the food away privately.
- ☐ Anorexic people often abuse laxatives. When they do eat (or are forced to eat), they quickly take a laxative, hoping to usher the food out the other end.
- ☐ Anorexics also abuse diuretic drugs. These "water pills" help get rid

of excess water in the body, making the person think she has gotten rid of a few more extra pounds.

☐ People with anorexia nervosa usually are compulsive exercisers. They are constantly over-exercising, and they even exercise "in secret" (late at night in their bedroom after parents have gone to bed) to avoid criticism for such vigorous activity.

☐ Men and women suffering from anorexia deny having a problem. They deny their symptoms and the need for any help.

☐ No matter how much weight they lose, these people believe that they are fat and need to lose more weight. They are terrified of gaining weight and getting fat.

Bulimia nervosa:

☐ People suffering from bulimia nervosa go on eating binges in which they will consume unbelievable amounts of food, such as whole pizzas, followed by a cake and a whole carton of ice cream. Afterwards, they induce vomiting to get rid of the food they just consumed.

☐ These people also use laxatives, diuretics and vigorous exercise to prevent gaining weight.

☐ People with bulimia nervosa often crash diet in between binges to avoid gaining weight from the last binge episode.

☐ People with this disorder often look "normal." They don't resemble the sickly, wasted appearance of those suffering from anorexia. Bulimics often go to great lengths to hide their binge-cycle behavior, so no one suspects anything is wrong.

Many psychological experts and psychiatrists suggest that many people with eating disorders are struggling with self-identity, self-respect and self-control.

Many seem to fear losing the security of childhood and are afraid of the insecurity and responsibilities of adulthood. The eating disorders might be an attempt to control something in their lives.

However, not everyone with self-confidence problems develops an eating disorder. In order for an eating problem to be considered anorexia nervosa or bulimia nervosa, the American Psychiatric Association suggests the following guidelines.

Anorexia nervosa:

☐ Refusal to maintain body weight over a minimal normal weight for age and height, or person fails to make expected weight gain during certain periods of growth, leading to a body weight 15 percent below what is expected.

☐ Intense fear of becoming fat or gaining weight, even though they may be grossly underweight.

☐ Misperception about how she looks, feels or weighs. Anorexics "feel fat" even when they are thin, and they believe that areas of their bodies are "too fat" even when they are underweight.

☐ Women with anorexia nervosa miss at least three monthly periods in a row.

Bulimia nervosa:

☐ Recurrent episodes of binge eating—eating a large amount of food in a short period of time.

☐ Feeling of being "out of control" of their eating habits during the eating binges.

☐ Self-induced vomiting, strict dieting or fasting, regular use of laxatives or diuretics or extremely vigorous exercise to control weight gain after the binges.

☐ Two binge eating episodes per week for at least three months at a time.

☐ Compulsive overconcern with body shape and weight.

People who develop these eating disorders usually have more than weight problems to worry about. The stress the illnesses place on the body could have long-term, dangerous effects.

Conditions that can be caused by anorexia nervosa include:

☐ Abnormal or disturbed sleep patterns or inability to sleep soundly
☐ Inability to concentrate
☐ Serious mood swings
☐ Periods of severe anxiety, irritability or depression
☐ Inability to make decisions

☐ Hypothermia — always feeling cold, inability to get warm
☐ Swelling in the legs and ankles
☐ Abnormally slow heart beat
☐ Unusually low blood pressure
☐ Growth of fine hair everywhere on the body
☐ Infertility
☐ Osteoporosis
☐ Heart failure
☐ Increased risk of infection due to suppressed immune system

Conditions that can be caused by bulimia nervosa:

☐ Fluid and electrolyte imbalances due to excess vomiting
☐ Magnesium deficiency
☐ Irritation and bleeding of the esophagus and stomach due to excess vomiting
☐ Abnormalities of the large colon due to laxative abuse
☐ Fluid retention that leads to swelling and edema
☐ Extreme fatigue
☐ Swelling of the parotid glands (a type of salivary gland in the mouth)
☐ Erosion of the enamel on the teeth due to the stomach acid from vomiting
☐ Gingivitis and other gum disorders and dental problems
☐ Calluses on the knuckles from inducing vomiting using the fingers
☐ Abnormal menstrual periods caused by damage to the ovaries

If you recognize any of the characteristics or symptoms listed above in a friend or family member, talk to your family doctor.

Eating disorders are complicated problems, but doctors are experiencing successful treatments when they combine medical therapy, individual counseling, family counseling and support groups to help treat those with the illness.

Medical Sources ————————————————

The Western Journal of Medicine (157,6:658)
The Lancet (340,8821:723)

Light therapy offers hope for some bulimia sufferers

Are you trapped in the binge and purge cycle of bulimia?

If so, there may be a "light" at the end of the tunnel.

Canadian researchers are offering encouraging news for some people suffering from bulimia.

Bulimia seems to become more severe for some people during the winter months, perhaps because winter's shorter days disrupt their internal clocks.

To see whether an increased amount of light could cut down on the frequency of the overeating/vomiting episodes that characterize bulimia, researchers exposed bulimics to daily light therapy.

The bright, white-light therapy cut their number of bulimic episodes nearly in half.

White-light therapy might be most beneficial to those whose bulimia is more severe in the winter months.

Because eating disorders are dangerous to your health, talk to your doctor if you think you have an eating disorder.

Medical Source ———————————————————————

Medical Tribune (33,10:3)

Healing your body from head to toe

Skin care
Eye care
Ear problems
Mouth and
  teeth problems
Joints and
  muscles
Foot problems

Skin care

Feeling itchy? Don't do anything rash

If you've got an itch, you've probably got a rash, right? Not so fast. A general itchy feeling can also be due to a number of other causes, some of which are serious.

Any of the following can trigger prickly itchiness:

- [ ] **Systemic disease** — Kidney failure, hyperthyroidism, Hodgkin's disease and liver disease are all possible reasons for itching. Polycythemia vera, a condition in which the bone marrow produces too many blood cells, can be another cause.
- [ ] **Drug reaction** — A number of drugs, including antibiotics such as penicillin and sulfa, might start an itching reaction in some people. Other drugs like gold, birth control pills, estrogen, aspirin, morphine and codeine sometimes cause itching.
- [ ] **Insect bites** — Fleas, mites and scabies can produce intense itching. Curing your pet's infestation with mites or fleas can eliminate the problem for you. Scabies, on the other hand, passes from person to person through infested clothing, sheets or blankets and through close personal contact. Scabies tend to burrow in between fingers and around the wrists, elbows, nipples, genitals and navel. Scabies itching never lets up and gets worse in the evening. A good scrub and medicine prescribed by your doctor will cure scabies, and a thorough laundering will rid affected clothing, sheets and blankets of this pest.
- [ ] **Dry skin** — This is a problem for many people in the wintertime, and for elderly people all the time. Low humidity, hot showers or baths and drying soaps can make your skin itchy.
- [ ] **Fiberglass insulation or fabrics** — Contact with insulation and some fabrics can cause an itchy reaction.

Until you determine and treat the source of the itch, try these tips to lessen the urge to scratch:

> ➤ Bathe with lukewarm water and a mild soap.
> ➤ Pat your skin dry instead of rubbing it.
> ➤ Limit bathing frequency.
> ➤ Use a moisturizer after your bath.
> ➤ Apply an ice pack to the itchy area.
> ➤ Try menthol lotions.
> ➤ Take an antihistamine if allergies plague you.
> ➤ Avoid steroid creams. They can cause side effects.
> ➤ Run a humidifier in your home.

See your doctor to determine the cause of your itch. He might run a series of tests and ask you about your medicines, allergies, family history, bathing habits, pets, sexual and travel histories.

Medical Source ———————————————
Emergency Medicine (25,5:19)

Fighting an acne attack

Acne can happen to anybody at any age, but don't give up. There are some things you can do to help prevent and treat it.

There are two basic kinds of pimples: whiteheads and blackheads. They occur when a plug of oils and skin becomes lodged in a follicle (place where hair grows out).

Researchers believe acne may be caused by stress, heredity or the way your body reacts to bacteria on your skin.

Another common cause of acne is hormonal activity. During puberty, the adolescent body begins producing large amounts of a hormone called androgen. This hormone causes the sebaceous glands to overproduce oil. Bacteria accumulate with the excess oil and result in pimples.

Acne can also be caused by constant external irritation to the skin. For example, using chin straps on football helmets, constantly cradling the telephone against your cheek, or frequently supporting or rubbing your face with your hands are common factors behind pimple flare-ups.

Acne can be a side effect of some medications, such as birth control pills, lithium, halides, azathioprine (Imuran), dantrolene sodium (Dantrium), hydantoins and rifampin (Rifadin and Rimactane).

The majority of teens who suffer from occasional acne flare-ups have what is known as "noninflammatory acne." It causes a few pimples to spring up every now and then, but the pimples do not cause infections and scarring. Noninflammatory acne is not a serious medical condition.

If you have acne that covers your face or involves your chest, shoulders, back or groin area, if one or both of your parents have scars from acne, or if your pimples have already left bad scars, you need to see a dermatologist. You could have the serious, hereditary, "inflammatory acne," and you need professional treatment to avoid further scarring.

Try these tips to help fight acne:

- ☐ **Don't sweat it.** Anytime you sweat you should rinse your face, shoulders and back as soon as possible.
- ☐ **Come clean.** Wash with a grease-free soap every day, even if your skin tends to be dry. If it is dry, use a moisturizer, but use one that says noncomedogenic (won't promote acne) on the label.
- ☐ **Fight back.** Try one of the many acne treatments available that contain benzoyl peroxide, salicylic acid or resorcinol. Ask your doctor for advice on which is best for you.
- ☐ **Switch medicines.** If you are taking birth control pills or other hormone medications, ask your doctor or pharmacist if your brand can cause pimples. You may be able to change brands.

Listed below are some no-nos if you have acne.

- ☐ **No hands.** No matter how badly you may be tempted to, don't squeeze pimples — it can cause infection.
- ☐ **No hair.** Try to avoid hairstyles that touch your face.
- ☐ **No heat.** Stay out of the sun. Too much harsh sunlight will irritate your skin and aggravate acne.
- ☐ **No grease.** Use water-based soaps and makeup. Oil-based makeup can contribute to acne.

❏ **No wool.** Prolonged contact with wool can aggravate acne on your back and shoulders.

Medical Sources —————————————————

The Physician and Sportsmedicine (20,8:100 and 93,5:289)
Postgraduate Medicine (92,5:181)

Retinoic acid: fountain of youth for your skin?

Crow's feet and laugh lines got you down? Chances are you can slow down or even reverse these signs of aging with retinoic acid derived from vitamin A.

A popular and effective treatment for acne, retinoic acid comes in a gel called Retin A that can be applied to your skin. And though Retin A has been approved by the Food and Drug Administration (FDA) for the treatment of acne, it is also becoming a friend to aging baby boomers.

As your face ages, the skin becomes thinner and less elastic, and your expression lines deepen. If you are fair-skinned and have exposed yourself to sun, wind, cigarette smoke and other chemicals over the years, your facial skin will look even more wrinkled, leathery and tough as you grow older.

Retin A can actually reverse these signs of aging and lower the number of liver spots you will have in future years. Researchers are also hoping to prove that Retin A offers protection against the formation of some skin cancers.

Retin A might cause uncomfortable side effects for some people. Typical side effects include:

> ➤ Peeling
> ➤ Blistering
> ➤ Dryness
> ➤ Pinkness

You probably won't be overly sensitive to Retin A if you have dark skin like people from the Mediterranean region. But experts warn that you might be sensitive if you're one of these people:

❏ People who have eczema, rosacea and other skin problems

❐ Middle-agers who have dry skin and who have used cosmetics heavily

❐ People who blush when they drink alcohol or get embarrassed easily

❐ Fair-skinned, blue-eyed, freckled people who sunburn easily

People who use Retin A should use sunscreen and moisturizers regularly. If side effects become too severe, you can try using Retin A less often.

Because your body does not absorb Retin A gel from your skin, there is no risk of systemic side effects or birth defects from Retin A.

Retin A is currently a prescription drug. If you think you could benefit from Retin A, see your dermatologist for an evaluation.

Medical Source ———————————————
Postgraduate Medicine (92,6:191)

Vitamin D cream relieves psoriasis discomfort

You get it from milk and vegetables every day in your diet, but it wasn't until three ladies rubbed it on their skin that they were believers.

Rub milk and vegetables on your skin? you ask in disbelief.

No, not exactly. But milk and some vegetables contain an important vitamin that has rescued at least three women from severe pain and suffering.

The vitamin is vitamin D, and it is the important ingredient in a new cream that seems to be effective in relieving much of the pain and discomfort of psoriasis.

Psoriasis is a chronic skin disease that causes flaking, thickening, itching and pustules (blisters) of the skin. There is no cure for the disease, and if the blisters cover too much of the body, it can become life-threatening.

Up until now, people suffering from psoriasis have used medicated tar and creams and steroids to try to relieve the symptoms. These methods are successful in some people, but not in others.

Three elderly women were recently hospitalized (on different occasions) because of their pustular psoriasis, and doctors could not find any medication to help them, according to a medical report. Until they found calcipotriol, that is.

Calcipotriol is a new cream that contains a form of vitamin D.

Doctors began treating the three suffering women with daily doses of calcipotriol on their pustular skin, and within a 48-hour period, each of the women experienced relief from the pustules.

In fact, in all three cases, the calcipotriol cream treatment caused the pustules to resolve completely after just two days.

Scientists are not sure how the new cream helps clear up the dangerous psoriatic pustules, but the active ingredient seems to be the vitamin D.

Calcipotriol offers other advantages over traditional psoriasis drugs — the cream is colorless and odorless, so it doesn't smell and stain the skin like some other psoriasis creams and tars do. And it doesn't cause the serious side effects that steroids can cause.

Scientists warn that calcipotriol can irritate the skin, and this irritation seems to occur more in three groups of people: those who have fair, easily sunburned skin; people who have been using the drug etretinate; and people who have been using long-term steroids to treat their psoriasis.

However, the skin irritation clears up when the cream is discontinued, and those people can try the cream again after a few weeks.

For people who do not experience side effects, calcipotriol cream seems to bring relief within two to three weeks, and sometimes as quickly as 24 hours.

If you suffer from psoriasis, especially the pustular type, talk to your doctor about the vitamin-D cream.

Medical Source ——————————————————
British Medical Journal (305,6858:868)

Protect your skin from razor bumps

Face it — shaving can be an unpleasant experience, especially if you have sensitive skin.

But you might find comfort in knowing that there are ways you can help reduce the pain and prevent its return.

Razor bumps are increasingly common among men. Black men are more likely to experience these bumps, which are caused by sharp-edged hairs curving back into the root. Razor bumps can cause a variety of problems, such as a rash or scaly skin, or they can even develop into an infection.

Genetics is not the only factor contributing to razor bumps or painful shaving. The way you shave also can cause problems. Stretching your skin while shaving against the grain of your beard can cause the hair to go under your skin.

Below are a few steps you might want to try for treatment of razor bumps:

☐ If you develop razor bumps, stop shaving immediately. Most people can resume shaving in four to five weeks.

☐ After resuming shaving, do not use an electric razor — they encourage the hair to go under your skin. Instead, use a safety razor or an electric clipper.

☐ Use shaving cream containing benzoyl peroxide. This will prevent the acne, peeling and skin dryness associated with razor bumps.

☐ Use hair removal creams or lotions. They remove hair if you do not want to risk shaving. Be sure to read the directions before applying. After the treatment is complete, use a wooden tongue depressor to scrape the loose hair off your face.
Use cold compresses if the treatment causes your face to burn or chap.

Talk to your doctor if your razor bumps continue or worsen.

Medical Source ————————————————
Emergency Medicine (24,15:143)

Don't get burned by aerosol hairsprays

Having a bad hair day? Using aerosol hairsprays near heat or fire could really make you hot under the collar, warns the Food and Drug Administration.

The FDA's warning comes in response to recent reports of injuries and deaths resulting from aerosol-hairspray-related fires.

A woman in Kansas suffered fatal burns after lighting a cigarette before the spray had completely dried on her hair.

Hairspray-related fires can seriously burn your hair and upper body. Anyone near may also be injured.

When using hairspray, be sure to follow these guidelines:

☐ Stay away from matches, lighters and lit cigarettes.
☐ Wait until your hairspray is completely dry before using curling irons or blow dryers.
☐ Be sure to keep all hairspray products out of children's reach.

Most aerosol hairsprays carry some variation of this warning: "Flammable. Avoid heat, fire and smoking during use until sprayed hair is fully dry."

Aerosol hairsprays often contain hydrocarbon propellants and SD alcohol 40 solvent. This combination, which has been used to replace banned chlorofluorocarbons (CFCs), is responsible for the flammability of most aerosol hairsprays.

Medical Source ───────────────────────
    FDA Consumer (27,4:2)

Dying to color your hair?

Every two out of five women and a smaller number of men dye their hair. If you're among that number, recent studies examining possible links between hair dye and cancer may color the way you look at these products.

While some studies link hair dye to an increased risk of cancer, other studies don't. However, it's important to keep in mind that most hair dyes, unlike other cosmetic color additives, are not tested for safety before they are marketed.

Manufacturers have removed many compounds in hair dyes that researchers have found to cause cancer in animals. However, scientists speculate that many of the replacement compounds will not significantly decrease cancer risk because they are very similar to old compounds.

Some small, short-term studies have linked hair dye use to cancer in humans. However, these studies did not take into account other possibly contributory factors to cancer such as smoking.

Even though these studies raise some questions, "there's no basis for us to say that hair dyes pose a definitive risk of cancer," concludes John Bailey, Ph.D., director of the FDA's colors and cosmetics program.

If you choose to use hair dyes, there are ways to reduce possible cancer risks.

- ❑ Use as little hair dye as possible. Don't change your hair color every week, for example.
- ❑ Consider using henna, which offers a variety of colors from dark brown to reddish-blond. This product does not fall into the coal-tar category and has been tested for safety.

You can identify and avoid coal-tar hair dyes, which can cause allergic reactions in some people, by looking for the following warning found on the label of most coal-tar hair dyes:

"This product contains ingredients which may cause skin irritation in certain individuals. A preliminary test according to accompanying directions should first be made. This product should not be used for dyeing the eyelashes or eyebrows; to do so might cause blindness."

Before using a hair dye:

- ❑ Test the dye by placing a small amount behind one ear. Leave dye on for two days. If you do not develop any itching, redness or burning, you probably won't have a reaction to the dye. If you do have a reaction, test other brands until you find one you can tolerate.
- ❑ Wear gloves to apply dye.
- ❑ Follow directions carefully.
- ❑ Never mix different hair dye products. This can cause dangerous reactions and may result in an undesirable hair color.
- ❑ Don't leave dye on longer than recommended.
- ❑ Rinse scalp thoroughly after dyeing hair.
- ❑ Never dye eyebrows or eyelashes. This can cause blindness.

Since most hair dyes have not been proven risk free, the FDA recommends that you "proceed with caution when selecting a hair dye," until further information about links between hair dye and cancer is available.

Medical Source ————————————————————
   FDA Consumer (27,3:31)

Choosing a hair dye

If you are considering changing the color of your hair, you have four basic types of hair colors to choose from. They are classified according to how they color hair and how long they last. Some products in all the categories except gradual dyes contain coal-tar ingredients, which may cause cancer.

Temporary hair colors — These dyes sit on the hair surface. They come out in one to three washings. If hair with this type of dye gets wet, the dye may run onto face and clothing.

Semi-permanent dyes — These dyes penetrate into the hair shaft. Twenty to 40 minutes after application, these dyes are worked in like a shampoo and then rinsed out. They last through five to 10 shampoos.

Permanent dyes — These dyes contain hydrogen peroxide and can be used to lighten hair, which other dyes cannot do. Permanent dyes will not wash out with shampoo.

Gradual or progressive dyes — These dyes gradually darken hair. They are normally applied daily until the desired color is attained. Once the desired color is achieved, they are used periodically to help maintain that color. Unlike temporary dyes, these dyes won't wash off quickly or run when they get wet.

Medical Source ————————————————————
   FDA Consumer (27,3:31)

A close-up look at permanent eyeliner

Some women are now opting to have their eyes permanently tattooed with eyeliner. It allows women who are allergic to makeup to wear eyeliner and saves time for women who wear eyeliner every day. Imported from the Orient over 10 years ago, tattooed eyeliner is now a popular service offered in many beauty salons.

The procedure can take from 20 minutes to an hour. A local anesthetic is often given for pain. Disposable needles are used to implant pigment, taken from vegetable products, into the base of the upper or lower eyelashes. Swelling may occur and scabs may form. Scabs usually disappear within a week.

The procedure has yet to undergo formal safety testing although the FDA is considering such tests. At this time, there are no known risks of permanent eyeliner, but FDA chemist John Bailey warns that this does not mean the procedure is completely safe. Investigators caution that allergic reactions could damage the eyes and eyelids and perhaps be difficult to treat. Surgery might be necessary to remove the tattoo, possibly harming the eye or leaving scars.

Medical Source ───────────────────────────

FDA Consumer (27,3:31)

EYE CARE

Over-the-counter eye products provide relief

If your eyes are burning, itching, stinging, watering and turning red, you may want to take a peek at some over-the-counter eye medications at your local pharmacy.

Minor eye irritation and inflammation, tear deficiency and corneal edema are the only three eye conditions you can safely treat with over-the-counter eye products.

Irritated and inflamed eyes often burn, itch, sting, turn red and water. Common causes include foreign particles that become lodged in the eye, chlorinated water and allergens (any substance that triggers an allergic response such as pollen, dust, perfume or smoke).

Foreign particles are the most common cause of eye damage. If you suspect that a foreign particle is causing your eye irritation, flush the eye with clean water or with an eyewash solution.

Eyewashes contain the same elements as tears and are available over the counter. If the irritation persists, see a doctor. The fragment could have damaged the eye or still be lodged there. Large objects that become lodged in your eye should always be removed by a doctor to prevent further eye damage.

If any chemical is splashed into your eye, rinse the affected eye for 20 to 30 minutes in warm water. Do not put any medicine in the eye and see a doctor immediately.

Eyewashes and eye products that contain astringents, demulcents or emollients are often useful in alleviating eye irritation.

- ❐ Eyewashes are good for removing allergens, chlorinated water and loose foreign material. They relieve the discomforts of burning, irritation, itching and stinging.
- ❐ Astringents reduce tissues' ability to absorb water and cause them to dry and shrink. They are often used to treat watering of eyes due

to minor irritation.

☐ Demulcents soothe or soften the area to which they are applied. They provide relief for eyes that have been irritated by exposure to wind, sun and allergens.

Demulcents may leak out of the eyes onto the lashes and eyelids and dry. The crusty remains can be removed with a washcloth soaked in warm water.

☐ Emollients form an oily film that prevents loss of moisture and helps protect against irritation by airborne pollutants.

☐ Vasoconstrictors help decrease excessive eye redness. On rare occasions, if enough of the drug is absorbed into the body's circulatory system, vasoconstrictors can be poisonous. This problem is usually associated with prescription vasoconstrictors. If you have glaucoma, consult your doctor before using this product.

In tear deficiency or dry eye, the eyes do not produce enough water, causing eyes to burn, feel dry and turn red. The exact cause of this disorder is not known, but it commonly occurs with aging.

People with this condition are at increased risk of eye infections. The problem needs to be diagnosed by an eye professional, but over-the-counter eye products containing demulcents and emollients are usually the recommended treatments. Moist compresses and the use of a humidifier can also help.

In corneal edemas, fluid collects in the cornea, the main lens of the eye that does most of the focusing. This disorder is characterized by swelling, local irritation, foggy vision, light intolerance, seeing halos around lights and extreme pain.

Corneal cell degeneration, glaucoma, infection, inflammation of the iris or any other part of the eye, and excessive wear of contact lenses can result in a corneal edema.

Because of the wide variety of possible causes, this condition should be diagnosed and monitored regularly by an eyecare professional. Once diagnosed, it is safe to treat with over-the-counter eye products.

Hypertonic agents, which come in liquid or ointment form, remove the excess fluid and temporarily improve eyesight and relieve eye pain. The liquid form is better for people who wear contact lenses because it will not stick to the lenses and impair vision like ointments can. If you do not wear contacts, some ointments are more effective than liquid solutions. Ask your pharmacist for recommendations.

Sties, granulated eyelids and pinkeye can often be successfully treated at home without medication. At present, there are no effective over-the-counter treatments for these problems.

A sty is a small pus-producing abscess that forms near the eyelashes. It is characterized by swelling, acute pain, tenderness and redness. Normally the infection resolves itself. Warm, moist compresses are helpful in alleviating the condition.

Granulated or inflamed eyelids are characterized by redness, irritation and scaly skin at the lid edges. They result from bacterial infections or increased production of oils on the face and scalp.

This condition is accompanied by a burning or gritty feeling in the eye, itching and a crusty buildup on the eyelid edges. If this problem is caused by too much oil production, scalp dandruff and excess face oils must be controlled.

The crusty buildup along the edges of the eyes can be removed with warm cloths or with cloths that have been soaked in watered-down baby shampoo.

If the condition does not respond to treatment, see a doctor. You may have a bacterial infection. An antibiotic eye ointment is usually effective in treating the problem. Continue medication a week after symptoms disappear.

Pinkeye results from inflammation of the conjunctiva, the clear membrane that covers the white of the eye and lines the inside of the eyelids. It is commonly caused by allergies or bacterial or viral infections.

This disorder causes eye redness, drainage and a gritty feeling in the eye. It doesn't affect vision. If the pinkeye is due to allergies, a vasoconstrictor can eliminate the eye redness.

Pinkeye due to a bacterial infection often clears up on its own. If the condition does not clear up within a reasonable amount of time, you may need antibiotics.

Stop using any of these over-the-counter products or home therapies if you have eye pain, vision changes, continued redness or irritation.

Do not use over-the-counter eye products for conditions that worsen or persist longer than 72 hours. Although over-the-counter eye products can provide temporary relief, the best solution is to treat the underlying problem causing your discomfort.

The symptoms of these eye disorders often overlap and make self-diagnosis difficult. Misdiagnosis that leads to incorrect treatment can cause vision loss.

If you are in doubt about the condition causing your eye discomfort, consult your doctor or pharmacist.

Medical Source ————————————————————
U.S. Pharmacist (18,2:23)

Things you should know before using over-the-counter eye products

- ❒ If you have vision loss, eye pain or discharge, do not use any over-the-counter eye products until you consult your doctor.
- ❒ Do not use an over-the-counter eye product if you are already using a prescription eye medicine unless you check with your doctor.
- ❒ Use only those products that have been specifically recommended for treatment of eye disorders.
- ❒ Do not use products after their expiration date has passed.
- ❒ Do not use liquid treatments that are cloudy or discolored. Do not use ointments that look or feel gritty.
- ❒ Throw away unused liquid medicines that have been open for more than four weeks. Throw away unused ointments that have been opened more than three months. Do not open products until you are ready to use them. Close products immediately after use to prevent contamination.
- ❒ Do not use eye makeup or other cosmetics around your eyes while using eye medication.
- ❒ If symptoms persist or worsen, stop using medicine and consult

your doctor. Do not use over-the-counter products for longer than 72 hours unless your doctor recommends it.

Medical Source
U.S. Pharmacist (18,2:23)

Getting maximum benefits from eyedrops

- ☐ Wash and dry hands before applying medicine.
- ☐ Check medicine for expiration date, discoloration or contamination.
- ☐ Tilt head back. Gently pull down lower eyelid with index finger. Using the same hand, place middle finger alongside the inside corner of eye and apply slight pressure. This will keep medicine from draining out of your eye.
- ☐ Hold medicine container above eye or lay across bridge of nose so the tip is directly above your eye. Squeeze recommended number of drops into eye. If you have trouble telling if you are getting drops in your eye, store your eye medicine in the refrigerator. The cold sensation will make it easier to tell how many drops have been administered.
- ☐ After applying drops, wait a few seconds. Then look down and lift lower eyelid to touch upper eyelid.
- ☐ Release eyelid, but keep eyes closed for one to two minutes. Blink several times to spread medicine over entire eye.
- ☐ Do not allow tip of medicine bottle to touch eye.

Medical Source
U.S. Pharmacist (18,2:23)

Easing eyedrops into your child's eyes

If you've had it up to your eyeballs trying to get eyedrops into your child's eyes, here are some eye-opening tips that just might help you get some results.

- ☐ Gently wash your child's face, especially around the eyes.
- ☐ Place the child on his back with his face up.

❑ Tell your child to close his eyes.

❑ Dry away any tears and place the correct number of eyedrops on the closed eyelids creating a puddle over the inner corners of the eyelids (next to the nose).

❑ Tell your child to open his eyes. The eyedrops should naturally flow into his eyes. You might have to help him open his eyes.

Medical Source ⸻
Postgraduate Medicine (92,3:73)

Easy way to put eye ointment in your eye

❑ Pull lower eyelid down gently.

❑ Hold tip of tube between the section of your lower eyelid and eyeball. If you have trouble keeping your hands steady, you may want to sit in front of a mirror with your arms propped on a hard surface.

❑ Squeeze 1/4 to 1/2 inch of medicine inside lower eyelid. Do not let tube touch eye.

❑ Release eyelid and close eye.

❑ Eye medications can cause temporary blurry vision. Blinking your eyes a few times will help bring things back into focus.

Medical Source ⸻
U.S. Pharmacist (18,2:23)

Prevent blindness with a simple test

A simple wall calendar may keep you from going blind, if you know how to use it. Place your hand over one eye and look at the calendar. Do the lines look broken, distorted or wavy? Now try the other eye.

If you're over age 50, you should use the calendar to test your eyes every day. You may be able to save your sight.

Age-related macular degeneration (ARMD) is the most common cause of vision loss in people over 50. The macula is located in the center of the retina. It's the part of the eye that is most sensitive to light, and it helps you focus in on all of life's little details.

After 50 or 60 years, the macula begins to break down, causing your central vision to become blurry. You'll see a grayness or a blank spot in the center of your field of vision, words may be blurry, straight lines will look broken or distorted, and things may seem smaller than they are.

You may need more light to read by, and your eyes may take longer to adjust when you come in out of the bright sunlight.

There are two types of macular degeneration — "wet" and "dry." The dry type, where the tissues in the macula just waste away, accounts for 70 percent of all cases. You can't stop or do anything about the dry type, but it progresses slowly. You'll be able to read with the use of high-powered reading glasses or a magnifying glass.

The wet type is far more serious. The blood vessels in the macula begin to grow and leak fluid. This leakage can severely damage your eyesight in a matter of days. But if you test your eyes every day, you'll be able to tell if your vision is changing.

If you catch the degeneration early enough, your doctor may be able to stop the growing and leaking blood vessels with laser surgery.

Your eye doctor can give you an Amsler grid to use to test your eyes instead of a calendar if you wish. The lines on the grid are closer together than calendar lines.

Remember to cover one eye while you check the other. Otherwise, one good eye may compensate for an eye that's becoming damaged. Macular degeneration often affects only one eye.

Medical Sources ───────────────────────
  Senior Patient (2,9:39)
  The Johns Hopkins Medical Letter, Health After 50 (2,2:2)

Microwave popcorn can damage the eyes

Never open a freshly popped bag of microwave popcorn near your face. Microwave popcorn bags are designed to hold in heat and allow the oil inside to reach temperatures high enough to pop the kernels.

When you open the bag, the rush of steam released could burn any exposed skin and is especially harmful for your eyes.

One 29-year-old man quickly opened a bag of microwave popcorn, looking inside to see if all the kernels had popped. Steam rushed out and scalded his right eye. After wearing a patch for five days and treating his eye with antibiotic ointment, his vision returned to normal. Two months later, the man had to be treated again because his cornea kept sloughing off, but he eventually healed.

Use caution when opening microwave popcorn bags. Your skin and eyes are at risk.

Medical Source ————————————————
The New England Journal of Medicine (323,17:1212)

Choosing contact lenses — convenience or safety?

Researchers are saying that you probably can't have both — when it comes to contact lenses, that is.

If you choose the convenience of disposable soft contact lenses, you might be compromising your eyes' safety.

In fact, people who wear disposable soft contact lenses have up to 14 times the risk of developing the dangerous eye infection, ulcerative keratitis.

Ulcerative keratitis is usually caused by bacteria that enter the eye through nicks and scratches in the surface of the cornea that can be caused by the lenses.

If caught in time, the infection is curable — but depending on the location of the infection in the eye, serious scarring may develop. Infections that are not caught and treated early enough can lead to permanent blindness.

Disposable lenses have grown in popularity largely because of the convenience they offer: You put them in on Monday, leave them in all week, then take them out at the end of the week and throw them away. You put in a fresh, brand-new pair on Monday.

There's none of the hassle of taking them out every night and putting them in the next morning. And that means the hassle of all the cleaning solutions is gone, too.

All you need is some saline solution to put in your eyes in the morning and occasionally throughout the day if your eyes feel dry.

The manufacturers of the disposable soft contact lenses thought that the minimal amount of handling would cut down on the amount of eye infections that contact lenses sometimes cause.

And they thought that throwing away the dirty lenses each week and replacing them with a fresh, uncontaminated pair would lower the risk of eye infections. According to the latest research, the manufacturers thought wrong.

Wearing contacts overnight was the most significant risk factor in developing ulcerative keratitis. The problem with sleeping in disposable soft contact lenses might be that the lenses don't allow enough oxygen to get to the eyeball when the lids are shut.

If you wear contact lenses of any kind and you develop red, painful or blurry eyes, take out your contact lenses immediately and call your ophthalmologist. Early treatment is the best way to help avoid long-term vision problems and blindness.

Medical Sources
The Journal of the American Medical Association (269,5:579)
Medical Tribune (33,23:3)

Making your contact lenses more comfortable

Contact lens wearers — has your dream of inconspicuous corrective vision turned into an itchy, bleary, red nightmare?

After just a few hours of wear, does it feel like grains of grit are grinding between you and your contacts?

Do you wake up in the morning with your eyelids crusted shut?

If you're nodding yes, you might be suffering from "giant papillary conjunctivitis" (GPC or conjunctivitis, for short). Don't worry, it is curable.

GPC is an allergic reaction to all the "gunk" that has built up on your contacts. As a result, the inner surface of your eyelids look like they've been paved over with little white cobblestones. This "gunk" your body is reacting to is mainly protein deposits from the tears that constantly flow to keep your eyes moist.

Seasonal allergies, dried-out lenses (which can trap debris), lenses with harsh edges and eye surgery can also irritate the conjunctivitis condition.

Some signs and symptoms of GPC include:

> tearing
> crust on eyelids when you wake up
> eye irritation
> mucous discharge
> pain after wearing contacts for just a few hours
> contacts slipping on your eyes
> deteriorating or cloudy contacts
> deposits on your contacts that just won't come off

Whether your contact of choice is hard or soft, daily or extended-wear, and regardless of whether you've been wearing contacts for three weeks or three years, GPC will get you — if you don't "wash out" your lenses, that is. Poor hygiene habits can lead to potentially dangerous eye problems.

The quickest way to get rid of GPC is to permanently get rid of your contacts. But, most contact wearers don't like the idea of switching back to glasses, even for a little while.

So, the next best thing is to give your eyes a two-week rest from your contacts. Or, at the very least, cut down your lens wear to a couple of hours a day until the GPC clears up. However, switching to disposable lenses might be a more attractive offer.

Disposable contacts allow GPC sufferers to basically start over with a brand-new lens, free of deposits, every week or two.

If you do continue to wear your contacts, it is important that you give them a vigorous daily cleaning. You might want to ask your doctor for a special "sponge" to clean your contacts. It works better than using your hands.

In addition to day-to-day washings, your contacts need to be deep-cleansed in enzymes at least once a week. Your doctor may recommend you do this more often, until the GPC goes away.

Enzymes are necessary to clear off the deposits that your everyday cleaning regimen doesn't dissolve.

To ease your discomfort during the day, try using saline drops in your eyes before you put your lenses in, after you take them out, and every two hours in between.

Other treatment options include replacing your old contacts or changing to a contact with a smoother shape.

It helps if you avoid cleaning solutions containing thimerosal or chlorhexidine. Many people are allergic to these substances.

You might also try "scrubbing" your eyelids. This procedure should only be done under the supervision of an eye-care professional:

- ☐ Apply one to two drops of baby shampoo to a wet cotton-tipped applicator, lather and dilute with water.
- ☐ Grasp the lower lid firmly from the lashes and pull down.
- ☐ For five to 10 seconds, gently rub the lid margin just above the lashes with the cotton-tipped applicator.
- ☐ Grasp the upper lid firmly from just below the lashes and raise the lid.
- ☐ For five to 10 seconds, gently rub the lid margin just below the lashes with a fresh cotton applicator.
- ☐ Rinse lids with warm water and repeat the procedure on the other eye.

It is recommended that you perform this procedure twice a day for several weeks. If there is no improvement in the GPC condition in that period of time, discontinue lid scrubs and see your eye doctor immediately.

GPC is an uncomfortable condition, and it may take a few weeks or even a few months for it to clear up. But, once you're cured, if wearing contacts is still a dream come true for you, follow this advice:

To prevent GPC from becoming a recurring nightmare, follow directions for keeping your contacts clean and disinfected at all times.

Medical Source ————————————————
U.S. Pharmacist (17,9:68)

A guide to common contact lens-related disorders

Listed below are the names, symptoms and probable causes of some common contact lens-related disorders. If you think you have developed any of these problems, contact your eye doctor immediately.

Disorder	Symptoms	Probable cause
Ulcerative keratitis	Rapid onset and progression of pain, redness and discharge.	Using disposable or extended-wear soft contact lenses.
Acute epithelial necrosis (overwear syndrome)	Blurred vision before the onset of problem due to swelling of the cornea. Delayed pain.	Trauma to the eye due to lack of enough oxygen in the eye.
Tight lens syndrome	Overwear, starting in the morning after wearing lens overnight and not getting enough oxygen to the eye during the night. Usually affects vision.	Lens tightening in the eye.
Microcystic epitheliopathy	Recurrent, brief episodes of pain and epiphora (overflow of tears due to obstruction of the tear ducts).	Seen in 80 to 100 percent of users of extended-wear soft contacts. Due to impaired metabolic activities. Leads to formation of small cysts on eye.
Epithelial edema (swelling)	Blurred vision after several hours of wear. May clear up after removing lenses. May progress to necrosis (death) of many cells.	Death of epithelial cells on surface of the eye.

Disorder	Symptoms	Probable cause
Corneal abrasion	Sudden onset of pain and epiphora. May resolve in several hours.	Trauma caused during insertion or removal of lenses; foreign bodies (dust, sand, etc.) get trapped behind lenses; protein deposits on lenses.
Enzyme/toxic keratopathy	Severe pain after inserting a lens after soaking in a proteolytic enzyme or chemically preserved soaking or cleaning solution.	Response to the compounds lenses were soaked in; soft lenses are especially prone to this problem.
Thimerosal keratopathy	Long-term irritation and redness soon after inserting lenses each day. May affect vision in severe cases.	Preservatives or enzymes may cause hypersensitivity reaction (allergic reaction).
Lens-related red eye	Chronic redness, discomfort. May cause blurred vision.	Lens spoilage.
3 and 9 o'clock strain	Redness. Discomfort is rare.	Surface of the cornea dries right next to edges of lenses.

Medical Source
Archives of Ophthalmology (110,11:1601)

Choosing sunglasses for maximum eye protection

You probably know that invisible ultraviolet B (UVB) and ultraviolet A

(UVA) rays from the sun age your skin and cause skin cancer.

But did you also know that too much UVB and UVA radiation can damage the retina of your eyes and cause the clouding of the eye lens that we call cataracts?

Unfortunately, just any old pair of sunglasses won't provide the protection your eyes need. Good sunglasses should protect your eyes in sunlight without distorting your vision or color perception.

However, the two most important criteria for choosing safe sunglasses are how well they filter ultraviolet rays and visible light. To find this out, you'll have to read the label on the sunglasses you buy. The Food and Drug Administration has suggested this system for labeling sunglasses:

- ☐ **Cosmetic sunglasses** are appropriate for shopping or business. They filter out less than 60 percent of visible light, 70 percent of UVB rays, and 20 percent of UVA rays.

- ☐ **General purpose sunglasses** provide more protection, filtering out 60 to 93 percent of visible light, 95 percent of UVB rays and 60 percent of UVA rays. You might use general purpose sunglasses for outside activities like driving, flying, hiking or boating.

- ☐ **Special purpose sunglasses** provide serious protection for people in ultra-bright surroundings like ski slopes or beaches. These glasses filter out 99 percent of UVB rays, 60 percent of UVA rays, and at least 97 percent of visible light.

Be sure you read the label and understand what you are buying. Dark-tinted lenses that filter out most of the visible light should also block ultraviolet rays. Otherwise, too much UV light will enter your dilated pupils and damage your eyes.

Consider these features when buying sunglasses:

- ☐ Gray, green or brown-colored lenses are best. Other tints distort your color vision.
- ☐ Dark frames are preferable to clear or light-colored frames that can cause bright spots.
- ☐ Plastic lenses are more impact-resistant than glass, but they scratch more easily.

❏ Gradient lenses are dark on the top and light on the bottom —
good for situations when most of the light comes from above.

❏ Double gradient lenses are dark at the top and bottom and lighter
in the middle. These are helpful when you're in an environment
where light comes from above and is reflected from below, such as
out on a lake boating or fishing.

❏ Polarizing lenses are popular with drivers, boaters and fishermen
because they cut down on light reflected from flat, horizontal
surfaces.

❏ Sunglasses cannot protect your eyes from the UV radiation of
tanning lamps. You need special goggles for that purpose.

So, just because summer is over — don't pack your shades away with the
beach chairs. You still need your sunglasses for optimal enjoyment and safety
outdoors.

Medical Source ————————————————————————
   U.S. Pharmacist (18,6:18)

Over-the-counter reading glasses — an economical alternative

If you're having trouble focusing in on life's little details, over-the-
counter reading glasses may be just what you're looking for.

As you approach 40, you may have trouble reading or doing close-up
work. If so, you're probably experiencing presbyopia or "old vision."

It's an inevitable part of aging in which your ability to see objects less than
20 feet away gradually decreases. You may first begin to notice this when you
have to hold printed material farther and farther away to read it.

You may also have problems shifting your focus from a distant object to
a near one. These changes may be accompanied by eyestrain, headaches and
spells of dizziness.

Your eye lenses change shape to bring objects into focus. As you grow
older, your lenses become thick and rigid and can't change shape as easily.

This is what causes your focusing problems. By age 70, the lens probably will have lost all its power to bring near objects into focus.

People often buy prescription bifocals for this problem.

However, prescription glasses will probably have to be changed several times between the ages of 40 and 60 because the ability to focus continues to decline during this period.

Since prescription glasses are so expensive, over-the-counter reading glasses, which normally cost less than $15, are an economical alternative if presbyopia is the only problem you have with your eyes.

Over-the-counter reading glasses don't correct vision; they merely magnify things. The lenses in these glasses, which may be either plastic or glass, meet or exceed the same federal standards for prescription glasses against impact.

They are optically correct, will not distort vision and come in a wide range of magnification strengths. They are really just magnifying glasses made portable.

Many people are hesitant about using over-the-counter reading glasses, fearing these glasses may damage their eyes.

The American Academy of Ophthalmology offers assurance that non-prescription reading glasses are safe and will not damage the eyes even if they are used incorrectly.

The displays containing over-the-counter reading glasses normally have charts to help you choose the correct level of magnification for your eyes.

Take a few extra minutes to find the right pair for you. Otherwise, you may end up with glasses that cause eyestrain and give you a headache.

Once you find a pair of glasses that improves your near vision, care for them as you would prescription glasses:

> Wash them with a moist cloth or use lens cleaner.
> Keep the lenses from getting scratched.

Use these glasses for reading or detail work. They aren't safe for driving or other activities that require accurate far vision.

Never substitute reading glasses for regular visits to a qualified eye doctor. Sometimes over-the-counter reading glasses won't correct loss of close-up sight.

Most reading glasses have the same magnification in each lens and may not help a person who has a different level of vision loss in each eye.

Headache and eyestrain may occur if a person's line of sight does not coincide with the optical center of the lenses. This type of eyestrain will not damage the eyes and will go away once the person removes the glasses.

If you're burned out on blurriness, take a peek at some over-the-counter reading glasses. They may give you a whole new perspective.

Medical Source ─────────────────────
U.S. Pharmacist (18,1:19)

Spinach can save your eyesight

A big medical study indicates that eating a lot of spinach, broccoli, sweet potatoes and winter squash can shield your eyes from blinding cataracts.

You also get added anti-cataract protection by taking vitamin-C supplements — 250 to 500 milligrams a day — for more than 10 years, the researchers suggest. That's about four to eight times the official Recommended Dietary Allowance of 60 milligrams for vitamin C.

The big boost in eye protection seems to come from the vitamin A and carotene compounds in the vegetables. Three surprises: Carrots lose out as cataract preventers, and the better-known carotene — beta carotene — is not the star of this study.

Carrots are among the richest sources of beta carotene, a nutrient in vegetables that your body turns into vitamin A as needed.

And the third surprise: Taking regular multivitamin supplements doesn't seem to help fight cataracts. Foods are your best bet, along with high-C tablets. Most multivitamins include only enough vitamin C to meet the RDA.

Cataracts cloud the lens, the clear part of your eye. That blocks out light and causes the light that reaches the retina to be unfocused and blurred.

People with diabetes run a big risk for cataracts. Getting older, smoking, getting too much sun, and eye injuries also increase your risk. Now, scientists are beginning to wonder whether eating the right things can slow down or halt cataract formation.

The researchers studied only women for eight years. More than 50,000 nurses ages 45 to 67 took part in the survey across 11 states. So, the scientists can't predict for sure that the results hold true for men.

But they are sure of this: Women who took in the most vitamin A — by eating high-A foods, rather than by taking vitamin-A supplements — cut 40 percent off their risk of developing cataracts.

Researchers also saw a small protective effect from riboflavin, one of the B-vitamins, but they couldn't measure enough of a boost to be statistically certain.

What happened to carrots for eyesight? Maybe it's because other carotenes besides the beta variety provide the protection against lens-clouding cataracts. Spinach is naturally high in carotenes known as lutein and zeaxanthin, while carrots are low in these nutrients.

Previous studies have suggested that riboflavin and the antioxidant nutrients — vitamin C, vitamin E and beta carotene — can help reduce cataracts. A deficiency of vitamin A leads to vision problems, ranging from night blindness to loss of sight.

Now, some cautions. Don't overdose on vitamin A. This is a so-called fat-soluble vitamin, meaning that it doesn't dissolve well in water. Your body stores excess vitamin A in the liver. Too much of this vitamin can cause liver and bone damage.

The RDA for vitamin A is one milligram for adult males and 800 micrograms for adult women. Many people start feeling the toxic effects of vitamin A at about five to 10 times the RDA.

Although vitamin C is considered to be among the least toxic of all vitamins, megadosing yourself with vitamin C can cause diarrhea and digestive upsets.

The RDA for riboflavin ranges from 1.2 to 1.7 milligrams for adults. No poisoning from overdoses has been reported, maybe because the body can absorb only about the amount it needs, no matter how much goes through the intestines.

But improving your nutritional intake isn't the only thing you can do to help prevent cataracts. Try these tips to help save your sight:

> ➤ Protect your eyes by wearing goggles or glasses when using machines, lawn or garden tools and shop equipment.
> ➤ Wear sunglasses that block at least 99% of UV rays.
> ➤ Keep diabetes under control.
> ➤ Get regular eye exams.

Medical Sources ────────────────

British Medical Journal (305,6849:335)

Recommended Dietary Allowances, 10th Edition, National Academy Press, Washington, D.C., 1989

Simple tips to relieve computer screen dry eyes

Do your eyes feel unusually tired or scratchy after a long day at the computer? If so, try "lowering your sights."

You blink as little as seven times a minute when working at a computer screen, compared to 22 times a minute while relaxing. Blinking helps keep your eyes moist.

Besides blinking less, when you use your computer, you tend to keep your eyes open wider, which also causes evaporation of eye moisture and dries out your cornea, making your eyes tired.

Changing your position, literally "lowering your sights," forces you to lower your eyelids a little so that you expose less of the cornea, which prevents your eyes from drying out so quickly.

To do this, lower your terminal and tilt the screen upward so that you are looking down on the screen. You can also accomplish this by raising your chair.

Try to stop working several times a day and close your eyes for a few seconds. This allows your eyes to remoisturize themselves.

Regular use of artificial tears, available in the form of eye drops, can help. If nothing seems to relieve your dry eyes, ask your optometrist about glasses specially designed for this problem.

Remember to take "blink breaks" throughout the day. More blinks a day keep dry eyes away.

More simple tips for those common computer screen complaints: dry or burning eyes, eye fatigue, blurred vision and aches in the neck and back:

☐ Use good room lighting. Adjust the room lighting levels and position your computer so that it is most comfortable for you. The typical office lighting may be too bright for computer work.

☐ Eliminate sources of glare. Use drapes and blinds on windows. Don't sit facing a bright window. If necessary, use screen hoods or glare shields over the screen. If you have adjustable lights, you might want to turn them down to reduce glare.

☐ Adjust the screen brightness and contrast so that it is comfortable for you.

☐ Rest occasionally during periods of intense concentration. The National Institute of Occupational Safety and Health recommends taking a 15-minute rest break every hour from your computer. Don't forget to blink frequently to reduce dryness and irritation. Looking at a distant object can relax your eyes. Closing your eyes can also help.

☐ Maintain a good viewing distance. Getting too close to your computer can cause your eyes to become tired. Adjust your workstation so that your keyboard, screen and paper copy are an equal distance from your eyes with the screen slightly (about 20 degrees) below eye level. It might be helpful to use a copy-holder to hold your papers. A good viewing distance is 22 to 26 inches.

☐ Keep your work environment free of dust. Dust can make your eyes tear, feel gritty or turn red. Proper humidity and ventilation are important. Be sure to clean your computer screen to remove dust and to keep from straining your eyes.

Medical Sources ⎯⎯⎯⎯⎯⎯⎯⎯⎯⎯⎯⎯⎯⎯⎯⎯
FDA Consumer (25,8:18)
The New England Journal of Medicine (328,8:584)

EAR PROBLEMS

Earwax — natural protection for your ears

Most of the time, earwax (cerumen) acts as an invisible friend, working out of sight to keep the skin in your ear canals moist and to defend against infection. But when earwax becomes impacted or trapped in your ears, it can become a very sticky subject indeed.

Ordinary earwax is made up of several materials: secretions from two types of skin glands, skin cells that have been shed from your ear canals, dust and other debris. Normally, the movement of your jaw while chewing and talking helps cerumen migrate to the outer ear where it can be easily washed away.

However, cerumen sometimes becomes impacted or stuck deep in the ear, causing these annoying and sometimes serious symptoms:

> ➤ hearing loss
> ➤ ringing in the ears
> ➤ earache or a feeling of fullness in the ears
> ➤ dizziness
> ➤ reflex cough (through stimulation of the vagus nerve)

Those most likely to suffer from impacted cerumen are very young children with narrow ear canals and older people whose earwax becomes drier with age. Older men are especially vulnerable because their ear hairs become coarser and longer and hold the wax inside the ears.

The use of cotton swabs to clean the outer ear can interfere with the normal outward migration of earwax. In fact, the use of cotton swabs to clean the ears can start a vicious cycle in which you damage the skin inside the ears, making the ears stop producing cerumen. The skin of the ear canal then dries out and starts to itch, which makes you want to clean your ears again.

Hearing aids and the earpieces on a doctor's stethoscope can also push earwax back into the ears, causing impaction.

If you suspect that wax is stuck deep in your ear canal, consult your doctor about softening agents such as olive oil and other products available at your drugstore.

You should not try to remove an impaction yourself by using an electrically powered water jet device.

Machines like the WaterPik are designed to clean your teeth, and they are much too strong for your ears. In fact, even when a WaterPik is set at one-third its full power, about 6 percent of the people who use this machine for rinsing wax from their ears perforate their eardrum.

So don't injure your ear further with a water-jet device. See your doctor for removal of a stubborn wax impaction.

And remember — ear wax is usually normal and helpful, and generally takes care of itself.

Medical Sources ───────────────────────
Journal of the Royal Society of Medicine (85,6:346)
Health Gazette (15,10:3)

Ringing in the ears — what you need to know

Do you wish you could turn off the ringing in your ears as easily as you turn off the TV or stereo?

If you can't turn off tinnitus completely, there are ways you can tone it down. Ringing or other noises within your ear, technically known as tinnitus, can range from mildly annoying to incapacitating.

Approximately 36 million Americans experience tinnitus, seven million so severely that it interferes with their daily lives.

Many people with tinnitus hear ringing, but other sounds heard include buzzing, whistling, hissing, sizzling, humming, the chirp of crickets and the roar of the ocean.

Although tinnitus can occur in one or both ears, two out of three people with tinnitus have it in both.

Tinnitus is a very common problem in middle-aged and older people. Sometimes it's only temporary — once the underlying problem is identified and treated, tinnitus disappears.

Tinnitus can be caused by a number of conditions that may or may not originate in the inner ear, such as:

> ➤ Wax buildup (See your doctor about removing the excess wax.)
> ➤ High blood pressure
> ➤ High cholesterol
> ➤ Dental problems
> ➤ Colds or flu

Permanent tinnitus is usually caused by damage to the inner ear hair cells. The cells normally vibrate at specific frequencies to transmit sounds to the brain.

Damaged cells cannot transmit the correct sound messages to the brain. They simply forward random sounds, which the brain interprets as the noise of a ringing bell, chirping cricket, etc.

The cells responsible for transmitting high frequencies are the most commonly affected.

Once damaged, these cells cannot be repaired. Inner ear hair cells sustain damage for many different reasons.

> ➤ Exposure to loud noises
> ➤ Age-related hearing loss
> ➤ Certain medications (Taking 10 to 20 aspirin a day can lead to tinnitus.)
> ➤ Allergies
> ➤ Tumors
> ➤ Thyroid problems
> ➤ Diabetes

Tinnitus can be an exasperating and even frightening experience. With no place to escape from the sound, you may feel as if you are going crazy.

Despite your doubts, the sounds really exist. Sometimes, even other people can hear the noise in your ears.

They usually hear clicking or cracking sounds, which are caused by blood vessel abnormalities or muscle spasms within the middle ear.

Most noticeable during quiet times, tinnitus can interrupt your sleep, making you irritable, stressed and tense, which often worsens the condition.

However, there are ways you can relieve tinnitus and keep it from interfering with your daily life.

❐ Stop smoking and limit caffeine. These substances can cause blood vessels to narrow, which can make noise in your ears worse.

❐ Try relaxation techniques. Biofeedback teaches you to control muscle tension in order to reduce stress, which can aggravate tinnitus.

❐ Consider physical therapy. Bone or muscle problems, such as osteoarthritis, can aggravate your tinnitus.

❐ Use hearing aids or noise screens. These provide background noise that drown out the sounds of tinnitus. Leaving a stereo or television on at low volume may help.

Some people find that tuning into static, easily found between stations, is less distracting. You may want to consider a white noise machine, which produces a low, continuous sound.

❐ Avoid loud noises and use earplugs when necessary. Loud noises can make tinnitus worse or cause it to move from one ear into both. Wear earplugs when using firearms or power tools. Do not listen to loud music.

Make sure your place of work meets the federal Occupational Safety and Health Administration (OSHA) guidelines for noise limits. You can receive information on these guidelines and request a brochure called *Hearing Conservation* by writing to OSHA's Office of Information at 200 Constitution Ave. N.W., Room N-3647, Washington, DC 20210.

❐ Seek support. To receive a list of local support groups, send a self-addressed envelope and $1.75 to The American Tinnitus Association, P.O. Box 5, Portland, OR 97207. They also publish a quarterly newsletter.

If you experience tinnitus, you should have a hearing and general medical exam immediately. The noises in your ears may signal a serious disorder.

Medical Sources ─────────────────────
Emergency Medicine (24,15:165)
Cecil Textbook of Medicine, 19th Edition, W.B. Saunders Company, Philadelphia,
   PA, 1988

Sound advice for hearing problems

If you've heard that hearing loss is an inevitable part of aging, don't
believe it. Have a complete ear and general health exam if you experience any
hearing problems.

The most common cause of hearing loss is exposure to loud noises, but
hearing loss can be related to medication or to some other underlying cause.
Often the problem can be corrected.

Certain drugs can irreversibly damage your ears, especially in large doses.
If you take any of the following medications and you experience hearing
problems, ask your doctor for alternate recommendations.

> ➤ Antibiotics, especially aminoglycosides such
>   as streptomycin, neomycin and gentamicin
> ➤ Diuretics
> ➤ Anticancer drugs
> ➤ Salicylates, such as aspirin
> ➤ Quinine

Sometimes, for no apparent reason, disorders develop that impair your
hearing. Doctors can treat many of these conditions and restore hearing to
normal.

❑ Otosclerosis. One of the most common causes of deafness, it
   usually occurs in later years. The disorder affects 10 to 14 percent
   of all white adults, although it almost never occurs in blacks or
   Asians.
   Twice as many women as men are affected, and sometimes the
   disorder runs in families. Tinnitus, ringing in the ears, is an early

sign of the disorder. Deafness occurs when one of the small, moveable middle ear bones, which amplify sound vibrations, becomes fixed to the bony covering of the inner ear. Surgery returns hearing to normal.

❑ Buildup of earwax. Men tend to have more buildup than women because they frequently have hair in their outer ear canals that catches and holds wax. If you suspect wax buildup, see a doctor. Don't use over-the-counter medications to remove the wax. They frequently cause infection and irritation.

❑ Obstructions in the ear canal. Swimmers often develop harmless bone growths in their ears.

❑ Infections of the middle ear.

❑ Ruptured eardrum. Infections of the middle ear often cause a ruptured eardrum. Other possible causes: blow to ear or head, putting sharp object into ear, nearby explosion or fracture to the base of the skull.

❑ Ruptured inner ear membranes. Strenuous physical activity and even ordinary daily events, such as lifting, coughing or sneezing, can cause these ruptures.

❑ Barotrauma. Changes in atmospheric pressure, such as you may experience when flying or scuba diving, can sometimes damage the middle ear. Damage is usually temporary.

❑ Bone, nerve, brain or blood disorder. Disorders that have nothing to do with your ears can affect your hearing. To help your doctor with a diagnosis, report any recent upper respiratory tract infections, colds or flu.

Also let your doctor know if you have a history of any of the following conditions:

➤ High blood pressure

➤ High cholesterol

➤ Diabetes

➤ Thyroid gland disorders

➤ Atherosclerosis, commonly known as hardening of the arteries, or any other cardiac disorder

Some natural loss of hearing does occur with age. Known as presbycusis, it makes sounds less clear, especially high frequencies. Hearing loss can be hastened by heredity, illness, certain medications and exposure to loud noises. Some ears just wear out faster than others.

Even if you're getting older and suspect that your hearing loss could be a result of natural deterioration, don't turn a deaf ear to your problems. Always have a complete medical examination if you experience any sudden hearing loss, whether it's mild or severe.

Many times, hearing can be restored to normal or to the point that a hearing aid would be helpful.

Medical Source —————————————————————
Emergency Medicine (24,15:165)

Don't let this report fall on deaf ears: How to prevent noise-induced hearing loss

When we were teen-agers, we thought it was funny to come home from a loud concert with ringing ears, barely able to hear each other speak. We knew our ears would be back to normal the next morning.

But we were wrong.

Our ears probably didn't bounce back to how they were before the concert. Some of the sensory hair cells in the inner ear were destroyed by the noise.

There were enough healthy cells left for our hearing to return to normal, but every time we were around loud noises, more inner ear cells were destroyed. We were on the road to lasting hearing loss, along with the one-third of all Americans who have significant hearing problems by age 65.

You would think we would know better now that we're older, but we still destroy our hearing with loud leisure activities. Engineers are working on reducing noises in the workplace, but recreational and home activities can be just as loud or louder than factory machinery.

Compare these common noises (a noise that an average young adult can barely hear is zero decibels; the pain threshold is about 140 decibels):

Activity	Sound pressure level (in decibels)
Automobile interior	60-92
Firearm	130 or higher
Lawn mower	80-95
Manufacturing plant	85-105
Motorcycle/snowmobile	80-110
Music	
Rock concert	90-115
Stereo headset	60-115
Symphonic concert	80-110
Busy office	70-85
Power saw	95-110
Vacuum cleaner	70-85

Any noise over 85 to 90 decibels is hazardous when you're exposed to it for several hours a day. Very loud noises, such as firearms and fireworks, can cause "acoustic trauma," which means your ears are damaged immediately.

How can you know when you're hurting your ears? Hearing loss isn't often painful, so people tend not to notice the damage.

Plus, a noise that causes severe hearing loss in one person may not cause any damage at all to another person.

Be aware of these warning signs of hearing loss that may last a few minutes or a few days after exposure to loud noises:

- ❐ Ears feel full or under pressure.
- ❐ Voices sound muffled and far away.
- ❐ You hear a ringing sound in your ears when all is quiet.

Even if you don't have these symptoms after a noisy activity, some of your inner ear cells could still be destroyed. A noise is too loud if:

- ❐ You have to shout to be heard above the noise.
- ❐ You can't understand a person speaking to you when they're less than two feet away.
- ❐ A person standing near you can hear sounds from your stereo

headset when it's on your head.

You'll first know that you've started a decline toward deafness when you can't understand high-pitched noises — singing birds, the voices of women and young children.

Eventually, men's voices and other lower-pitched noises will become hard to understand. It's particularly difficult to hear what others are saying to you when you're surrounded by loud background noises.

You can take steps to avoid noise-induced hearing loss:

☐ Choose quiet leisure activities instead of noisy ones such as hunting or woodworking with power tools, especially if you work in a noisy place or drive to work in loud city traffic.
Never start a loud activity immediately after a noisy workday. Your ears need time to rest and begin to recover their hearing ability. They don't need total silence, but they do need a low-noise environment.

☐ Wear earplugs when you know you'll be around loud noises. Disposable foam earplugs, around $2 a pair, can shut out 25 decibels of sound. That can make the difference between a safe noise and one that causes hearing loss.
Always use earplugs when riding snowmobiles, motorcycles or other loud vehicles and when using power tools, lawn mowers or leaf blowers. Hunting without protecting your ears can be extremely harmful. If you aren't willing to wear earplugs while in the woods, purchase a headset or earmuffs you can quickly pull on and off.

☐ Reduce noise at home and work with sound-absorbing materials. Put rubber mats under loud dishwashers, computer printers and typewriters. Hang heavy curtains at the windows and quilts, decorative rugs or blankets on the walls. Thick, plush carpets over dense padding absorbs indoor noises well. Storm windows or double-pane windows reduce outdoor noises.

☐ Break the habit of loudness. Get used to a lower volume when using the television set, stereo or headset. Don't use several noisy machines at once.

☐ Don't use loud noises to drown out other, unwelcome noises. Don't crank up the volume on the car radio to drown out traffic noises, or turn the TV volume up so that you can hear it over the vacuum cleaner.

☐ Get your hearing checked. You should have your hearing tested every year if you're regularly exposed to loud noises. Children should have their ears checked before they start kindergarten, especially if they have chronic ear infections or a family history of hearing problems.

No surgery or medical device can restore hearing loss due to loud noises, but if you think you're losing your hearing, you can take extra precautions to save the hearing you have left.

Medical Sources ———————————————
American Family Physician (47,5:1219)
Emergency Medicine (24,15:165)

Hear what you're missing with hearing aids

One out of every 10 Americans has some hearing loss, but many of us would rather live in a world of muffled sound than buy a hearing aid.

The Better Hearing Institute in Washington, D.C., reports that you probably have a hearing problem if you:

> ➤ Shout in conversations
> ➤ Turn the TV or radio too loud
> ➤ Ask people to repeat themselves
> ➤ Favor one ear
> ➤ Strain to hear

A hearing aid amplifies and shapes sound waves that enter your ear, and it can dramatically improve your quality of life and your ability to communicate. Here are some tips on where to buy hearing aids and what kinds are available.

Where to buy

Keep your ear to the ground for great deals on hearing aids, but don't get caught up in price if you're a first-time buyer.

You need to buy your first hearing aid from an otolaryngologist (an ear, nose and throat doctor) or an audiologist (a licensed professional trained to identify and measure hearing problems) even though it may cost you more than going to a hearing-aid dealer.

Dealers, even though they have a lot of practical experience in fitting hearing aids, can't tell you if you have a serious health problem that's causing your hearing loss or if you have a type of hearing loss that hearing aids won't help.

If you have totally lost the ability to hear certain frequencies, a hearing aid will not help you understand speech clearly again. It will only make the sounds you can hear louder. Hearing aids do help when you've partially lost the ability to hear certain frequencies.

If you have trouble distinguishing between D's and B's and between L's and R's, you probably have a problem with low frequencies and would not benefit from a hearing aid.

Audiologists will refer you to a physician if they suspect a health problem is causing your hearing loss. Deafness can be a symptom of middle ear disease, multiple sclerosis, a brain tumor and other serious illnesses.

A qualified audiologist will have a master's or doctoral degree in audiology, and a Certificate of Clinical Competence from the American Speech and Hearing Association. Check the telephone directory for a hearing specialist near you.

You can buy your hearing aid from a dealer if you first visit an audiologist or doctor to determine the type of hearing loss you have and to rule out hearing loss that can be treated medically or surgically.

Always visit a doctor if your ear is deformed (from birth or in an accident), if your ear drains fluids, if you lose your hearing suddenly, if you are dizzy, if you have excessive earwax, or if your ear hurts or is uncomfortable.

What kind to buy

The most popular hearing aid today is the easy-to-hide, in-the-ear type. However, if you don't have good vision and you're troubled by arthritis, the second-most popular type, the behind-the-ear aid, may be for you.

The in-the-ear type is so small that you need to be able to see and use your fingers well to insert and adjust it. Using a mirror may help.

When they don't work

Hearing aids don't always work perfectly. They make sounds louder, but they don't necessarily help you understand speech. The amplified sound may seem unnatural.

You will probably have to visit your doctor or hearing specialist several times before you're satisfied. Most hearing specialists will give you a 30-day free trial before you pay for the hearing aid.

If your hearing aid quits working, check the batteries first. Another common and easily-solved problem is a buildup of earwax in the ear or on the hearing aid itself.

Expect a period of adjustment. You will hear sounds differently once they are amplified by the hearing aid. Check your community activities center to see if programs for new hearing aid users are offered.

Medical Sources ————————————————
U.S. Pharmacist (18,4:101)
American Family Physician (46,3:851)

Help for the hard of hearing

Don't let hearing loss cut you off from the outside world. Many mechanical devices can improve your ability to communicate.

Try various brands before you purchase a piece of equipment. Some brands work better than others.

- ☐ Amplifiers for telephones, televisions, VCRs, dictating machines and microphones.
- ☐ Loud bells, buzzers and ringers for telephones, doorbells, security alarms and smoke alarms.

❏ Flashing lights, vibrating devices, fans and bed shakers for alarm clocks, doorbells and smoke alarms.

❏ Closed-caption television receivers, relay services, message centers and other devices to keep you informed.

You can learn more about these mechanical devices through local groups that assist the hearing-impaired or through national groups such as:

➤ **National Association of the Deaf**, 814 Thayer Avenue, Silver Spring, MD 20910 (telephone: 301-587-1788; telecommunication device for the deaf [TDD]: 301-587-1789).

➤ **Alexander Graham Bell Association for the Deaf**, 3417 Volta Place N.W., Washington, D.C. 20007 (telephone and TDD: 202-337-5220).

➤ **National Information Center on Deafness**, Gallaudet University, 800 Florida Avenue N.E., Washington, D.C. 20002-3625 (telephone: 202-651-5051; TDD: 202-651-5052).

Medical Source ————————————————————
American Family Physician (46,3:851)

Two tips for people with hearing problems

❏ When conversing, position yourself in a corner or some place where you have two walls behind you that can reflect sound. Cupping your hand around your ear and turning your ear in the direction of the speaker can also help.

❏ Check your community calendar for programs in lip reading and counseling. These are often useful in helping you cope with hearing problems.

Medical Source ————————————————————
Emergency Medicine (24,15:165)

Mouth and teeth problems

Simple steps to keep your teeth and gums healthy

Are you among the 25 percent who require 60 percent of the dental care? Even if you're not, you can still lower your risk of tooth decay and gum disease.

- ☐ Regular visits to your dentist are an important part of a preventive tooth decay plan. Your dentist can tell you if you are at high risk for tooth decay and make appropriate suggestions for lowering your risk.

- ☐ Dentists typically use fluorides to make teeth more resistant to plaque, the chief cause of tooth decay. If your community doesn't provide fluoridated water, your dentist can recommend the following fluoridated products: salt, milk, fluoride tablets or drops. Using fluoride toothpastes and mouthwashes are also excellent ways of increasing your teeth's resistance to plaque.

  Fluoride mouthwashes, if used regularly and for the exact amount of time recommended, are reported to reduce tooth decay by 20 to 50 percent. The best toothpastes and mouthwashes to use are those with maximum fluoride concentration.

  Ask your dentist for his recommendations. In addition to these fluoride treatments, your dentist may also give you fluoride treatments at his office.

- ☐ Many dentists recommend sealants for teeth that have recently come in and for teeth with numerous pits and cracks on the chewing surface. This treatment makes teeth more resistant to plaque by sealing them to prevent decay. Sealants can be expensive, but they will probably save you money in the long run by making other dental repairs unnecessary.

❑ Your dentist may also suggest that you reduce the amount of sugar in your diet to decrease the amount of plaque produced. You might want to try satisfying your sweet tooth with artificially sweetened snacks. If you do eat sugar, chewing sugarless gum for 15 minutes afterwards might reduce your risk of cavities.

❑ If you can't brush after every meal, rinse your mouth out with water. This helps get rid of food particles on your teeth. And, be sure to floss your teeth every day.

❑ Babies are also susceptible to "baby-bottle tooth decay." This is often caused by permitting a baby's teeth to be exposed for long periods of time to a bottle containing fruit juice, syrup, soft drinks or milk.

Medical Source ————————————————————
Journal of the American Dental Association (123,5:68)

Frozen fruit juice satisfies sweet tooth but promotes tooth decay

Christmas may not be the worst time of year for tooth decay anymore. The bad tooth fairy gleefully notes that a favorite tooth-rotting summer treat is gaining in popularity — frozen fruit juice. You can buy frozen fruit juice products or make your own at home.

This seemingly harmless and even healthy frozen treat is so acidic that it can dissolve your tooth enamel much more quickly than regular fruit juice. Plus, you have to hold the cold lump in your mouth until it melts, making matters worse for your teeth.

Researchers took some apple, grape, strawberry, apricot, pear, peach, orange and black-currant juice, froze them, then tested the juice that melted first. This juice was so acidic that your saliva, which normally protects your tooth enamel by neutralizing acid, would have to work overtime and still not get the job done.

Especially bad for your teeth is that irresistible habit of sucking the juice out of a frozen treat and throwing away the tasteless ice that's left. Try to eat the ice, too. It helps water down those strong fruit acids.

The researchers recommend that you don't make frozen fruit juice a daily summer treat. Drinking juice without freezing it first is better for your teeth.

Medical Source ————————————————————
Journal of Dentistry for Children (60,3:223)

Fight plaque with any type of dental floss

Regular flossing helps remove plaque between your gums that can lead to soreness and swelling.

So, which kind of dental floss should you use? Regular use of dental floss is more important than the type of dental floss you use.

Investigators found no significant differences in a five-week study between waxed, nylon floss made by Johnson and Johnson and Glide expanded polytetrafluoroethylene floss (PTFE) made by W.L. Gore. Both were equally effective in removing plaque and reducing gum swelling and bleeding.

The only difference that the investigators found was that almost 75 percent of the 57 people participating in the study preferred the PTFE floss because it didn't fray during flossing.

The best kind of dental floss is dental floss that is used.

Medical Source ————————————————————
Clinical Preventive Dentistry (14,3:14)

Artificial sweetener might help prevent tooth decay

Artificial sweeteners satisfy our cravings for sweets without the risk of extra pounds or cavities associated with sugar. One artificial sweetener, xylitol, seems to actually help prevent tooth decay.

Studies indicate that small amounts of xylitol can effectively reduce tooth decay. Xylitol, like other artificial sweeteners, helps remineralize tooth enamel, making it more resistant to plaque.

Xylitol also stimulates the secretion of saliva which reduces the number of bacteria in the mouth, which, in turn, leads to a reduction in plaque formation.

Xylitol also seems to make fluoride toothpastes more efficient.

Fruits and vegetables such as plums, raspberries, strawberries, endive, cauliflower and eggplant naturally contain small amounts of xylitol. For commercial use, it is extracted from birch tree bark.

Since xylitol is the most expensive of the artificial sweeteners, it will most likely be used only in gums, hard candies and toothpastes. Less expensive sweeteners will still be needed to sweeten products such as soft drinks, jellies and ice creams.

Medical Source ───────────────────────────────
Journal of the American Dental Association (111,5:745 and 123,5:68)

Mouthwashes help reduce plaque

Want to save yourself some money this year? Then head over to the drugstore and pick up a toothbrush, toothpaste, dental floss and plaque-fighting mouthwash.

Researchers say that mouthwashes play an important part in dental care.

Recognized before only as a way to freshen breath, some mouthwashes actually reduce plaque — the number one cause of tooth decay and gum disease.

Plaque is a soft, sticky coating invisible to the naked eye which gives teeth that furry, unbrushed feeling. It's made up of saliva, bacteria and bits of food. It forms mostly during the night, and, if not removed in 24 hours, it hardens into tartar.

Tartar is difficult to remove and usually must be done during a professional cleaning. Plaque and tartar together cause tooth and gum disease.

Gum disease can range from gingivitis, in which the gums become infected, tender and swollen, to periodontitis, in which the tissue and bone that support the teeth start to erode. If untreated, the teeth will loosen and fall out. The best way to avoid these problems is to keep plaque from building up.

Researchers speculate that mouthwashes work by decreasing the amount of bacteria in the mouth.

Fewer bacteria mean that less plaque can be produced, which leads to fewer cavities and less gum disease.

Not all mouthwashes work, however, and some are too irritating for regular use. The ingredients that make up a mouthwash determine its effectiveness against plaque.

- ☐ One effective plaque fighter is cetylpyridinium chloride, found in the mouthwash Cepacol. One two-week study found that people who used a cetylpyridinium chloride mouthwash for 15 seconds before breakfast and after dinner decreased their plaque formation by half.
- ☐ Fluoride, found in the mouthwash Listermint with fluoride, is also effective in reducing plaque. In addition, fluoride strengthens tooth enamel and makes it more resistant to plaque.
- ☐ Sanguinarine, also known as the "Nigerian chewing stick" because it was often used by African cultures to clean teeth, does a good job reducing and preventing plaque formation. It also makes plaque more visible so that it is easier to remove. Sanguinarine is the main ingredient in Viadent mouthwash. Continue to brush your teeth regularly when using a mouthwash containing sanguinarine. Otherwise a yellowish-brown stain may develop on your teeth.
- ☐ Volatile oils, which include thymol, eucalyptol, menthol and methyl salicylate — the combination found in Listerine mouthwash, fight plaque very effectively. Volatile oil mouthwashes also work well in controlling gingivitis.
- ☐ Chlorhexidine gluconate, found in Peridex, is effective against plaque and is also used to treat gingivitis. It currently can be used only under a doctor's supervision.
- ☐ Researchers are investigating the plaque-fighting action of hydrogen peroxide, carbamide peroxide and phenolic compounds. Phenolic compounds are reported to reduce gingivitis by 25 to 35 percent.

Here are a few tips to help you get the best results from your mouthwash:

- ☐ Do not use a mouthwash if your mouth is irritated or has sores.

❒ Do not use a mouthwash that continues to irritate your mouth.

❒ Do not swallow mouthwash.

❒ Keep mouthwash out of the reach of children — its high alcohol content can be deadly.

❒ Use mouthwash twice a day for 30 seconds each time.

❒ Use one to two tablespoons unless mouthwash instructions or your dentist tells you otherwise.

❒ Circulate the mouthwash throughout your entire mouth, especially between your teeth.

❒ Do not eat, drink or smoke for at least 30 minutes after using mouthwash.

If you're uncertain about the mouthwash that's best for you, ask your pharmacist or dentist for his recommendations.

Medical Source ───────────────────────
U.S. Pharmacist (17,12:27)

Effective tips to slay 'dragon breath'

If people turn their faces away or wrinkle their noses when you come close for a private chat—you may need to "Scope out" this news about bad breath.

One of the top causes of bad breath is mouth dryness. Normally, your mouth cleans itself with a constant flow of saliva. When you don't have enough saliva, food particles and bacteria don't get washed away properly.

Below are some effective tips to help you slay your "dragon breath."

❒ Chew sugar-free gum. Chewing gum does more than just briefly freshen your breath. It helps get your juices flowing and prevents dry mouth. Chewing gum also makes you move your jaws and mouth. The movement works with saliva to get rid of food particles and other debris that may be causing your bad breath.

❒ Don't regularly use deodorizing sprays or antiseptic mouthwashes like Listerine or Scope unless your dentist recommends it to help control gum disease. Using a mouthwash daily can actually make your bad breath worse by upsetting your mouth's delicate balances and drying out your mouth. Mouthwashes and deodorants will only temporarily cover up bad breath.

☐ Drink plenty of water. Water will help keep your mouth clean and odor-free. If you can't brush your teeth after a meal, swish water around in your mouth to wash away food particles. Other beverages, especially coffee and alcohol, tend to linger unpleasantly on your breath. After your body absorbs beer, whiskey or wine, your lungs spend hours trying to get rid of it.

☐ Don't eat garlic if you have an important meeting later in the day or early the next morning. Garlic may be good for you, but it definitely stays on your breath. Onions, garlic and heavy spices are absorbed by your body and released through your lungs.

☐ Brush your tongue. Your tongue can contribute to bad breath by gathering food particles and bacteria. If your tongue becomes coated or furry, gently brush it when you brush your teeth. But don't get carried away — some people have brushed off taste buds and injured their tongues by brushing them too hard and too often.

☐ Relax. You may have noticed that you have a problem with bad breath right when you want to make the best impression, such as during a job interview or when you're meeting your future in-laws for the first time. Anxiety or stress can cause a dry mouth and bad breath.

☐ Clean your dentures regularly and soak them in a denture cleaner at night.

☐ Kick the smoking habit. The smell of cigarette smoke is offensive to most people, and smoking causes dry mouth.

☐ Breathe through your nose at night. Mouth-breathing usually makes "morning breath" worse because it dries out your mouth even more than usual. At night, your mouth moves very little and doesn't make much saliva, so food particles and bacteria tend to stay put. These particles break down while you sleep and cause morning breath. This is why it's so important to brush your teeth thoroughly at bedtime.

☐ Finally, make sure your bad breath isn't all in your head. Doctors have found that an amazing number of people, particularly depressed people, think they have bad breath when they really don't. To test your own breath, cup your hands in front of your mouth, breathe out through your mouth and in through your nose. If you have halitosis (the medical term for bad breath), you'll know it right away.

Bad breath that never goes away may be more than embarrassing. It could be a sign of a serious health problem that needs a doctor's care.

Something as simple as sinusitis can cause bad breath, and treatment with antibiotics may be all you need. Or, bad breath could indicate something as serious as diabetes, kidney or liver failure, a lung infection or Sjögren's syndrome (a chronic inflammatory disease in which collagen — the connective tissue in skin, ligaments, cartilage and the mouth and gums — breaks down). A mouth ulcer or infection, gum disease or a dry socket left after you've had a tooth pulled also can be culprits behind bad breath.

Some prescription drugs, such as antidepressants or medication for angina pectoris, can cause your breath to smell bad. Many of these drugs cause dry mouth which can lead to bad breath. You can defeat the effects of these drugs by drinking more water.

If your breath constantly smells sweet and fruity or like ammonia or urine, see your doctor. This could signal serious medical problems.

Medical Source ————————————————————
Dental Update (20,2:57)

Giving gum disease the brush

Giving gum disease the brush-off is not hard if you practice good oral hygiene, identify your risk factors, watch for warning signs and visit your dentist at least once a year for a professional cleaning.

If plaque and tartar build up and are not properly removed, you may develop gingivitis or periodontitis. Gingivitis is caused by a buildup of plaque and tartar along the gum line.

Untreated gingivitis will eventually lead to periodontitis. This happens when the built up plaque and tartar move below the gum line. If left alone, they will destroy the tissue and bone supporting your teeth until your teeth loosen and fall out.

Correct brushing is essential to remove plaque and tartar. Try these brushing tips:

- ❏ Choose a toothbrush with soft, round ends or polished bristles. It should be small enough to reach and clean every tooth.
- ❏ Use fluoride toothpaste.
- ❏ Brush every morning and every evening before bedtime.
- ❏ To effectively remove plaque and tartar, brush with short sideways strokes, then with up-and-down strokes. Brush the back of your teeth with vertical strokes.
- ❏ To clean the groove between your teeth and gums (a good place for bacteria to settle and multiply), hold your brush at a 45-degree angle to the outer surfaces of your teeth.

Flossing is also important because it removes the plaque and food particles between the teeth and along the gum line that brushing often misses. Flossing tips:

> - ➤ Use either waxed or unwaxed floss. Both work well.
> - ➤ Pull off about 18 inches of floss and wrap the ends around each index finger, stretching floss tight.
> - ➤ Insert the floss between two teeth.
> - ➤ Bend the floss around each tooth in a sideways "U" shape. With an up-and-down motion, rub the sides of the teeth, pushing the floss into the gum line, but only until you feel a slight resistance. Pushing too hard can damage your gums.

Some risk factors for gum disease include:

- ❏ **Heredity** — Genes influence your gums' susceptibility to decay-causing bacteria. You may want to look into your family's history of tooth decay to determine your genetic risk.
- ❏ **Medicines** — Some over-the-counter and prescription drugs decrease saliva and cause a dry feeling in your mouth. Without sufficient saliva, plaque and tartar build up more rapidly.
- ❏ **Alcohol** — Drinking alcohol can also reduce your saliva and cause

more plaque and tartar buildup.

☐ **Smoking** — Smoking slows your gums' ability to replace tissue destroyed by bacteria, resulting in a longer healing time.

☐ **Hormonal changes** — Hormonal changes, such as those that occur in pregnant women and diabetics, can make teeth and gums more vulnerable to plaque.

☐ **Extended illness** — Being sick for long periods of time weakens your immune system, making you more susceptible to infections, which can lead to gum disease.

Schedule an immediate trip to the dentist if you suffer from one or more of the following.

> ➤ Gums feel sore and soft, swell up, and/or bleed easily.
> ➤ Breath regularly smells bad. This may be accompanied by an unpleasant taste in the mouth.
> ➤ Gums change color from pink or brown to a reddish-purple color.
> ➤ Teeth's roots become exposed due to receding gums.
> ➤ Pus pockets develop between teeth.
> ➤ Bite shifts.
> ➤ Teeth feel loose.

Dentists check for gum disease by measuring the depth of your sulcus (groove between gum and teeth) and/or by X-raying your teeth.

Your dentist will check the sulcus at various points in your mouth. Sulcus deeper than 1/8" indicates infection pockets. The deeper the infection pocket, the more serious the gum disease. Dentists use X-rays to reveal bone loss, also a good indicator of gum disease.

Gingivitis usually clears up after a professional cleaning if it is followed by good daily oral hygiene. If your gingivitis has developed into periodontitis, you may require scaling and root planing or antibiotic therapy.

Scaling involves the use of a sharp scraping instrument or an ultrasonic device with a high speed vibrating tip to remove tartar and bacteria from your teeth and from under your gums.

If root planing is also necessary, then tartar will be removed from the root surface, and the root surface will be smoothed.

Antibiotics are also used to treat mild periodontitis. Researchers can now identify specific bacteria that help cause gum and tooth decay. Your dentist may prescribe specific antibiotics to knock out those troublesome bacteria.

Several surgical options are available to treat advanced periodontitis.

> ➤ Flap surgery—To make scaling and planing more effective, the affected tooth's root is exposed by surgically folding up a flap of gum.
> ➤ Bone grafting — Sterilized bone fragments or coral pieces are used to replace destroyed bone so your teeth will stay securely in place.
> ➤ Guided tissue regeneration — New bone is encouraged to form by placing "biocompatible" material between your tooth and the existing bone.

Researchers continue to study new ways to prevent dental decay.

Antibiotics may soon be applied directly to infection pockets instead of being given by mouth, thereby avoiding unpleasant side effects.

Another procedure under consideration involves the measurement of enzymes whose presence indicates that gum disease is in progress. This method would give dentists time to stop gum disease in its early stages.

You can meet the future with your own bright smile, even without these new developments, if you follow a good oral hygiene program and watch for early warning signs of gum disease.

Medical Source ——————————————————
Mayo Clinic Health Letter (12,12:4)

How to comfort sensitive teeth

Do your teeth shudder at the sight of food or scream when they see a toothbrush? If so, you may be among the 40 million Americans who suffer from sensitive teeth.

Fluid-filled tubes run from the outside of your teeth to the inside nerves.

The outside openings of these tubes are normally closed off by a protective layer.

If this layer is eroded, various irritants can cause movement of the fluid which stretches or compresses the tooth's nerves — causing pain.

These particular toothaches are often triggered by hot or cold air, pressure on teeth, or by consuming hot, cold, sweet or sour foods or drinks.

Teeth most commonly affected are the canines (the sharply pointed teeth near the front of your mouth), sometimes referred to as eye teeth. The premolars, directly behind the canines, are also a frequent site of pain.

There are several situations which can temporarily erode the protective layer and cause sensitivity.

Discomfort following a routine dental cleaning is common but will usually disappear after a few days.

If you've undergone a more complicated procedure, such as root planing (removal of plaque and tartar buildup on your teeth roots), it may take 14 to 20 days for your teeth to feel normal again. If you wear braces, expect periods of soreness.

Acids commonly erode the protective layer over the fluid-filled tubes. Most of your teeth's exposure to acid comes from food and drinks.

Listed in order of acidity are some of the substances that can erode the protective layer:

> Ginger ale
> Limes & lemons
> Wine
> Cranberry sauce
> Coffee
> Vinegar
> Pickles
> Cola
> Citrus drinks
> Apples
> Rhubarb

Don't brush your teeth immediately after eating acidic foods. Teeth can be very sensitive at that time, and brushing may make the pain worse.

Certain jobs are associated with increased teeth sensitivity. Approximately 23 percent of people working in chemical plants experienced dental hypersensitivity believed to be caused by exposure to vapors that erode the teeth's protective layer.

Obesity and pregnancy are often associated with acid reflux, which causes stomach acid to back up into the esophagus. This may result in increased tooth sensitivity.

You can also erode your teeth's protective layer and cause your gums to recede by brushing too hard.

If you have the unshakable habit of hard brushing, follow these toothbrushing tips to make your teeth less tender:

❑ Use the softest brush you can buy.
❑ Brush only twice a day. Do not use extremely abrasive toothpastes.

You may want to brush with special toothpastes designed for sensitive teeth. The only FDA-approved active ingredient for such toothpastes at this time is potassium nitrate.

Toothpastes that contain potassium nitrate as their active ingredient include Denquel Sensitive Teeth, Promise with Fluoride, Sensodyne-F and Sensodyne Mint.

The following guidelines will help you get the best results from these toothpastes.

❑ Apply a one-inch strip of toothpaste to your brush.
❑ Brush for at least one minute in the morning and again in the evening.
❑ Pay attention to sensitive areas.

Children under 12 should not use these toothpastes — some do not contain fluoride.

Sensitive teeth can cause other problems besides pain. If your teeth keep you from eating, you could develop nutritional deficiencies.

If your sensitive teeth cause you to neglect regular brushing, flossing and trips to the dentist, you may have serious dental problems later.

If your teeth are sensitive for more than four weeks, see your dentist.

Other problems may be causing your tooth sensitivity.

Medical Source ————————————————
   U.S. Pharmacist (18,1:29)

Make toothache pains bite the bullet

Have a toothache that's a real pain? The ancient Roman scholar Pliny the Elder suggested scratching those painful gums "with the tooth of a man who has suffered a violent death." To avoid future toothaches he recommended eating two mice a month.

But if you're not sure you can swallow this advice, an even better suggestion is to make an immediate trip to the dentist. If you have to wait a couple of days for your dental appointment, here are some toothache remedies from medical specialists that you can try at home.

As an alternative to medicated pain relief, you may want to try ice massage. There is no guarantee you'll get results, but it is safe with no side effects.

- ❏ Massage the back of either hand between the thumb and forefinger with ice.
- ❏ Massage the arm near the elbow on the opposite side of the pain with ice.
- ❏ You may also want to try a normal dose of the standard painkillers: aspirin, acetaminophen or ibuprofen. Do not place aspirin directly on or even near the affected area. It won't help the pain, and it can irritate the lining of your mouth.

Being able to identify the cause of your toothache and the type of pain you're experiencing will help you choose the best toothache medicine for you.

Sources of toothache:

- ❏ Breakdown of tooth enamel, the hard outer layer that covers and protects inner structures
- ❏ Cracked teeth
- ❏ Infected or irritated pulp, the soft tissue in the middle of each tooth that

contains the nerves and blood vessels — the "life center" of a tooth

- ❑ Pulp that contains excessive amounts of blood
- ❑ Temperature changes
- ❑ Electrical shock — as when a tooth filling comes into contact with a piece of aluminum
- ❑ Infection
- ❑ Pain that has its origin in the eyes or ears may be felt in the teeth. This occurs when different parts of the body are served by the same nerve. Sensations reaching the brain from one of these areas may feel like it comes from the other. A pain in one tooth can also cause another tooth to feel pain.

Certain disorders can also cause toothache:

- ❑ Malaria
- ❑ Leukemia
- ❑ Flu
- ❑ Sinus infection. If your teeth hurt when you clench them, you could have a sinus infection. Pain is worse in the morning or when the head is tilted.
- ❑ Menstruation, pregnancy and menopause may also make the teeth feel more sensitive than usual.

Toothaches, like many other types of pain, can vary with a person's emotional and mental state. Toothache pain is not the same as teeth that are overly sensitive.

Real toothaches arise from problems with the pulp. Some pulp damage is reversible. It is characterized by intermittent pain. Irreversible pulp damage is signaled by constant throbbing pain.

If neither aspirin, acetaminophen, ibuprofen or ice massage relieves your toothache, you may want to try some over-the-counter toothache products.

Suggestions for using over-the-counter toothache remedies:

- ❑ Carefully follow product instructions. Misused medicines can damage healthy pulp and dentin, the bonelike tissues that surround and protect the pulp.

❑ Do not use with children under two years; supervise children under 12 who use an over-the-counter toothache remedy.

❑ Use only for pain that is caused by an open tooth cavity.

❑ Use only for continuous throbbing pain. Using for intermittent pain can permanently damage the pulp and may necessitate a root canal.

❑ Do not use for more than seven consecutive days unless so advised by a doctor or dentist.

❑ Stop using product if irritation continues or if swelling, redness or fever develops.

❑ Before buying toothache relief medicine, tell the pharmacist what type of pain you're having, as well as what you think may be causing the pain, and get her recommendations.

Be sure to see your dentist as soon as possible whether or not the pain goes away. Waiting will more than likely only make the problem worse and the cost of treatment higher.

Medical Source ————————————————————
U.S. Pharmacist (17,11:26)

Coping strategies for canker sores and fever blisters

Can't eat, can't drink, can't bear to talk? Does your tongue bounce around in your mouth to check out all its sore spots?

If you feel mouth ulcers have settled in for a siege, medical authorities suggest coping strategies for two common ulcers, the canker sore and fever blister.

More than 80 percent of recurring mouth ulcers are canker sores. They affect men and women equally and may develop at any age.

Although these ulcers are not serious disorders or contagious, they can be very painful.

Below are some symptoms of canker sores:

❑ Sores may develop on the tip of your tongue or inside the linings of your cheeks and lips.

☐ Canker sores create a round, shallow hole about one-half inch wide, which is usually surrounded by a red border.

☐ The inside of the ulcer appears whitish-yellow.

☐ They don't form blisters and generally don't grow together.

☐ After seven to 14 days, these ulcers generally heal without scarring.

Doctors don't agree on one particular cause of canker sores, but some possibilities include stress; viral or bacterial infections; food allergies; mouth injury caused by dental work or brushing teeth too vigorously; or nutritional deficiencies of iron, vitamin B12, folic acid or zinc.

If both your parents have had canker sores, your chances of getting them are high — about 9 in 10. If neither of your parents had them, there is only a 1-in-10 chance that you will. Nothing seems to cure canker sores except time.

The first three or four days are painful, and local pain might be accompanied by an overall feeling of achiness, fatigue and fever.

However, there are some over-the-counter medications that will relieve pain and shorten a canker sore's natural life span. These include wound-cleaning products that contain carbamide peroxide or hydrogen peroxide.

Pain relievers containing benzocaine also can be helpful although these products should not be used for longer than seven days.

Applying a topical anesthetic (Anbesol, etc.) mixed with water as an oral rinse will provide quick relief, and covering the ulcers with an over-the-counter dental protective paste or gel will prevent trauma from eating or talking until the ulcers heal.

Listed below are some foods you should avoid if you have canker sores:

➤ pineapple and citrus fruits, such as oranges, grapefruit and lemons

➤ chocolate

➤ spicy foods

➤ foods with sharp edges, such as potato chips and crackers

➤ colas and juices (Try using a straw when drinking these beverages to prevent the substances from touching the canker sore and making pain worse.)

Below are some symptoms of a fever blister or cold sore:

☐ They are often preceded by swelling or a feeling of tightness, soreness or burning in the general area where the ulcer develops.
☐ They may occur on your lips, gums, roof of your mouth or nose.
☐ These sores may burst and grow together to form large sores that produce fluid.
☐ The skin may also crack or separate.
☐ Scabs form and healing generally occurs in 10 to 14 days with no scarring.

Fever blisters are caused by the herpes simplex virus type 1, which has an average incubation period of seven days.

Once you are exposed to and infected with the virus, attacks may continue throughout life, although you are less likely to be affected after age 35.

The virus lodges deep within a nerve between fever blister outbreaks and cannot be destroyed. You may reduce your risk of future fever blisters if you avoid conditions that tend to reactivate the virus.

Tanning booths, overexposure to sunlight, stress, excitement, exhaustion, extreme cold, windburn, fever, illness, injury, dental work and menstruation may trigger the virus.

Fever blisters are contagious. Once infected, you can transmit the virus to other people or objects other people might touch. To avoid transmitting the virus, do not touch the sores; do not kiss others; do not share drinking glasses or straws.

Some simple tips for relief of fever blisters include:

☐ Over-the-counter products that contain benzocaine, camphor or menthol will help ease the discomfort.
☐ Medicines that contain phenol help destroy bacteria and prevent infection.
☐ Petroleum jelly and cocoa butter can relieve pain, soften skin and prevent the cracking that often accompanies fever blisters.

If you have numerous ulcers (100 or so) throughout your mouth or if any ulcer recurs often, persists longer than three weeks or leaves scars, see your doctor. Occasionally, ulcers signal serious underlying problems.

Medical Source ————————————————
  U.S. Pharmacist (18,5:37)

JOINTS AND MUSCLES

Arthritis: easing the pain

If you suffer from joint pain, a combination of exercise, physical therapy and pain relievers may be all you need to get you back into the swing of things.

Knowing what type of arthritis you have can help you live more comfortably.

Osteoarthritis is far more common than rheumatoid arthritis. It causes the cartilage between the joints to degenerate, causing pain, stiffness and, occasionally, loss of function in the affected joint. Joints that experience the most wear — your neck, lower back, knees and hips — are most commonly affected.

If osteoarthritis has you feeling out of joint, here are some suggestions to get you back in shape.

- ❑ Get fit and stay fit. Regular exercise, such as swimming in a heated pool, or physical therapy helps alleviate pain, increases mobility and prevents muscle loss. Exercise and physical therapy can improve your cardiovascular condition and your mental outlook as well.
- ❑ Watch your posture. People with poor posture run a higher risk of developing OA.
- ❑ Establish good eating habits. Obesity puts greater stress on your joints, while eating healthy, balanced meals will provide you with strength and energy.
- ❑ Use canes or walkers. This technique, called joint unloading, takes pressure off the affected joint which, in turn, reduces pain. You might also ask your doctor about relieving pain with braces or insoles.

    If you're a regular cane user, try expanding the cane's grip area with a firm yet spongy material. Gripping a hard, narrow cane head can make your fingers stiff and painful. It may eventually cause "trigger finger," in which one or more fingers become locked in a bent position and can only be straightened with considerable force. A larger grip will help prevent this problem.

☐ Try pain relievers. Capsaicin cream, distributed under the name of Zostrix, seems effective in relieving pain associated with osteoarthritis and rheumatoid arthritis. Applied locally to the painful area, capsaicin is absorbed through the skin and works by deadening local nerves. It has no serious side effects and may be helpful during intensely painful periods of osteoarthritis.

Another useful and safe pain reliever is acetaminophen. Available over-the-counter, it is widely distributed under the name of Tylenol. Acetaminophen and capsaicin used together can provide extra relief.

☐ Check with your doctor about corticosteroid injections. Studies have shown that these drugs provide only short-term relief. Researchers are currently experimenting with other compounds that may provide more long-term benefits, but none are yet available in the United States.

☐ Consider joint replacement therapy. It effectively alleviates pain and restores function to the affected joint. Normally, doctors recommend putting off this procedure for as long as possible. If advanced osteoarthritis requires surgery, over 90 percent of people undergoing the operation experience excellent results.

Rheumatoid arthritis, a disease in which your immune system runs out of control, is far more serious. Although it can affect your whole body, it particularly strikes your joints.

This form of arthritis often starts with fatigue, followed by inflammation and swelling of the synovium, a membrane that surrounds your joints. RA usually develops on both sides of your body, striking your wrists, hands, feet and knees most often.

RA can also affect your heart, lungs and blood vessels. In rare cases, RA can even twist or deform your joints. The cause of rheumatoid arthritis is unknown.

People with RA often feel depressed because they believe they are powerless against the disease. However, you can control the symptoms, and there are treatments available that actually stop the progress of RA in many people.

The building blocks of a program to treat RA include:

> ➤ Education — to help you understand RA.
> ➤ Rest — either for your whole body or for your sore joints. Your doctor or physical therapist may recommend splints to rest certain joints when you're not exercising them.
> ➤ Physical therapy — to help you keep the muscles around the joints strong and to keep your joints working well.
> ➤ Occupational therapy — to help you learn how to manage at home and work and how to protect your joints.
> ➤ NSAIDs (Nonsteroidal Anti-Inflammatory Drugs) — such as over-the-counter or prescription strength ibuprofen to control pain and inflammation in your joints.

Your doctor may also need to prescribe drugs to help stop the progress of rheumatoid arthritis. People with rheumatoid arthritis can live longer, healthier lives with the help of new treatments.

Try to relax and avoid stressful situations. Stress might cause RA to flare up. Married people with RA suffer less disability than single people with RA, probably because of the support offered by a spouse.

Apparently, even your family situation can affect how well you live with your rheumatoid arthritis.

If you suspect that you have rheumatoid arthritis or osteoarthritis, talk to your doctor. He can give you more information about caring for your joint problems.

If you have trouble remembering all your questions about exercise and medication, write them down and take them with you to your appointment. With your doctor's help and support from your family and friends, you'll be able to live a more active life with osteoarthritis or rheumatoid arthritis.

Medical Sources ————————————————
> *Postgraduate Medicine* (93,1:89)
> *The Physician and Sportsmedicine* (21,2:31)
> *Health Gazette* (16,3:3)

Try exercise to decrease arthritis pain and improve mobility

If arthritis is your excuse for not exercising, you'd better think of a new one. Regular exercise can decrease pain and improve mobility in people with osteoarthritis or rheumatoid arthritis no matter what their age or level of fitness.

Rheumatoid arthritis progressively destroys joints, causing them to become stiff, sore and even deformed. Exercise helps people with rheumatoid arthritis maintain joint mobility.

Osteoarthritis causes degeneration of the cartilage that lines your joints. It most commonly affects weight-bearing joints, such as the knees. Exercise helps people with osteoarthritis gain strength. This often means they can reduce the amount of painkillers and nonsteroidal anti-inflammatory drugs (NSAIDs) they take.

Other benefits of regular exercise include stronger muscles and connective tissues, increased flexibility and bone mass and a higher aerobic fitness level.

Ask your doctor or physical therapist to help you set up a realistic exercise program, taking into account your age, arthritis severity and possible areas of injury. Try to develop a program that considers your interests and incorporates a variety of exercises. You're more likely to stick with exercise you enjoy.

Whatever type of arthritis you have, begin exercising slowly and increase your pace gradually. The type and severity of your arthritis may dictate how far and how quickly you proceed.

Although you can expect some muscle soreness, pain should generally subside when you stop exercising. If pain continues into the next day, you've probably overdone it.

When that happens, back off a little and then slowly build back up. It is important to keep exercising and not stop completely. You may want to try exercising in a warm pool until the pain stops.

If your arthritis flares up, modify your exercise program, but don't stop exercising. You can lose strength and mobility if you stop completely. Anti-inflammatory drugs can relieve the pain so that you can continue to exercise during flare-ups.

The following types of exercises will slowly improve your flexibility and strength without causing joint damage.

☐ Range of motion exercises put your joints through the widest range of movements possible. There are two types, passive and active. Passive range of motion exercises improve flexibility but do not involve the use of the muscles surrounding the affected joint. For example, you would use your right hand to move your left wrist through all possible movements. You would generally do 10 to 15 repetitions once or twice a day.
Active range of motion exercises improve strength and involve the use of the muscles surrounding the affected joint. You may begin these exercises once pain and inflammation subside. Begin with two or three of these exercises and progress to 10.

☐ Stretching exercises improve your flexibility. Stretching lengthens, loosens and relaxes muscles.

☐ Isometric exercises don't involve joint movement, and they are a good way to build up and maintain strength without causing further damage. An example is pressing palm to palm or palm to wall. Isometric exercises are especially important for people with rheumatoid arthritis.

☐ Isotonic exercises, such as weight lifting, sit ups and water exercises, help to preserve and increase strength. You may advance to isotonic exercises if you have no pain or inflammation and have built up sufficient strength.

To avoid causing any joint damage, start with low weights and increase them slowly. If you do leg lifts or knee stretches with weights, start with one pound, adding a pound each week until you have reached 10 pounds. You may want to try a resistance training machine if your arthritis is not severe and you have no joint deformities.

❐ Aerobic exercises will keep your whole body healthy and should be done for at least 30 minutes three times a week. Swimming, stationary bicycling and exercising on cross-country skiing and rowing machines put the least stress on joints.

Walking, bicycling, dancing, skating, cross-country skiing, gardening, table tennis, bowling, golf and jogging are all acceptable if you experience little or no pain. If you have joints with ligament tears or cartilage damage, do not walk or jog. Basketball, volleyball and other sports that involve jumping may aggravate arthritis.

Check with your doctor to find the right exercise program for you. The Arthritis Foundation in Atlanta (1-800-283-7800) can also provide you with additional information.

In treating and controlling the pain of arthritis, a little exercise can go a long way.

Tips for staying on top of your exercise program

Once you and your doctor have decided on a safe routine, make your exercise program part of your weekly schedule. Here are a few hints to help you avoid injury while exercising.

❐ Have your doctor or physical therapist demonstrate exercises they've recommended. Try the exercises yourself before leaving the office.

❐ Use smooth, not jerky, movements when exercising.

❐ Alternate joints that you exercise to prevent overstress. For example, work your upper body 10 minutes, then exercise your lower body 10 minutes.

❐ Limit the number of strengthening and stretching exercises that you do.

- [ ] Don't compete with others. Exercise at a pace that is comfortable for you.
- [ ] Modify your exercise program if you have pain for several hours or the next day, if you feel unusually tired, weak or stiff or if any joints turn red and swell.

Exercise often means less arthritis pain in the long run, but the pain that accompanies arthritis can be a powerful obstacle to getting started. Try these tricks to sidestep pain.

- [ ] Exercise immediately after a hot bath or shower. Pain is often least noticeable then. You may want to apply ice or warm compresses to sore areas or take a pain reliever such as acetaminophen or ibuprofen. Pain relievers may be needed less often as you become accustomed to your exercise routine.
- [ ] Try exercising in the morning if you have osteoarthritis and in the evening if you have rheumatoid arthritis.

If you're not used to exercising regularly, try these tips to keep yourself on track.

- [ ] Make a list of exercises you plan to do.
- [ ] Try a combination of exercises, such as weight lifting, swimming, bicycling and walking. Variety will keep you interested in exercising.
- [ ] Involve your family.
- [ ] Ask a friend to exercise with you.
- [ ] Try group exercise, such as water aerobics.
- [ ] Exercise to music.

Using the right equipment can add to your enjoyment in addition to preventing injury.

- [ ] For walking, jogging or aerobics, wear supportive, well-cushioned shoes. A cane or walker may be helpful if you have arthritis of the hip or knee. Knee immobilizers and back braces can also be useful. Exercise on surfaces that have some give, such as unpaved trails or boardwalks for walking or jogging and floor mats for aerobics.

☐ Swim with a snorkel and mask to avoid having to turn your head if you have arthritis in your back.

☐ Try the special handles available for gardening tools, rackets and golf clubs. If arthritis affects your hand and wrist, a splint may help.

Let your doctor know about any unusual pain or problems you experience.

Medical Source ───────────────────────
The Physician and Sportsmedicine (21,4:104)

Women: Slash your risk of osteoarthritis

If you're a woman, you're going to develop arthritis as you get older, and you'll just have to learn to live with it, right?

Wrong, say the authors of current medical studies.

It is true that the majority of people with arthritis are older females. But one authority on the subject says that there are 100 different kinds of "arthritis," and the disease can strike men and women of all ages.

One form of arthritis that is particularly troubling for women is osteoarthritis of the knee. This painful and disabling form of arthritis sometimes even forces people to resort to surgical replacement of the knee joint for relief.

Women who become overweight as they grow older greatly increase their risk of osteoarthritis of the knee. If you are overweight, losing as few as 11 pounds will slash your risk of developing arthritis of the knee by more than half.

Suppose you already have arthritis of the knee? In the past your doctor probably would have advised that you avoid weight-bearing exercise. However, new findings challenge that advice.

Arthritis sufferers who joined a patient-education class and tried a program of supervised-fitness walking with light stretching and strengthening exercises felt no increase in the painful symptoms of arthritis. In addition, these women were able to use less pain medicine and felt happier and less tense.

The message to women is clear: Losing those extra pounds can help prevent osteoarthritis of the knee.

And if you already have this painful condition, participating in an appropriate exercise program can help you live more comfortably.

Before starting an exercise program, consider these precautions:

- ❏ Talk with your doctor about the right exercise program for you.
- ❏ Don't exercise if you have any inflammation.
- ❏ Try breathing exercises. Inhale and exhale slowly while you stretch.
- ❏ Don't push yourself too hard. Let pain be your warning to stop.
- ❏ Try taking a warm shower or bath just before you exercise. It can help relax your joints and muscles.

Medical Sources ———————————————————

Annals of Internal Medicine (116,7:529, 535)
The Johns Hopkins Medical Letter, Health After 50 (4,4:6)

Smoking linked to arthritis

Lighting up a cigarette may set your joints on fire later.

In the first study to link arthritis to smoking, a Finnish research team reports that smoking seems to increase men's chances of developing rheumatoid arthritis.

After studying more than 57,000 men and women, the researchers found men who smoke to be eight times more likely to develop rheumatoid arthritis than men who do not smoke.

Ex-smokers are four times more likely to develop this condition than men who have never smoked. If you already have rheumatoid arthritis, smoking may aggravate the symptoms. Women who smoke do not appear to have an increased risk of developing this disorder.

Rheumatoid arthritis is the most severe form of joint disease. It occurs when a person's body attacks its own joints and surrounding tissues. Finger, wrist, toe, shoulder, neck, hip, knee or other joints then become red, warm, painful, swollen, stiff and, in severe cases, deformed.

Researchers speculate that exposure to tobacco smoke may trigger the production of rheumatoid factor. This substance is found in 50 to 95 percent of adults diagnosed with rheumatoid arthritis. When rheumatoid factor combines with male hormones, it may contribute to the development of rheumatoid arthritis.

An estimated 15 million men worldwide have rheumatoid arthritis. This number might be reduced to two million if all men were nonsmokers.

Medical Source ——————————————————
   Medical Tribune (34,1:13)

Fish oil — relief for achy, arthritic joints?

If you have arthritis, fish oils may be beneficial for you. These oils contain omega-3 fatty acids and are available in some cold-water fish.

Researchers speculate that these acids help suppress your body's production of prostaglandins, which have been linked to the inflammation that accompanies arthritis.

Fish oil supplements are available over-the-counter, but you should not begin taking them until you talk to your doctor. These supplements may decrease blood clotting ability, raise vitamin A to dangerously high levels or react with other medications.

It is better to eat fish that contain omega-3 fatty acids, such as cod, tuna, salmon, halibut, shark and mackerel.

Medical Source ——————————————————
   FDA Consumer (27,6:35)

Back pain: How you can avoid surgery

You reach down to pick up your grandchild and, ouch, there goes that pain in your back again. If this scenario is all too common, you're not alone.

But you don't have to lie flat on your back for weeks to get relief, and most people with back pain do not need surgery to correct the problem.

Most back pain is due to overuse or trauma to the muscles, but structural deformities such as arthritis and herniated discs may also cause back pain.

A herniated disc refers to a fibrous disc between each vertebrae in the spine. These discs are filled with a jelly-like substance that cushions the vertebrae. If you strain your back or a disc degenerates because of age, the pressure may squeeze some of the soft substance out of a disc.

Then you lose the cushion between vertebrae and feel painful pressure on nerves in the spinal cord. The most vulnerable discs are those in the lower back.

But even if you have a herniated disc, you might not need surgery. Your doctor may choose from nonsurgical treatments such as these to ease your back pain:

- ❏ Limit your physical activity for two or more days. During this time you'll need to lie flat on your back with your legs stretched out or slightly bent at the knees. Resume walking and normal activity as soon as possible to avoid losing muscle strength and to keep your heart in good condition.

- ❏ If your pain is limited to a small area, your doctor might inject a local anesthetic at the site of the pain. Not only does this reduce pain, it relieves muscle tension that contributes to the pain. If you have an injection, you will have to cut back on your activities afterward to avoid injuring the area further.

- ❏ Take a nonsteroidal anti-inflammatory drug (NSAID) that reduces inflammation and relieves pain, such as aspirin, ibuprofen, etc. The main drawback to NSAIDs is that they irritate the stomach and can cause indigestion, ulcers, bleeding and even perforation of the stomach.

- ❏ If the muscles in your lower back are contracting so strongly that they're causing your back pain, you might also need a muscle relaxant in addition to an anti-inflammatory. Possible side effects from muscle relaxants include drowsiness, headache, dizziness, blurred vision or dry mouth.

- ❏ If strained ligaments are causing your back pain, ask your doctor about prolotherapy, an injection of glucose, sodium morrhuate and procaine at the place where the ligament is strained. The mixture causes the ligaments to shorten and tighten and reduces strain on the back muscles.

❏ Manipulations that stretch and relax the back muscles are for people whose back problems are muscular in origin.

Chances are you will be able to recover from back pain without having surgery. Ask your doctor to recommend therapy that will give you relief from your aching back.

Medical Sources ───────────────────
Drug Therapy (22,10:93)
Medical Tribune (33,21:2)

Caring for your back

❏ Keep your back muscles flexible and in shape. If you stretch and exercise regularly, you won't have to worry that a weekend spent gardening or playing tennis will send you to bed with an aching back.

❏ Give support to your lower back. You may need a small pillow for your car seat and your chair at work.

❏ Don't bend and twist your back when you rake, vacuum or mop. Keep your back straight, and move your arms and legs smoothly. Your job may take longer, but your back will appreciate it. Buy lightweight gardening tools and cleaning equipment with long handles.

❏ Move around and stretch as much as possible when you're sitting in your chair at work. Try to stand up when you talk on the phone.

❏ Relieve tension by breathing deeply, talking to friends and walking. Stress can lead to tense muscles and backache.

❏ Never bend from your waist when you lift an object, even if it doesn't seem very heavy. Bend your knees and lift with your legs instead.

❏ Don't sleep on your stomach. If you absolutely must, put a small pillow under your stomach to keep your back straight. Put a pillow under your knees if you sleep on your back. The best sleeping position is on your side with a pillow between your knees.

☐ Work slowly and take a break every 20 to 30 minutes. And don't even start the project if you're already tired.

☐ Lose excess weight, especially if you have a potbelly. Stomach fat strains the lower back and throws your spine out of alignment.

☐ Don't wear high heels. They push your pelvis forward which might strain your back muscles.

☐ Take aspirin or ibuprofen if you wrench or strain a back muscle, and put an ice bag on your back for 15 to 20 minutes. For the next two days, ice your back muscles two or three times a day.

Medical Sources ————————————————
Mayo Clinic Health Letter (10,4:7)
Joy of Health (2,1:4)

Knotted muscles cramp your style

When your muscles are working properly, you hardly think about them. But sometimes a muscle will contract into a painful spasm called a muscle cramp, and you won't find relief until the muscle relaxes.

Although the calf muscle in your leg is the most likely spot for a muscle cramp, you can get a cramp in any muscle — whether you are in shape or not.

No one really knows what causes cramps, but we do know some of the factors that contribute to cramping:

☐ Dehydration (lack of fluids) is probably the biggest contributor to muscle cramping.

☐ Muscles that are injured, overstressed or exposed to extreme heat or cold are more likely to cramp.

☐ An imbalance of the essential minerals potassium and sodium can be a factor in cramping. We call these minerals electrolytes because they carry the electrical charge that signals muscles to relax or contract. If you're an athlete who sweats excessively and doesn't replace fluids, your electrolytes can get out of balance. The electrolyte balance won't return to normal until you replace fluids.

☐ A lack of the minerals calcium and magnesium also contributes to muscle cramping.

☐ Pregnancy has been linked to muscle cramps.

☐ A hidden disease such as diabetes or atherosclerosis (clogged arteries) might be a factor in cramping.

When you get a cramp, gentle stretching is the best way to relieve pain. While stretching, press on the muscle, ice it for up to 15 minutes and massage it.

Relieve muscle cramps in your calf by sitting on the ground with your legs stretched out in front of you and gently pulling your toes and the ball of the foot toward your kneecap.

You can help prevent cramps by drinking plenty of water. When you are exercising in hot weather, you can lose up to two quarts of water per hour.

If you want to see how much water weight you've lost during exercise, weigh yourself before and after. A loss of one pound of weight generally means that you lost one pint of water due to perspiration.

In addition, you can ward off cramps by taking these precautions:

☐ Maintain a good balance of electrolytes by eating oranges and bananas for potassium. We usually get more than enough sodium in the food we eat.

☐ Get enough minerals by eating calcium-rich foods, such as milk, yogurt, salmon, sardines, shrimp, dark-green leafy vegetables and dried beans and peas.

☐ Include plenty of foods high in magnesium in your diet: Almonds, cashews, apricots, whole grains, dark-green leafy vegetables and soybeans are good magnesium sources.

☐ Avoid clothing that is too tight because it could cut off blood circulation to your muscles. Protect your muscles from extreme cold with adequate clothing.

☐ Get your muscles ready for exercise by warming up and stretching slowly.

If you continue to have trouble with muscle cramps, talk to your doctor.

Medical Source —————————————————
The Physician and Sportsmedicine (21,7:115)

Leg cramps strike at night

They usually arrive in the night, unexpected — those nightmarish lower leg cramps, lasting from 10 minutes up to several hours.

Who gets leg cramps? A recent report says that almost everyone has experienced a leg cramp at one time or another. Some people, however, suffer from them quite often.

Athletes and others who exercise seem to be more prone to leg cramps, especially if they neglect to stretch and warm up before exercising. People with poor circulation are also affected. Women are more likely to have leg cramps than men, especially pregnant women as the growing fetus interrupts the blood flow to the lower legs.

Being overweight and standing for long periods of time can also increase your chances of developing leg cramps. Leg cramps tend to increase with age. Researchers believe that having arthritis or Parkinson's disease may also contribute to the development of leg cramps.

Leg cramps usually occur when you are resting or sleeping, but they can also follow exercise or heavy activity.

Here are a few techniques to help prevent leg cramps:

☐ Elevate the foot of your bed. If this is not possible, place pillows at the foot of your bed under the bedcovers so you don't fully stretch your legs out during the night.

☐ Do calf-stretching exercises on a daily basis. With your shoes off, stand two to three feet from a wall. Place your hands on the wall and lean forward, being sure to keep your legs and back straight. Press your heels into the floor. You should feel a pulling sensation in the back of your lower legs. Hold this position for 10 seconds, relax five seconds, and then do the exercise once more. Repeat the exercise three times a day.

If you get a leg cramp, try lying down and flexing the foot of your affected leg toward your knee.

If this doesn't work, get up and stand on both feet. Press the heel of the cramping leg firmly into the floor while raising the front half of that foot toward the ceiling. If these methods don't work, try massaging the muscle.

See your doctor if you have leg cramps often or if they are so severe that they interfere with your sleep or daily activities.

Medical Source ————————————————————
   U.S. Pharmacist (17,6:23)

Get a grip on hand injuries

Does a hand disorder have you in its painful grasp? If you have grip gripes, you're not alone. More and more workers are suffering from repetitive strain injuries (RSIs), which range from painful to disabling.

If you regularly use your hands to perform repeated motions, you could develop carpal tunnel syndrome (CTS), trigger finger or nerve spasms. Carpal tunnel syndrome, also known as washerwoman's thumb, telegrapher's arm and writer's cramp, is the most common hand disorder.

Most people with CTS are over age 40. The disorder is almost twice as common in women as men.

The carpal tunnel is a small passageway made up of bones and ligaments just beneath the skin of your wrist.

Repetitive motions cause swelling of the membrane lubricating the nerves and tendons that pass through this tunnel. This constricts the median nerve, which controls the muscles of the forearm and hand. When that happens, you feel the pinch of CTS and often have numbness, tingling and pain in your thumb, index and middle fingers.

Underlying medical conditions, such as osteoarthritis and rheumatoid arthritis, may influence the development of carpal tunnel syndrome. You also may be more likely to develop CTS if you've sprained your wrist.

If you suffer from trigger finger, one or more of your fingers becomes locked in a bent position. Trying to straighten the finger usually results in an audible clicking sound.

Trigger finger occurs when repetitious movements irritate finger tendons, causing them to develop swollen knots. These knots then get caught in the lubricating membrane and the finger sticks in one position.

Nerve spasms occur when nerves are squeezed together by physical pressure or swelling. After a while, the nerve becomes irritated and goes into spasms. Pain is similar to severe muscle cramps.

To prevent hand disorders, learn to work with your hands so that you don't put undue pressure on them. The most stressful wrist actions include wringing movements or movements used when playing a musical instrument, knitting, using vibrating power tools, typing or tightly gripping a steering wheel for long periods of time.

People who are at risk for developing carpal tunnel syndrome from their jobs include:

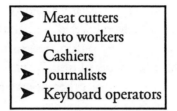

➤ Meat cutters
➤ Auto workers
➤ Cashiers
➤ Journalists
➤ Keyboard operators

Jobs that require repetitive hand motions account for half of all hand disorders. If you use repetitive hand motions at work, you might want to ask your employer to consider implementing strategies that could help workers avoid hand disorders and work more comfortably.

☐ Use height-adjustable tables.
☐ Provide chairs that offer back support and adjustable workstations that allow workers to adjust screens and keyboards.
☐ Allow injured employees enough time to recover completely.

If you have any of the following symptoms, rest your hands until the symptoms subside and see your doctor as soon as possible.

➤ Tingling or numb feeling
➤ Pain
➤ Burning
➤ Weakness
➤ Pins and needles sensation when your wrist is tapped
➤ Stiffness
➤ Swelling
➤ Tendency to drop things

Many times RSIs can be treated before they do irreversible damage. There are various treatment options if you develop one of these disorders:

☐ Rest your hands as much as possible.

☐ Use your hands in outstretched positions instead of twisting and turning them. This puts minimum stress on joints, tendons and muscles. An occupational therapist can teach you techniques, including the use of adaptive equipment, such as jar openers and knob turners, to improve your condition and eliminate pain.

☐ Ask your doctor about wearing a lightweight plastic splint on the affected wrist for several weeks, either all day or only at night. Splints prevent you from putting pressure on your wrist, but allow you to use your hand for most daily tasks.

☐ Use aspirin, ibuprofen or other nonsteroidal anti-inflammatory drugs to relieve pain.

If you have any pain that lasts longer than several weeks, see your doctor. If your regular doctor is not able to relieve your symptoms within a couple of weeks, see a hand disorder specialist. The earlier a diagnosis is made, the greater the likelihood of recovery and the less chance of a disability.

For more information about repetitive strain injuries and arthritis call the National Institute for Occupational Safety and Health, 1-800-356-4674. The Arthritis Foundation's National Hotline number is 1-800-283-7800.

Medical Source ───────────────────────
    FDA Consumer (27,6:35)

Handy tips for avoiding repetitive strain injuries

With these hints at your fingertips, you can prevent repetitive strain injuries (RSIs) hands down.

☐ Take short rest breaks every half hour when doing work that requires extensive use of your hands.

☐ Stretch your hands during your rest period.

☐ Don't keep your hands in one position or bend your wrists for long periods of time.

❏ Use your whole hand and all of your fingers, instead of just your thumb and index finger, to pick up objects.

❏ Never sleep on your hands.

❏ Hold the steering wheel gently when driving.

❏ Protect and care for your joints.

❏ Rest your hands when they hurt.

Typing is one of the most common activities that requires repetitive hand actions. If you type a lot, altering some of your typing habits can go a long way toward preventing any of these gripping disorders.

❏ Keep your wrists even. Do not bend them up or down.

❏ Use a foam pad when typing so that your wrists have support. These pads are available at many office supply stores.

❏ Type lightly.

❏ Do not rest your wrists on the keyboard.

Medical Source ————————————————
The Johns Hopkins Medical Letter (5,4:6)

How to s-t-r-e-t-c-h your hands

Stretch your hands each morning before beginning work and take regular stretch breaks throughout the day.

❏ Make loose fists, then gently stretch your hand to its full length.

❏ Press your hand palm flat at the edge of a table. Extend your fingers. Bend your wrist 90 degrees. Hold position five seconds.

❏ Place your forearm on a table and hang your wrist over the edge. Stretch fingers out. Lift hand up and back as far as possible. Using other hand, gently pull back on your outstretched fingers. Hold five seconds.

Medical Source ————————————————
Medical Update (5,4:42)

Heating pads for achy muscles

Here's a hot flash for weekend warriors. Whether you've strained your back gardening, or your calf muscles are aching from a long walk, relief is close at hand.

The warmth from a heating pad or a reheatable gel/clay pack helps to alleviate pain from minor injuries.

For the first 48 hours after your injury, follow the RICE rule: Rest, Ice, Compression and Elevation. Then, on the third day, warm up the gel/clay pack or plug in the heating pad and apply heat to your injury for 20 to 30 minutes several times each day.

Heat will help your injury by enlarging the blood vessels that bring extra blood into the tissues.

Your injured tissues receive more of your body's natural defenders: antibodies, leukocytes, nutrients, oxygen and enzymes.

The extra blood flow also carries pain-causing metabolites and waste products from inflammation away from injured tissues. Heat helps collagen, a protein found in all your connective tissues, stretch better. This relieves your stiff tendons and muscles.

Local heat is particularly helpful with the following injuries:

- ❒ **Lower back pain** — Your risk of developing lower back pain increases if you drive, sit or stand for long periods of time. Don't lie on top of a heating pad to warm your injured back. The trapped heat might burn your skin.

- ❒ **Ankle injuries** — Sprained or strained ankles account for 10 percent of all emergency room visits. Basketball players are particularly vulnerable to ankle injury, but you can sprain your ankle just by missing a step.

- ❒ **Tendonitis** — It is an inflammation of your tendons. Participation in sports often causes tendinitis, but you can also develop tendinitis from many forms of repetitive work. Local heat helps tendinitis by elasticizing the collagen tissue, relieving stiffness.

- ❒ **Shin splints** — They are another form of tendinitis. Shin splints often result from running on a hard surface.

- ❒ **Strained calf muscle** — It is another common athletic injury.

For all of these injuries, follow the RICE formula for the first 48 hours, and then get out the gel/clay pack or the heating pad.

Remember, there are certain situations in which you should never use local heat including:

> ➤ if you have a fresh bruise
> ➤ when a vein has a blood clot
> ➤ when you have swelling without inflammation
> ➤ on a part of your body where blood flow is restricted
> ➤ if you have a hemorrhaging disorder like hemophilia
> ➤ if you have phlebitis
> ➤ on any sleeping or unconscious person
> ➤ on any person whose skin isn't fully sensitive
> ➤ if you have diabetes
> ➤ if you have poor circulation
> ➤ on an infant
> ➤ if you have used any cream or liniment sold for aching muscles
> ➤ if you suspect that you have a brown recluse spider bite
> ➤ on any open wound

If you follow these guidelines, heat can be an inexpensive, yet effective, way to relieve minor aches and pains. If your injury doesn't seem to be getting better, consult your doctor.

Medical Source —————————————
   U.S. Pharmacist (18,10:39)

Chilling danger from ice therapy

Treating athletic injuries with ice is easy, cheap and it's a proven remedy for swelling and inflammation. So why are some sports medicine experts cool to the idea of cryotherapy?

Diane Covington and Dr. Frank Bassett say there's a down side to ice therapy.

At the Duke University Medical Center, Bassett and Covington examined several athletes who had used ice therapy to treat injuries. These athletes later noticed numbness, weakness and shaking in the muscles below the original injury.

Too much cryotherapy had actually damaged nerves close to the surface of the skin, according to the report.

Fortunately, strength and feeling did return to the athletes' muscles, but recovery took anywhere from four days to six months.

Covington and Bassett advise that cryotherapy is still an excellent treatment for athletic injuries when it is used correctly.

You can avoid injury from ice therapy by following these tips:

> Use ice for less than 20 minutes at a time.
> Do not apply ice directly to your skin. Insulate your skin with a dry towel between ice and skin.
> Avoid compressing the injured area with ice.
> Use extra caution if you have very little body fat.

Medical Source —————————————————————
The Physician and Sportsmedicine (21,3:78)

Ease the pain of an ankle sprain

Ever stepped off a curb and turned your ankle? You feel foolish, but it hurts just as bad as when a pro basketball player comes down on the side of his foot after an impressive rebound.

Almost everyone who exercises has experienced a sprain on the outside of the ankle, called a lateral ankle sprain. After all, the ankle is constantly in motion and it bears all your weight.

If you're in a lot of pain after an ankle sprain, you need to see your doctor. Ankle sprains may be common, but they can be serious.

If the sprain is mild, you can ease the pain and keep the swelling down by using the RICE treatment — Rest, Ice, Compression and Elevation.

- ☐ Stay off your feet for the first two days after you sprain your ankle. If you have to walk, use a cane or a crutch on the side that's not injured so that you can take weight off the hurt foot.
- ☐ Put an ice pack on your ankle for about 20 minutes three or four times a day.
- ☐ Wrap your ankle in an elastic bandage to control swelling and to support and protect it, especially if you must walk around. Start wrapping at your toes, make a figure-eight at the ankle, and continue wrapping loosely about six inches up the leg.

  Don't wrap so tightly that your toes go numb or turn red. Wear the bandage as long as your ankle hurts when you try to walk.
- ☐ Prop up your swollen ankle above the level of your heart. Stretch out on your sofa with your foot on a pillow.

If your ankle is still swollen after a few days, use a "contrast bath" twice a day. Put your foot in a tub of cold water for one minute, then move to a tub of warm water for two minutes. Do this for 15 minutes, gently moving your foot up and down in the water.

Since you risk another sprain as long as your ankle is weak, continue to support it with sturdy shoes or boots even after the pain is gone. Wear a bandage or brace when you plan to walk or exercise vigorously.

Five to 10 times a day, do gentle exercises to strengthen the muscles that support your ankle.

First, remove any bandage or brace and let your leg hang freely off a bench, sturdy table or tall chair. Roll your foot in a circle at least three or four times. Make both clockwise and counterclockwise circles.

When your ankle begins to feel stronger, improve your strength, flexibility and balance with a "rockerboard" you can make at home:

- ☐ Cut a croquet ball (or other round, hard ball) in half and glue it to a small board.
- ☐ Find a short platform — the same height as the rockerboard. Stand with your uninjured foot on the platform and your injured foot on the rockerboard. Evenly distribute your weight between both feet.
- ☐ Rock your sprained ankle to the front and back and from side to

side several times, moving very slowly.

You'll notice that pointing your toes toward your head can be painful for weeks after a sprain. To regain flexibility, try to climb three flights of stairs a day, backward. Keep doing this until you're completely pain-free.

Some people spend half their lives in an ankle brace because they sprain it again and again. If you have a chronic ankle sprain, you may be pushing too hard and too long when you exercise.

If you walk or work out until you're exhausted or suddenly start to run faster than you normally do, you're putting yourself at risk for a sprain. The muscles that support the ankle are particularly vulnerable to fatigue.

Medical Sources ─────────────────────
Postgraduate Medicine (94,2:091)
The Physician and Sportsmedicine (21,11:43)
The American Journal of Sports Medicine (21,6:805)

Preventing ankle sprains

You can help prevent sprains by strengthening and stretching your calves and ankles. Here are a few useful exercises:

- ☐ Hold your foot in the air and write the alphabet with your toes.
- ☐ Put a tennis ball under the ball of your foot and step down on it. Hold it down for 10 seconds, then release for 10 seconds. Repeat 10 times.
- ☐ Sit on the edge of a chair and loop a bungi cord, a towel or surgical tubing (can usually be found at a pharmacy) around the ball of your foot. Hold your leg out and stretch your foot in every direction. Repeat 10 times in each direction.
- ☐ Sitting in a chair, use the side of your foot to push a paint can or another object weighing about 10 pounds on a hard floor. Keep your heel planted and use it as a pivot. First push to the right, then back to the left.
- ☐ Sitting on a chair, loop surgical tubing around your foot, run the stretchy cord under your other foot and hold the free end in your hand. Move your ankle up and out to the side. Don't move your

knee. Hold for five seconds, then bring your ankle back down. Repeat 10 times.

☐ Stretch the back of your lower leg muscles by leaning against a wall with one leg forward and knee bent. The back leg should be straight with the heel pressed to the floor. Lean into the wall for 10 seconds. Do this five times with each leg.

Do this exercise with the back knee bent as well as the front knee. This will stretch the muscles on the sides of your calves.

Medical Sources ————————————————
American Family Physician (45,3:1233)
The Physician and Sportsmedicine (21,11:43)

Exercise to end knee pain

Don't always blame your achy knees on arthritis. You may just need to exercise.

Normally, your thigh muscle holds your kneecap firmly against the knee except when you completely straighten your leg. The kneecap doesn't slip from side to side because it's connected to a tendon which runs in a groove at the end of the thigh bone.

If your thigh muscles become weak, that tendon is able to slip out of the groove and your kneecap loses its stability.

The kneecap moves around, rubbing against bones and ligaments, and you get a painful, swollen knee.

Exercising your thigh muscles is especially important if you've had a cast on your leg, if you've injured your knee or if you've been confined to bed for several days. Do not begin any exercise program without checking with your doctor or physical therapist first.

The knee exercises in the following article are excellent for building your thigh muscles and strengthening your knees.

If gentle exercise doesn't put a stop to your achy knees or if your knee pain is severe, you need to see your doctor.

Medical Source ————————————————
Postgraduate Medicine (93,3:75)

Avoid adding insult to injury: Rebuild your strength with exercise

"The most common injury is reinjury," physical therapists are fond of saying.

Have you:
- ❐ Been favoring one leg because of an old injury in the other?
- ❐ Had a broken or sprained limb locked in a cast or splint?
- ❐ Been trapped in bed by an illness for several days, especially if you're older?

If you said yes to any of the above questions, be prepared to twist a knee, sprain a wrist, turn an ankle, dislocate a shoulder or injure your hip, unless you work to build up muscles that have wasted away.

Exercise, particularly rehabilitation for a damaged limb, is the only way to fully recover from a long period of bed rest or an injury. Weak muscles lead to unstable joints and could make you an accident waiting to happen.

If you have an old knee injury, measure your thighs just above your knee. You may find that one leg is at least a half-inch smaller than the other, just because you've favored the less painful leg.

Both your thighs may lack good muscle tone if your hurt knee has caused you to quit exercising.

Because you often don't walk normally after a knee or ankle injury, your hip is at risk for injury, too. Your leg rehabilitation exercises should include exercises to restore strength and flexibility to your hip.

Exercising a sprained ankle as soon as two days after an injury can get you back on your feet twice as fast as not using the ankle until the pain goes away. The bones and ligaments in the ankle aren't stable unless the surrounding muscles are strong.

Use the exercises listed below to restore strength to an injured limb. A "set" means doing an exercise several times in a row without stopping. Rest between each set. You can make most of these exercises harder by strapping weights on your ankle or holding them in your hand.

Warning: Never begin exercising without checking with your doctor or physical therapist first.

Hip Exercises

☐ Hold on to a chair for stability and lift your knee to waist height. Lower and repeat. Do three sets of 10.

☐ While standing, lift your leg 30 degrees to the side. Repeat. Do three sets of 30.

☐ Lean with your hands on a table or flat surface. Lift your leg straight backward. Do three sets of 20.

☐ Standing, lift your knee to waist height. Move your knee out to the side and return to the middle. Repeat. Do three sets of 30.

☐ Lie on your back with your toes slightly pointed. Lift leg straight up 30 degrees and return. Do three sets of 10. (Also good for injured knee.)

Knee Exercises

☐ Lying on your back, tighten your thigh muscle. Hold tight for 10 seconds, then relax for 10 seconds. Repeat 10 times.

☐ Hold a barbell or broomstick behind your neck and squat until your knees are bent 30 to 40 degrees. Squatting more than 45 degrees is bad for your knees. Do three sets of 10.

☐ While lying on your stomach, bend your knee up to a 90-degree angle. (Your foot should face the ceiling.) Slowly lower leg to floor. Do three sets of 20.

☐ Sit on a table with your legs hanging off the side. Straighten your leg completely, then slowly lower it to 30 degrees. Repeat. Don't lower your leg more than 45 degrees or the underside of your kneecap may get irritated. Do three sets of 10.

☐ Lie on the floor and place a rolled towel under your knee. Straighten your leg, then return to resting position. Do three sets of 10. You can do this in place of the previous exercise.

Ankle Exercises

☐ Write the alphabet in the air with your toe.

☐ Step on a tennis ball with the ball of your foot. Press the ball down for 10 seconds then release for 10 seconds. Repeat 10 times.

☐ Sit on the edge of a chair and loop a bungi cord or other stretchy cord around the ball of your foot. Hold your leg out and stretch your foot in every direction. Repeat 10 times in each direction.

❐ Pivoting on your heel, use the side of your foot to push a paint can or another object weighing about 10 pounds on a hard floor. First push to the right, then back to the left.

Shoulder Exercises

❐ Lie on your back and hold a broomstick in both hands. Use your uninjured arm to pull your injured arm through a complete range of motion. Continue for three to five minutes.

❐ Hold a pocketbook or a light object with the hand on the injured side and support your body weight by leaning with your other hand on a table or chair.

Swing the pocketbook forward and backward for one minute, from side to side for one minute, and in clockwise and counter-clockwise circles for one minute.

❐ Stand at arm's length from a wall and walk your fingers up and down the wall. When your shoulder starts hurting, don't go any higher. Do this both facing the wall and with your arm toward the wall.

❐ Put your arm out to the side and bend your elbow 90 degrees. Rotating at the shoulder, move your hand toward your feet, then toward your head.

❐ Stand with your back to a table and hold on to the table with both hands. Bend your knees until your shoulder muscles begin to stretch.

❐ Standing with your arms hanging loosely, lift your arm out to the side — 90 degrees from your body. Hold it there, then lift above your head. Pause, then lower your arm. Do three sets of 10. Do the same exercise lifting your arm to the front.

All of these exercises can be done at home to build muscle strength after a period of bed rest or to restore strength and stability to a joint you've injured in the past.

If you've just twisted your ankle severely while exercising, heard your knee pop after a skiing fall or banged your shoulder in a car wreck, don't just grin and bear the pain. You need to check with your doctor to make sure you don't need a cast, a brace or even surgery to repair a torn cartilage or ligament.

Medical Source ——————————————————
American Family Physician (45,3:1233)

Don't let tennis elbow score with you

Just because you don't play tennis doesn't mean you can't get tennis elbow.

Weak muscles in your shoulder, hand or arm can lead to tennis elbow. It starts with an ache on the outside of your elbow or on the forearm opposite your palm. Your arm becomes tender, your wrists get weak and you may have difficulty grasping objects. And before you know it, you've been aced by tennis elbow, a form of damage to the forearm muscles.

People who play tennis usually get tennis elbow from a repeated forceful extension of the wrist as in swinging a racket. You can just as easily injure your arm gardening or raking leaves. Bowling, golfing, playing baseball and even carrying around a heavy briefcase can cause tennis elbow.

If you develop elbow problems while playing tennis, you may have a bad backhand. Bending your elbow during the backhand stroke puts too much stress on the muscles around your elbow.

To recover from tennis elbow, try these strategies:

- ❑ Rest your arm for four to six weeks, and don't return to the courts until your elbow pain is gone.
- ❑ Ice your elbow during the first five days of recovery for five to seven minutes, two to three times a day.
- ❑ Apply moist heat to your elbow after the first five days for 15 minutes, three times daily, and massage the muscles of your forearm.
- ❑ Begin stretching and strengthening exercises after the first five days.
- ❑ Ask a tennis professional about the correct racket grip size and string tension.

Stretching and strengthening exercises will help increase the flexibility of your muscles and prevent you from developing tennis elbow again.

This easy stretching exercise is good for prevention or treatment:

❑ Stand with your arm fully extended at shoulder height, palm up. With the other hand, stretch your fingers toward the floor. Repeat with your palm turned downwards.

❑ For an easy strengthening exercise, try squeezing a deflated tennis ball for five to 10 minutes three times a day. You can progress to squeezing an inflated ball — but stop if you feel pain.

Check with your doctor or physical therapist about other helpful exercises.

Medical Source ————————————————
The Physician and Sportsmedicine (21,7:21)

FOOT PROBLEMS

Step out on common foot problems

Having foot problems can be 'toe'tally horrendous, especially if you have one of the conditions known as bone spurs, hammertoe, claw toe or soft corns. These problems may sound serious, but they can actually be remedied by simple, nonsurgical procedures.

Bone spurs are inflammations of the tissue located in the ball of your foot. Taping your arch, or arch strapping, effectively relieves discomfort. Apply benzoin tincture (available without a prescription at your local pharmacy) to the ball and heel of your foot to help keep the tape in place.

After the benzoin is dry, place three strips of tape across the ball of your foot. Then, starting at the front of your foot, make a figure eight with a strip of tape, wrapping the ball, heel and arch.

Reinforce this with a second strip of tape, and cover that piece with three more strips across the ball of your foot.

Use self-adhesive wrap to make sure the tape stays put, and leave the wrap on your foot for a week. This will help give the tissue a chance to rest without interfering with normal walking.

Weak muscles in the base of your foot can cause hammertoe. Hammertoe usually affects the second toe, which is bent downward unnaturally, and leads to corns and ulcers at the tip of your toe. Claw toe is a related disorder, caused by muscle and nerve problems. Claw toe affects several toes at once, drawing them up into a curved position.

Both diseases require the same treatment:

❑ Don't wear shoes that force your toes downward or toward the ground. Use hammertoe pads. The pad balances the uneven pull of the tendon and allows the toe to return to its original shape.

❑ Don't wear tight shoes. These shoes can cause friction and rubbing between the fourth and fifth toes, leading to the formation of soft corns. To treat soft corns effectively, use a small, foam pad to separate the toes. Make sure the pad does not cause irritation or add extra pressure. Replace your current shoes with ones that have more room.

❏ Exercise your feet by picking up marbles with your toes and placing them in a bowl or by simply taking a barefoot walk on the beach.

Medical Source ———————————————
Emergency Medicine (24,15:34)

Foot fitness tips

❏ Examine your shoes if you begin to experience foot problems. A lack of proper space between your toes or laces that are too tight can contribute to your condition.

❏ Keep your toes clean, and dry them thoroughly after washing. This tip is especially useful for avoiding soft corns.

❏ Use a blow dryer to heal raw skin caused by ulcers or blisters. First soak the area, then use a blow dryer at a cool setting for 15 to 20 minutes. This allows the wound to heal faster with less chance of infection.

Medical Source ———————————————
The Physician and Sportsmedicine (20,12:6)

Put your foot down on fungal infections

Because of their moth-eaten appearance, fungal infections are commonly referred to as tinea, from the Latin word meaning moth. In describing such infections, the word tinea is followed by the Latin term for the part of the body affected: Tinea pedia affects the feet; tinea corporis affects the entire body; and tinea cruris affects the groin.

These infections are caused by dermatophytes, simple parasitic fungi that live on the skin, hair and nails. They grow best in warm, moist areas of the body. Only rarely do these microorganisms move beyond the skin.

Most of the time your body rejects these fungi. However, when your resistance is down, you can quickly become susceptible. Your ability to fight fungal infections may be lowered by:

> ➤ Problems with your immune system
> ➤ Poor nutrition
> ➤ Warm temperatures
> ➤ Excessive moisture, which can be caused by high humidity, heavy sweating or wearing closed shoes
> ➤ Skin damage, such as blisters, cuts or bacterial infections

Athlete's foot, also known as jungle rot and ringworm of the feet, is the most widespread fungal infection. Athlete's foot can last from a few weeks to many months. Some people complain that they have a constant infection. Symptoms include:

> ➤ Mild rash
> ➤ Itching
> ➤ Bad odor
> ➤ Peeling or cracking

If left untreated, athlete's foot can spread from between the toes and soles of your feet to toenails and other areas of your body. To prevent athlete's foot from getting worse:

❑ Keep feet as dry as possible.

❑ Wear loose-fitting or open shoes and light-weight socks.

❑ Change shoes and socks at least once a day.

❑ If the areas between your toes gets very wet, put rolls of gauze between toe tips to keep your toes from touching and to absorb moisture.

❑ Wear bath thongs when showering on rough concrete surfaces. Rough surfaces can scratch your feet, allowing fungi to lodge more easily in your skin and cause infection. Even when not showering on rough surfaces, you should wear sandals if you have blisters or other damage to your feet.

Ringworm produces ring-shaped sores with a clear center and a red, scaly border. The sores look this way because healing takes place from the center outward. The term ringworm also describes any fungal infection of the skin, hair or nails, even when the sores are not ring-shaped.

Jock itch, also known as tinea curis, usually affects men, although women may also develop this disorder. It spreads over the upper, inner thighs and may extend to the groin, pubic and anal areas.

Sores appear semicircular with well-defined, slightly elevated edges and light-brown centers. Jock itch is often a long-term, recurring infection.

As hard as it may be, try not to scratch when you have fungal infections. Prolonged, intense scratching damages the skin and increases your risk of developing a bacterial infection.

To keep the infection from spreading and to avoid contracting the infection again, don't share any personal grooming items, such as washcloths or towels. Wash all clothes, bed sheets and personal items in hot water or have them dry cleaned.

Medical Source ————————————————
   U.S. Pharmacist (18,4:20)

Be footloose and fungal-free with OTC products

Relief from fungal infections is as close as your local pharmacy. In most cases, you can treat athlete's foot, jock itch and ringworm just as safely and effectively with over-the-counter (OTC) medicines as with prescribed drugs.

However, OTC anti-fungal drugs won't effectively treat toenail or scalp infections because the nail thickness and depth of hair roots keep medicine from reaching the infected area.

Anti-fungal medicines are available as sprays, ointments, creams, powders and liquids.

   ❑ **Sprays** — Supply medicine to affected area quicker than any other medicine. They also relieve itching rapidly.
   ❑ **Ointments and creams** — Best for long-term treatment. Don't use ointments on cracked or very moist skin because they may prolong the infection. Creams and powders are safe to use on cracked or moist skin.
   ❑ **Powders** — Absorb excess moisture well. They don't provide high

concentrations of medicine.

☐ **Liquids** — Most effectively supply medicine to infected area.

You may have to use a product for two to three days before you experience relief. Continue treatment for two to four weeks until the infection is completely eliminated. You may experience irritation, skin redness and itching while using these drugs.

There are a number of anti-fungal drugs on the market that are safe to use, but not all are equally effective. Listed below are the active ingredients in anti-fungal drugs that have proven both safe and effective:

> ➤ Clioquinol
> ➤ Clotrimazole
> ➤ Haloprogin
> ➤ Miconazole Nitrate
> ➤ Povidone-iodine
> ➤ Tolnaftate
> ➤ Undecylenic acid in combination with zinc, calcium or copper salts. Zinc is reported to help reduce inflammation.

If you are using an OTC treatment that contains clioquinol and need to undergo a thyroid function test, show your doctor the medication you are taking. Clioquinal can interfere with these tests.

Here are a few general guidelines for using OTC anti-fungal products that will help you safely stamp out fungal infections:

☐ If you have diabetes, asthma or any other chronic health problem, see your doctor before attempting to self-treat your infection.

☐ Don't use on children age 2 years or younger unless your doctor so recommends. Supervise all children under 12 who use these medications.

☐ Don't use in or near your eyes, nose or mouth.

☐ Don't use for prolonged periods of time in areas that retain a lot of moisture, such as between your toes or near your groin. Too much of the medicine may be absorbed and cause adverse side effects.

- ☐ Use products exactly as directed.
- ☐ Wash infected area with soap and water, and dry thoroughly before applying medicine. Wash hands well afterwards.
- ☐ When using ointments and creams, apply the smallest amount possible and rub the medication in well.
- ☐ Shake sprays before using. Spray medicine evenly, holding can six to 10 inches from the infected area. Don't breathe fumes or use near an open flame.
- ☐ Treat all skin in the general area of the infection.
- ☐ If you miss a dose, apply medication as soon as you remember, then return to your regular dosage schedule.
- ☐ If the product you are using relieves some symptoms, but does not make the infection go away, try another brand.
- ☐ Stop using any product that causes persistent irritation or worsens the infections. Ask your doctor or pharmacist for alternate recommendations.

If your symptoms are not relieved after several weeks of treatment, see your doctor. You may have a bacterial infection, often indicated by an unpleasant smell and oozing blisters, or other disorder.

Medical Source ————————————————————
U.S. Pharmacist (18,4:20)

Treating everyday aches and pains

Anemia
Breathing
  problems
Burns
Colds and flu
Digestive disorders
Dizziness
Headaches
Hemorrhoids
Hiccups

ANEMIA

Eat healthy to avoid anemia

You feel tired, lightheaded and slightly woozy. In fact, you've felt that way for several weeks. You know you're not sick with the flu, so you can't understand why you always feel worn out. Even extra rest doesn't help. Sound familiar?

You're probably suffering from iron deficiency anemia.

Iron deficiency anemia occurs when the body does not have enough iron to work effectively. Iron is used to make hemoglobin, which forms a major part of red blood cells.

The hemoglobin in the red blood cells picks up fresh oxygen brought in through the lungs and carries it to all the tissues of the body. In other words, the hemoglobin in the red blood cells provides the entire body with the oxygen necessary for survival.

However, when iron stores are low or empty, the number of hemoglobin molecules decreases, which, in turn, decreases the number of red blood cells.

This means that all the tissues in the body, including the internal organs, muscles and brain, get less oxygen. The decreased amount of oxygen in the tissues causes the common symptoms associated with iron deficiency anemia:

> ➤ Headache
> ➤ Sore mouth or tongue
> ➤ Brittle nails
> ➤ Fatigue
> ➤ Dizziness
> ➤ Chills
> ➤ Inability to think or concentrate
> ➤ Breathlessness
> ➤ Chest pain

Iron deficiency occurs because a person isn't eating enough dietary iron or because he is losing too much in the form of blood. The body tries to protect against iron deficiency anemia by storing excess iron in storage molecules known as ferritin. When a person does not get enough dietary iron, his body can pull some iron out of storage for immediate use. Unfortunately, even the iron stores can be depleted over time. Some people are more prone to iron deficiency anemia than others:

☐ Women. Women who menstruate regularly or are pregnant or breastfeeding lose a great deal of iron, which often is not replaced through their diets.

☐ Children. Children can grow so rapidly that their bodies' requirements for iron exceed what they take in with their meals.

☐ People who use painkillers frequently. Regular use of aspirin or other anti-inflammatory medicines known as NSAIDs (nonsteroidal anti-inflammatory drugs) often causes irritation and bleeding in the stomach, which can lead to iron deficiency anemia.

☐ People with intestinal problems. Gastric or intestinal ulcers, hemmorhoids or intestinal tumors can cause minor blood loss that can lead to anemia. People who have undergone surgery for intestinal problems may also have trouble digesting iron.

People who are unable to absorb iron must receive monthly iron treatments from their doctors. If iron deficiency anemia is caused by intestinal bleeding, doctors can often correct the problem with medical treatment. Once the underlying problem is cured, the anemia usually disappears.

Although iron deficiency anemia can cause serious physical problems, it is a disorder that is relatively easy to overcome. Most anemia cases can be cured by increasing the intake of iron. However, iron supplements are not usually necessary and can even be dangerous. Iron supplements taken on a long-term basis can cause an iron overload in the body — a potentially life-threatening condition known as hemochromatosis.

Too much iron can also interfere with absorption of other essential nutrients such as copper, manganese and zinc. Also, iron supplement tablets often cause constipation, diarrhea, nausea and vomiting. Try to avoid iron supplements unless they are specifically prescribed by your doctor.

To avoid the dangers and side effects of iron supplements, most doctors simply recommend increasing the intake of iron-rich foods, such as:

> ➤ Braised beef liver
> ➤ Roasted chicken breast
> ➤ Roasted turkey breast
> ➤ Cooked flounder
> ➤ Baked potatoes
> ➤ Iron-enriched white bread
> ➤ Iron-enriched spaghetti noodles
> ➤ Whole-wheat bread
> ➤ Lima beans
> ➤ Light canned tuna
> ➤ Raisins
> ➤ Peanut butter
> ➤ Peas
> ➤ Pork tenderloin
> ➤ Broccoli spears
> ➤ Cooked oysters
> ➤ Eggs
> ➤ Iron-enriched cereals
> ➤ Fruits and fruit juices

You may also want to check labels for nutritional information on iron-fortified foods available at your supermarket.

Try these tips to help you get more iron from your food:

❒ Combine vitamin C-rich foods with iron-rich foods. For example, drink a glass of vitamin C-rich orange juice while eating an iron-enriched bowl of cereal. Vitamin C enhances the body's ability to absorb iron from dietary sources.

❒ Don't drink tea with your meals. The tannic acid in tea interferes with the body's ability to absorb iron.

❒ Don't take calcium supplements with your meals. The calcium supplements interfere with iron absorption. Taking calcium supplements between meals will help eliminate any interference.

If you are experiencing symptoms of iron deficiency anemia, ask your doctor to check your iron levels at your next office visit. Then talk with him about adding some iron-rich foods into a healthy diet to help cure or prevent iron deficiency anemia.

Medical Sources ————————————————
Postgraduate Medicine (93,4:181)
Tufts University Diet and Nutrition Newsletter (10,11:3)

Recommended Daily Allowances of iron

Children aged 1-10	10 milligrams
Females aged 11-50	15 milligrams
Females, pregnant	30 milligrams
Females, breastfeeding	15 milligrams
Females aged 51 and up	10 milligrams
Males aged 11-18	12 milligrams
Males aged 19 and up	10 milligrams

Medical Source ————————————————
Taber's Cyclopedic Medical Dictionary, Edition 17, F.A. Davis Co.,Philadelphia, 1993

BREATHING PROBLEMS

Asthma

Asthma can be a suffocating problem. In the past 20 years, the severity of asthma attacks in the United States has continued to worsen.

Researchers speculate that each year as many as 550,000 people aged 15 to 55 take a trip to the emergency room for severe breathlessness.

Trying to identify the triggers of asthma attacks can be mystifying. Your own home may hold the clues. Evidence indicates that dust mite, cat and cockroach allergens (common substances known to trigger asthma) are responsible for many asthma attacks. You may be sensitive to one or more allergens.

Researchers studied 228 people treated at an emergency room, half of whom had breathlessness as their chief complaint.

Thirty-eight percent of the people treated for breathlessness were allergic to dust mites, cat dander and cockroach allergens, compared with only eight percent of the people treated for other complaints. Constant exposure to such allergens may make people more susceptible to asthma attacks.

Cat dander was the most common allergen found in suburban homes, while cockroach dander was the most common in city housing. Dust mite distribution was similar in both areas.

Living in an overcrowded area or rundown house can increase your risk of asthma attacks. You can modify your housing conditions to reduce risks by maintaining low humidity and good ventilation and by eliminating as many carpeted areas as possible.

These measures will help keep dust mites, commonly found in bedding, furniture and carpets, under control. You may also want to consider using a miticide.

Pesticides can help control cockroaches, often found in your kitchen. Ask your doctor about ways to reduce levels of cat allergen without getting rid of your cat.

If you suspect your asthma attacks could be caused by common household allergens, you may want to be tested to determine which allergens activate your asthma. (See the Allergies chapter for many more tips on how to rid your home of dust mites and other common allergens.)

Finally, you may be able to breathe more easily about asthma attacks.

Medical Source ————————————————
American Review of Respiratory Diseases (147,3:573)

For people with asthma: how to survive bathing your cat

Unless you have a British Turkish house cat, which actually enjoys playing in water, your cat probably is not going to take kindly to the idea of a bath. Yet if you have a problem with asthma and keep a cat, bathing Kitty will probably reduce your asthma attacks. Washing your cat once a week can reduce the amount of cat allergen, produced by saliva, dander and oil glands in the skin, by 90 percent.

- ❑ Get your cat on a schedule of regular baths. If possible, start washing the cat while he's still a kitten.
- ❑ Wash him in a sink instead of a bathtub. This way you won't be bent over and at his mercy.
- ❑ Place a rubber mat in the bottom of the sink to give the cat something to grip so he can keep his balance.
- ❑ Fill the sink with 2 to 4 inches of lukewarm water before you bring your cat in to bathe him. Running water often frightens cats.
- ❑ Wait until your cat is relaxed before you attempt bathing him. Talk soothingly to him during the bath to keep him calm.
- ❑ Gently insert a cotton ball into each of the cat's ears to keep water from entering ear canals.
- ❑ Position your cat so he can see you and place him into the water slowly, hind legs first.
- ❑ Hold him securely. Some people find holding the cat by the scruff of the neck helpful.
- ❑ Wet fur completely, starting with his back and sides. Use a cup for

pouring water on him.

☐ Use a mild, moisturizing shampoo. You can get a special shampoo from your veterinarian or you can buy a baby shampoo and dilute it well. Do not use any soaps with chemicals or conditioners. Wash the cat's head last. Be very careful not to get any soap in his eyes, ears or mouth.

☐ If the cat starts to get chilled, pour some warm water over him.

☐ Be sure to rinse your cat until the water runs clear. You may use a spray hose, but keep the pressure low so you won't scare him.

☐ Towel him dry. You may want to use towels that have been slightly warmed in the dryer. Make sure they're not too hot. Don't let the cat get chilled.

☐ You may use a hair dryer to finish drying your cat after your have toweled him off. Keep the dryer on a low setting and keep it moving over his entire body. Don't dry one section at a time or you risk burning him. If he has long hair, brush it while using the dryer to keep it from tangling.

After the bath, soothe your cat's rumpled feelings with a good head scratch and a special treat.

If your cat absolutely refuses to let you wash him, you may want to consider having a professional animal groomer bathe your cat.

Medical Sources ————————————————

Mayo Clinic Health Letter (11,9:6)

The Tiger on Your Couch, William Morrow and Company, Inc., New York,1992

Asthma and sex

Asthma is one of the most common lung disorders known to man, affecting over 10 million people today. And although the disease probably has been around for centuries, scientists are just now discovering that asthma could be a sex-related disorder.

Yes, sex-related, but not in the human reproduction sense. Rather, your sex, or your gender, seems to be an important factor in determining the severity of the disease.

A group of scientists noticed that the number of hospitalizations for asthma seemed to increase in girls when they reached puberty, whereas they seemed to decrease in boys when they reached the age of puberty.

So, they began gathering information to determine the link between sex, age and asthma.

The scientists researched the hospital records from five counties in southeastern Pennsylvania and found a total of 33,269 admissions for asthma between the years 1986 and 1989.

They gathered all the necessary information from the hospital charts (age, sex, reason for admission, etc.) and then compared all the data. The results were remarkable.

The researchers discovered that before the age of 10, boys were admitted to the hospital twice as often as girls. During the teen years, however, male hospitalizations for asthma started to decrease, while the number of female hospitalizations began to rise.

Then, between the ages of 20 and 50, the female-to-male ratio rose to 3 to 1. In other words, three women were hospitalized for asthma for every one man.

Scientists suspect that the reason for this increase in the number of female hospital admissions for asthma during the adolescent years might be due to hormonal changes that begin at puberty.

When they compared the levels of three hormones in women with asthma and in women without asthma, they found that at least one of the hormone levels was out of the normal range in 80 percent of the women with asthma.

On the other hand, males experience an increase in the level of testosterone around the age of puberty. Scientists aren't sure if the elevated hormone levels influence the severity of asthma.

Some scientists admit that the hormone changes at puberty and the changes in the hospital admission records for asthma might be coincidental. But it seems to be one of the only key pieces of evidence they have so far.

Medical Source ————————————————
The Journal of the American Medical Association (268,24:3437)

Asthma sufferers should plan for a rainy day

The symptoms of an asthma attack can come on unexpectedly. One minute you're fine; the next you're wheezing and can hardly breathe at all.

You wonder what the culprit was this time. Then you remember: It rained yesterday.

Asthma sufferers learn early on to stay away from things that can trigger an asthma attack such as smoke, dust, heavy perfumes or other irritants. And many people say that their asthma tends to get worse after a heavy rainstorm.

So, what does the weather have to do with an asthma attack, you ask?

Well, pollen granules are known lung irritants. And when dry, these granules are sometimes too large to get down deep into the lungs. But when it rains, water causes these particles to swell and burst.

The rupture of the pollen then releases starch granules into the air. These starch granules are small enough to be inhaled deep into the lungs and cause the airways to narrow, triggering bouts of wheezing.

If you suffer from allergies and asthma you should try to stay indoors as much as possible the day after a rainstorm (when pollen usually ruptures) and use your air conditioners and air filters. You should also avoid venturing out into the woods, fields, parks and other areas during the pollen season.

Medical Source ————————————————
The Lancet (339,8793:584)

Deflating news for asthma sufferers

Asthma sufferers may not always bounce back from a car wreck that causes the automobile airbag to inflate. If you have asthma, your airways are likely to tighten when they react to the chemicals the inflated airbag gives off.

In one study, half the people with mild asthma had trouble breathing after sitting in a closed car with an inflated airbag for 20 minutes.

Try to roll down a window if you are trapped in a wrecked car, and remember to carry your inhaler with you when you travel.

Medical Source ————————————————
American Family Physician (48,4:643)

Exercise-induced asthma

Your child drags into the house complaining about a chest problem. Not finding any bumps, bruises or scrapes, your mind starts racing. ... What could be wrong?

It could be a case of asthma triggered by exercise.

When chest pain is related to energetic activity, exercise-induced asthma could be the culprit, according to Dr. Daniel Scagliotti of Children's Mercy Hospital in Kansas City, Mo.

Dr. Scagliotti believes that even if the pain seems unrelated to exertion, exercise-induced asthma shouldn't be ruled out, since the symptoms can develop hours after the exercise.

Undiagnosed, exercise-induced asthma can limit your youngster's activities, especially in sports. But chest pain from exercise-induced asthma can be easily treated and prevented.

Dr. Scagliotti and a team of researchers reported the results of a study of 88 children and adolescents. None of the youngsters had a history of heart disease or asthma, but several had reported cases of chest pain and shortness of breath.

Researchers placed them on a treadmill for six to eight minutes and asked them to reach a target heart rate of 180 beats per minute in the first few minutes of exercise. The volunteers could not warm up before they began exercising.

Researchers tested their breathing capacity before and after the treadmill test. Study results showed that the two main factors in determining the onset of exercise-induced asthma are the type of exercise performed and the intensity. Running, for example, is more likely to cause exercise-related asthma than biking or swimming.

Children who have been diagnosed with exercise-induced asthma should probably begin activities slowly and avoid abrupt moves from sedentary to very active states.

Inhaled albuterol also successfully relieves the symptoms of exercise-induced asthma. Albuterol is among a group of drugs called bronchodilators that widen the airways in the lungs. Treatment with such drugs may enable these children to lead more physically active lives, including participation in competitive programs.

But warm-ups before exercising are a must, researchers suggest.

Talk to your doctor if you have questions about chest pains in children and exercise-related asthma.

Medical Sources ─────────────────────────
Emergency Medicine (25,1:65)
Pediatrics (90,3:350)

Time your asthma medicine right to ease exercise

If you're an asthmatic, you know that it's easy to get in a vicious cycle of poor health. You don't exercise because of breathlessness. So your risk of obesity, high blood pressure and cholesterol increases because you're not getting enough exercise. And every time you try to start working out, you give up again because you wheeze and can't get your breath.

You can break this cycle by using your asthma medication before you begin your exercise program, claims Dr. Sally Wenzel, assistant professor of medicine at the National Jewish Center for Immunology and Respiratory Medicine in Denver.

A puff of an asthma reliever like albuterol, metaproterenol or cromolyn before you get going can prevent breathlessness and start you back on the road to aerobic fitness.

Dr. Wenzel also notes that swimming is a terrific exercise because asthmatics breathe humidified air more easily.

Your pharmacist can advise you about over-the-counter asthma remedies that will allow you to get back into an exercise routine.

Medical Source ─────────────────────────
Medical Tribune (33,9:10)

Asthma sufferers should jump in the lake

If you suffer from asthma, swimming could be a good form of exercise for you — if you don't swim too much, that is.

Swimming is an exercise that many doctors recommend for people who have asthma, because it's good exercise that causes very little respiratory discomfort (compared with other forms of exercise).

However, a recent study indicates that too much time in the water could aggravate asthma. A group of scientists began the study after noticing that symptoms of asthma, including wheezing and shortness of breath, are common among athletes who swim frequently.

The scientists surveyed 251 competitive swimmers to determine how common respiratory complaints were among swimmers. Over 90 percent of the swimmers they surveyed reported at least one respiratory complaint that seemed to be related to swimming.

Of the 251 study participants, 34 of them had asthma. And of those 34 swimmers, over 70 percent of them claimed that they had been diagnosed with asthma after they began swimming competitively.

The scientists believe that the swimmers suffered from respiratory problems such as wheezing and shortness of breath because of the chemicals in the pool water.

Chlorine and other chemicals that are used to keep pool water clean and free from bacteria can irritate the lungs and cause coughing, wheezing and other common lung problems. Poor ventilation in indoor pools seems to contribute to the irritation.

The scientists pointed out that the study participants all swam at least 12 miles each week, which is much more than a recreational swimmer would do. They think that the greater amount of time spent in the water might contribute to the lung irritation and that casual swimmers probably don't spend enough time in the chlorinated water to be bothered by the chlorine.

If you suffer from asthma and your doctor recommended that you swim to get some extra exercise without aggravating your asthma, continue to follow your doctor's advice.

If, however, you swim several miles per week and notice increased problems with your asthma, talk with your doctor about the possibility of chlorine irritation from the pool water. You could be spending too much time in the water.

Medical Source ————————————————
Medical Tribune (33,14:33)

Hot, hazy days may mean breathing trouble

If you live in the city, hazy summer days mean more than daylight-saving time. They also mean more respiratory illnesses.

In a recent study, researchers from New York University Medical Center's Department of Environmental Medicine gathered information on the number of people admitted to local hospitals for respiratory complaints during the summer months of 1988 and 1989.

The researchers then tracked the daily concentration of ground-level ozone from automobiles, which seems to be thicker in the air on hazy days. They matched up the days of hospital admissions with the levels of air pollution and found some remarkable results.

The research team discovered that there was a statistical correlation between respiratory problems and increased amounts of pollutants in the air on hazy summer days.

For example, on the haziest days when the pollution was the thickest, the number of hospital admissions for asthma went up 23 percent in New York City and 29 percent in Buffalo.

These results indicate that people with histories of respiratory illnesses and those who suffer from respiratory problems (such as asthma) that can be aggravated by air pollution should consider staying inside as much as possible on hot, hazy days.

Medical Source ⎯⎯⎯⎯⎯⎯⎯⎯⎯⎯⎯⎯⎯⎯⎯⎯
   Science News (143,4:52)

Wintertime wheezing in kids may be aggravated by air pollution

Wintertime. For most children, it's a time of snowflakes, snowmen, snow fights and "snow days" off from school. But, for some, the first snowfall can mean wheezing and asthma attacks.

Scientists now think it may be more than just the cold air that triggers your child's respiratory distress — it may be what's in the air he's breathing.

A study in the Netherlands found a link between even the slightest amount of pollution and noxious gases in the air and chronic respiratory problems in some young children.

Seventy-three elementary-school-aged children in two cities in the Netherlands were studied during the winters of 1990 and 1991. Every child in the study suffered from attacks of shortness of breath, chronic coughing during the fall and winter seasons or asthma. The chilly air they breathed outdoors contained sulfur dioxide, particulate pollution, nitrogen dioxide and black smoke.

Parents recorded their children's daily "peak expiratory flow" (how easily they were able to breathe), respiratory symptoms and medication use including bronchodilators — drugs that open the airways.

Pollution levels in the two towns climbed as the temperature dropped, keeping the frozen pollution particles suspended in air. To ensure that pollution was the only factor being measured, scientists adjusted the findings to account for the effects that cold weather alone, regardless of air contents, has on the human respiratory system.

According to the study, air pollution seemed to aggravate symptoms, rather than actually bring on a wheezing incident or asthma attack.

The observations made in the Netherlands support recent similar studies in Utah, Ohio and Spain. Higher concentrations of particle-laden polluted air in Utah and increased levels of sulfur dioxide and black smoke in Barcelona were associated with more people being hospitalized with respiratory trouble.

In Steubenville, Ohio, a decrease in the population's lung functions was shown to be related to a moderate increase in air pollution.

While there appears to be a definite link between the elevated levels of pollution in wintertime air and the prevalence of chronic respiratory symptoms in some children, experts are not clear on what action to take.

Making the public aware of the problem and encouraging parents to keep young sufferers indoors as much as possible may help.

Medical Source ————————————————
American Review of Respiratory Disease (147,1:118)

Cars pollute children's lungs

Heavy traffic passing through the local school district could be damaging your child's lungs.

According to German researchers, the effect of car pollution on children's lung health is comparable to the effect of passive smoking in children with parents who smoke.

All the fourth-grade children in the city of Munich, Germany, were given physical examinations throughout the 1989-1990 school year. The children's parents filled out a questionnaire about symptoms of allergies and asthma.

The researchers counted the number of cars that passed through each school district on weekdays. They determined the school districts which had fewer than 26,000 cars pass through every day, 26,000 to 48,000 cars and over 48,000 cars.

The more traffic the children were exposed to, the more wheezing and dyspnea they suffered. Dyspnea is the kind of loud, difficult breathing that's normal when you exercise vigorously.

The car pollution didn't seem to cause children to have asthma. But since traffic exhausts apparently cause inflammation of the air passageways, they could be dangerous for children with asthma.

The levels of pollution in Munich didn't exceed standards for air quality, according to air monitoring stations the researchers set up.

The American Academy of Pediatrics is calling for the U.S. government to tighten its pollution standards, particularly levels of ozone pollution. Ozone forms when sunlight reacts with automobile exhaust and gasoline vapors.

Ozone pollution levels are lower earlier in the day, so encourage your children to exercise then rather than in the evening.

If your child's school is in a heavy traffic area, ask the school to schedule physical education courses and outdoor activities in the morning, especially if your child has asthma.

Medical Sources ————————————————
British Medical Journal (307,6904:596)
The Atlanta Journal/Constitution (June 9,1993,E4)

Short of breath? Exercise can help!

Imagine feeling as if you had just run up five flights of stairs. You're gasping for air, and your body cries out for oxygen.

Now imagine you live with this breathless feeling all the time. This is what happens when the lungs lose their elasticity as a person develops emphysema, chronic bronchitis or another of the lung diseases called chronic obstructive pulmonary disease (COPD).

Most forms of COPD result directly from smoking tobacco. Although there are fewer smokers today, so many people smoked in the past that the number of people with COPD is still on the rise. In fact, COPD ranks fifth among all causes of death in the United States today.

There is no cure for COPD, although quitting smoking can help halt the progress of the disease. Most people with advanced COPD gradually give up working and exercising because they simply lack the breath to continue.

Until recently, researchers have studied only how aerobic exercise benefits healthy people.

We know that it can lower heart rate and blood pressure and improve the way our bodies transport oxygen. But according to Dr. Denis E. O'Donnell, assistant professor, division of respirology and critical care medicine at Queen's University in Ontario, Canada, doctors now believe that exercise training can also help people with COPD.

When researchers tested older people with COPD for eight weeks, they found that exercise training:

> Reduced breathlessness.
> Increased ability to exercise.
> Improved self-esteem.
> Led to greater independence.
> Enabled people with COPD to participate in a
  wider range of activities.

Dr. O'Donnell emphasized that to get the benefits of aerobic exercise, people with COPD must continue to exercise regularly.

Most exercise programs for people with COPD are based on one or more of these activities:

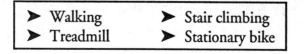

> Walking   > Stair climbing
> Treadmill   > Stationary bike

Dr. Denis O'Donnell says that some people with COPD will need to increase their strength with weight training before they can benefit from exercise training.

Some might also need to retrain themselves to breathe with a technique called pursed-lip breathing, which can ease breathing during exercise.

Pursed-lip breathing involves taking small breaths and then exhaling as long as possible through pursed lips. When you get ready to breathe out, position your lips as if you were about to whistle. This is the pursed-lip position.

Your physician can help you decide on an appropriate exercise routine and also help you learn pursed-lip breathing.

Medical Sources —————————————————
Geriatrics (48,1:59)
The Merck Manual, 16th edition, Merck Research Laboratories, Rahway, N.J., 1992

Proper nutrition relieves lung disorders

Chronic obstructive pulmonary disease, also known as COPD, affects between 15 and 20 million people in the United States today.

Chronic obstructive pulmonary disease is a medical term meaning that some portion of the airways leading to the lungs is blocked, leading to great difficulty in breathing and often resulting in serious infections.

COPD includes a range of lung conditions, including emphysema, asthma and bronchitis. These illnesses are serious enough by themselves. Unfortunately, many people with COPD also suffer from malnutrition.

In fact, between 26 and 47 percent of the people with COPD suffer from some degree of malnutrition. Malnutrition weakens the body even further, and it often causes more serious health complications or even early death in many patients with COPD who could have fared better by eating a balanced diet.

Up until now, most doctors thought that the weight loss and poor nutritional states that characterized most people with COPD were unavoidable conditions caused by the illness itself. However, doctor now suspect that malnutrition in COPD can be avoided.

A group of researchers tested the effects of increased nutritional support in people with COPD to see if better nutrition improved their health.

The scientists recruited 27 people with emphysema to participate in the study. Each of the 27 volunteers suffered from malnutrition and weighed less than 90 percent of their ideal body weights.

The volunteers were then divided into two groups. Group one (the control group) went home and continued to eat their meals as they had before they began the study. They did not receive any instructions for healthier eating nor any nutritional supplements for their diets.

However, the volunteers in group two (the intervention group) were admitted to the hospital where they received nutritionally balanced meals with increased calories and protein content. They were also offered various nutritional supplements, which were incorporated into their meal plans.

They stayed in the hospital and received this special treatment for about three weeks and then were discharged from the hospital, with instructions to go home and continue to eat well and try to gain weight.

Both groups maintained their usual medical care for COPD throughout the study. After four weeks, and then again after four months, both groups of volunteers were re-evaluated.

At the end of the re-evaluation periods, the researchers analyzed the information they had obtained from the volunteers during the study and found some encouraging results: The nutritional supplementation and well-balanced diets improved health status and even seemed to slow the progress of the disease.

The members of the "intervention group" enjoyed an average weight gain of about five pounds, whereas the members of the "control group" suffered weight loss during the test period.

Group two intervention volunteers experienced an increase in muscular strength (measured by hand grip strength and strength of the muscles used to exhale). However, members from group one lost muscular strength in the same time period.

Group two members also experienced improved stamina and were able to walk farther than they could before the study began. Members of the control group, however, lost stamina and could not walk as far after the study as they could four months earlier.

These results suggest that getting adequate nutrition can help improve health in COPD patients, whereas poor nutrition actually worsens a person's health more than the disease already has.

If you suffer from COPD, talk to your doctor about making sure your diet provides enough nutrients to keep you as healthy as possible to help lessen the effects of the disease.

Medical Source ————————————————
American Review of Respiratory Disease (146,6:1511)

BURNS

Taking the heat out of painful burns

Most burns are merely a painful nuisance that we know will heal in time. But each year, 2.5 million Americans burn themselves badly enough that they need to see a doctor or go to a hospital for treatment, and almost 12,000 people in the United States die from burns.

Sometimes it's hard to know if a burn is superficial or deeper and more damaging than it appears. Dr. Wayne F. Peate, of the University of Arizona College of Medicine in Tucson, explains how you can determine if your burn is serious enough to see a doctor.

Treatment for a burn depends on how the burn occurred. Most burns result from contact with one of these sources:

> Hot liquids
> Steam
> Flames
> Radiation
> Electricity
> Sunlight
> Hot solids (molten metal)
> Acid or alkali chemicals
> Explosions
> Liquid nitrogen

You should always see a doctor if you are burned by electricity or chemicals. Electrical burns can cause heart problems and damage tissues deep in the body.

Chemicals such as hydrofluoric acid, commonly used in the semiconductor industry, cause burns that are initially painless, but can severely injure deep body tissue.

You can also get information about the seriousness of a burn from its appearance. First- and second-degree burns that are smaller than a silver dollar on an adult and smaller than a quarter on a child can usually be treated at home. Burns covering a larger area should be examined by a doctor.

First-degree burns — These are the least serious burns. They involve only the top layers of skin and usually leave no scars. In a first-degree burn, the skin is red and turns white when touched. Sunburn is the most common cause of first-degree burns.

Home care — Apply cold water to the burn as quickly as possible. Don't use ice! Extremely cold temperatures can damage the skin as badly as extremely hot temperatures. Soak the burn in cold water or apply wet towels. Continue until the pain stops.

The sooner the temperature of your skin is returned to normal, the less skin damage you will have. Cover the burn loosely with gauze and let it begin healing on its own for at least 24 hours before applying lotions or ointments.

Apply a moisturizer such as aloe vera lotion to sunburned areas unless the burn blisters. Over-the-counter antihistamines may relieve itching. Pain killers, such as aspirin or acetaminophen, can help control any pain. See your doctor if your sunburn develops into blisters or if you experience fever or chills.

Second-degree burns — These burns vary in appearance depending on how deep they are. They often cause blistering. The more superficial second-degree burns look white or whitish red, and they feel wet or waxy dry to touch. Flames, oil or grease often cause second-degree burns, and they usually leave a scar.

Home care — Soak burned area in cool water, then gently dry the burn with a clean towel. Cover the burned area with antibiotic cream. Don't touch the burn with your fingers.

Use rubber gloves or a sterile tongue depressor blade (the kind the doctor uses) or even a cotton swab to apply the cream. Cover the burn with a nonstick dressing, such as gauze covered with petroleum jelly, and keep the dressing in place with more gauze.

Wash off, then reapply the antibiotic cream two or three times a day, covering the wound with gauze each time. Don't try to pop any blisters. If a blister pops on its own, clean the area with soap and water, then apply more antibiotic cream.

When the burn begins to heal and the blisters go away, you can use aloe vera or sunburn-relief spray to ease any stinging or burning.

Third-degree burns — They usually destroy the skin completely and look white or charred. You will only be able to feel deep pressure in a third-degree burn, and there will probably be some scarring. Some of the common causes for third-degree burns include fire, steam, scalding liquids, grease, chemicals and electricity. If you suspect a third-degree burn, see your doctor immediately.

General burn care:
➤ Bathe daily. Avoid overly hot showers or baths.
➤ Don't apply bandages too tightly. Some signs that you may be cutting off your circulation include numbness, tingling or a change in skin color.
➤ Have a tetanus shot if your immunization is not current.
➤ Remember that burned skin is sensitive to the sun for one year.
➤ Never apply butter, oil or grease to a burn.
➤ Don't use ointment on burns that have blistered.

Call your doctor immediately if:
➤ You have burns on your face, eyes, hands, feet or pelvic area.
➤ You develop signs of an infection, such as fever, chills, vomiting, swollen glands or if your burn begins to look infected. Your burn is probably infected if it starts to get warm, red and swollen again, or if you see any brown, yellow or green fluid or pus around the burn.
➤ You begin coughing, wheezing or have difficulty breathing or swallowing.
➤ Your burn does not heal in about 10 days.

Treating minor burns is usually a simple procedure. Of course, the best treatment is to avoid burns altogether. Follow these precautions to safeguard your family from burns:

- ❐ The most common burns are sunburns. Make sunscreen, hats and protective clothing a must for outdoor activities. Encourage your family to stay out of the sun from 10 a.m. until 4 p.m., when the sun's rays are the most damaging.
- ❐ Most fatal burns occur at home during the night. Install smoke detectors in your home and practice an evacuation route with your family. Teach your family to crawl before the smoke and to feel a doorknob for heat before opening it. Explain that people should wrap themselves in a blanket and roll on the ground if their clothing catches fire. Ask your local fire department to inspect your home for fire hazards. They can help you cut down on your risks of burns and household fire accidents.
- ❐ Turn your hot water heater below 120° Fahrenheit. Even brief exposure to water hotter than 120° can damage the skin.
- ❐ In the kitchen, turn pot handles away from the front of the stove. Use mitten pot holders, and consider installing a stove guard to protect young children. Test the temperature of all foods. Food heated in a microwave can be much hotter than its container.
- ❐ Wear rubber gloves and protective eye goggles when using household chemicals like oven cleaner.
- ❐ Keep chemicals and caustic agents like batteries stored up high and away from children.
- ❐ Throw out oily rags.
- ❐ Cover electrical outlets.

Medical Source ───────────────────────
American Family Physician (45,3:1321)

COLDS AND FLU

Cold comfort: how to ease your common-cold misery

A cure for the common cold? Feel free to be skeptical, but you probably will see a cure in your lifetime.

The "rhinovirus" causes most of the common colds. Scientists now know what a "rhinovirus" looks like and how it gets inside human cells. Armed with this information, drug designers should be able to develop medicines that will prevent a cold by keeping the viruses out of human cells.

Researchers are also improving the interferon drug — a common-cold "wonder drug" that's been around for a while but has too many side effects to be useful.

Scientists haven't yet nailed down a cure for the common cold, but they have figured out a lot about how and why people catch colds.

If you're stressed out, you need to chill out!

Have you ever noticed that when you're under a lot of pressure at work or when things aren't going right at home, you top it all off by coming down with a cold. People under mental stress are much more likely to catch a cold than calm, relaxed people.

A team of British and American scientists gave nasal drops containing a cold virus to 400 people. About 90 percent of the people judged to be under stress came down with a cold. About 74 percent of those who weren't stressed developed colds.

Stressed-out people tend to be busy people who get around a lot, so it could be that they just expose themselves to more infections. It's more probable, though, that stress actually weakens your immune system.

Mental or physical stress makes it easier for you to come down with a cold once you're infected, but how do you actually catch a cold?

Despite Mom's repeated warnings that "You'll catch your death of a cold" if you venture out without a jacket, swim in cold water, go out with wet hair, etc., those old tales just aren't true.

You can't catch a cold from cold weather, wet feet, wet clothes or drafts. It's a cold fact that you can only catch a cold from another person.

Doctors seem to be split about 50-50 on how colds pass from one person to another. Some doctors insist that colds pass by hand-to-hand-to-nose. That means that if you shake hands with an infected person or touch something an infected person has touched and then touch your nose or face, you're likely to catch their cold.

Other doctors believe that the common cold is passed through the air — you are contaminated when a person with a cold sneezes or coughs near you and the droplets land on you.

Either way, your best bet is to be a cold fish and stay away from people with cold symptoms. Try not to touch your face after you've shaken hands with a person with a cold, and wash your hands as soon as possible.

If you have a cold, be considerate of others: Try to avoid touching your face, particularly your nose and mouth, and scrub your hands often with hot, sudsy water.

Once you've caught a cold, all you can do is make yourself as cozy as possible and wait it out. Here are some hints to help ease your misery:

- ☐ Drink lots of nonalcoholic liquids, especially water! Most people think they're drinking enough when they really aren't. The best way to tell if you're getting enough fluids is the color of your urine. Drink until your urine is clear. If it's a deep yellow color, your body needs more liquids.
- ☐ Give a cold shoulder to cigarette smoke. Smoking not only makes cold symptoms worse, but it also makes you more likely to catch a cold. Cigarette smoke numbs the hairs in the nose that work to keep the nose clean.
- ☐ Ease a sore throat with warm beverages, like tea with honey and lemon. Gargling with warm salt water works well, too.
- ☐ Get plenty of rest.
- ☐ Suck on hard candy to relieve a dry throat and mild cough. Candy works about as well as medicated lozenges, and it's safer for you.

❏ Soothe chapped lips and nose with a petroleum-jelly ointment.

❏ Try a humidifier, a vaporizer or a pan of water on the stove to help relieve a stuffy nose and help loosen mucus in your throat. The moist air might relieve a dry cough, too.

❏ Don't mistake the flu or strep throat for a simple cold. If you feel exhausted and have a high fever, headache and severe muscle aches, you probably have the flu instead of a cold. You need to see your doctor for treatment.

With strep throat, you'll have a very painful throat plus a high fever, pus on your throat or tonsils and possibly a rash. You'll need antibiotics to cure strep throat.

❏ Get that chicken soup comfort. Mom was right about chicken soup, you know. Not only does the steam and aroma help relieve your stuffy nose, but the chicken soup also seems to work as an anti-inflammatory.

Spicy soups are especially good at unstuffing your head. The spicy foods loosen nasal mucus and make your nose drip, which can be helpful in treating chronic sinusitis.

Medical Sources ───────────────────────
Medical World News (34,3:31)
Postgraduate Medicine (91,6:55)
Medical Tribune (34,11:11)
The Lancet (338,8770:832)

Over-the-counter relief

When a cold is really getting you down, all the chicken soup, warm beverages and rest in the world just aren't going to cut it. You occasionally have to resort to over-the-counter medicines.

Just remember that, for now anyway, drugs can't cure a cold. They can only ease your symptoms and make you feel better.

The main rule for cold medicines is: Take specific drugs for specific symptoms. Avoid the combination drugs.

Decongestants and antihistamines. Don't take medicine to dry up your runny nose. It's your body's way of getting rid of a virus.

Nose sprays, drops or inhalers are the best way to ease a stopped-up nose. Don't use them for more than three days at a time, or you'll risk a rebound effect. They'll actually start making your nose stuffier. Don't share the containers with other family members — you'll spread the infection.

You can take an oral decongestant for your stuffy nose, but nose sprays and drops work faster and are safer.

Oral decongestants can raise your blood pressure, so be especially cautious with them if you have high blood pressure, heart disease, thyroid problems or diabetes.

Antihistamines relieve allergy symptoms, but they aren't particularly useful for cold sufferers.

Aspirin and acetaminophen. Plain, generic aspirin or acetaminophen is the cheapest and best way to treat the all-over achiness that can accompany a cold.

However, if you're under 40, don't use aspirin if you have a high fever or you think you may have the flu. You'll increase your risk of getting Reye's syndrome.

Sore throats are best eased by warm liquids, but occasionally you may need something stronger. Try plain aspirin or acetaminophen. Throat lozenges and sprays, mouthwashes and gargles don't work very well, and some contain ingredients that aren't safe.

Cough medicines. If you're coughing up phlegm and mucus, you have a "productive" cough and you should let it run its course. You can take a medicine called an "expectorant" that helps you cough, but they aren't very effective.

If you have a dry, hacking cough, you may want to take a cough suppressant so you can get some rest. Cough suppressants are also called "antitussives." Try to find a cough suppressant with just one ingredient called "dextromethorphan." This drug is the safest and most effective on the market.

Hang in there, cold sufferers. A common-cold cure is finally in sight.

For now, do all you can to make yourself comfortable — stock up on single-ingredient cold medicine, sip on chicken soup, get plenty of rest, and drink, drink, drink!

Medical Source ————————————————
Public Citizen Health Research Group's *Health Letter* (9,2:1)

Cure for the common cold may be just around the corner

No more sniffling, sneezing, coughing, aching colds to drive you crazy or drive up your doctor bill when they develop into bronchitis, laryngitis or sinusitis. Is it possible? Well, researchers think they're on the right track.

The nonsteroidal anti-inflammatory drug naproxen reduced cold symptoms by 29 percent in 79 college students purposely infected with colds. Naproxen consistently relieved headaches, coughs, muscle aches and general listlessness.

Although naproxen relieves cold symptoms, it does not kill or halt the progress of the cold virus. However, researchers now believe that a combination of the drugs naproxen, interferon and ipratropium could possibly destroy the cold virus.

At this time, the only known drawback to this treatment is the high price of interferon.

The Center for Innovative Technology has applied for a patent to further develop this combination of medicines. It could be available in five to 10 years.

Medical Source ————————————————
Annals of Internal Medicine (117,1:37)
Medical Tribune (33,14:20)

Fighting the flu

Grandma may have griped about the "grippe," but today most people complain about the flu. Spread by coughing or sneezing, influenza is an infection of the nose, throat, bronchial tubes and lungs. To complicate matters, the symptoms of colds and flu often overlap. In fact, the same virus that causes flu can also cause a cold.

If you're feeling stuffy, sniffly, weak and achy, how can you tell if it's a cold or the flu that has you in its grip?

The biggest difference between a cold and the flu is the severity of the symptoms. Generally speaking, you feel much worse when you have the flu than when you have a cold.

Flu symptoms develop rapidly. If you were feeling great a few minutes before and suddenly feel as though you've been run over by a truck, chances are you have the flu. Other symptoms include:

> ➤ Fever. Your temperature may be 101° Fahrenheit or higher. If you have a fever, you probably have the flu instead of a cold.
> ➤ Chills
> ➤ Headache
> ➤ Tiredness
> ➤ Muscle aches and pains, especially in arms, back and legs
> ➤ Loss of appetite
> ➤ Cough
> ➤ Sore throat
> ➤ Runny nose
> ➤ Hoarseness

If you're 65 years or older or have a history of diabetes, lung or heart disease, see a doctor if you suspect you have the flu.

Once you've been diagnosed with the flu, go home and get into bed. Rest will help your body fight the virus. Here are some other helpful hints:

☐ Make sure the room you choose to recuperate in is warm and well-ventilated.

☐ Keep a humidifier in your room. The moist air will help you cough up throat mucus more easily.

☐ Take over-the-counter painkillers, antihistamines or decongestants to relieve aches and reduce fever. Don't take aspirin if you have a fever and are under age 40. Some studies have indicated a link between the use of aspirin to relieve the symptoms of a viral illness and the development of Reye's Syndrome (a disorder that causes brain and liver damage and can be fatal).

☐ Drink plenty of liquids. If you don't drink enough liquids, you can actually prolong your illness. You'll know you're drinking enough if your urine is clear-colored. Fruit juice, tea and carbonated drinks can help reduce the amount of mucus in your lungs.

☐ Inhale steam to soothe painful lungs.

☐ Gargle with warm or cold double-strength tea to relieve a sore throat.

☐ Use salt water drops, made with 1 teaspoon of salt added to one quart of water, to relieve a stuffy nose.

Although your fever will disappear after two to five days, your cough and sore throat may persist for a while longer. You may also feel weak and depressed.

Your body will completely rid itself of the flu in seven to 10 days. You can get out of bed once your fever is gone, but take life easy for a while. Gradually return to normal activities once you've regained your strength.

Sometimes the flu develops into a more serious disorder, such as bronchitis, a middle-ear infection or pneumonia. These illnesses can be fatal to people who have heart or lung disease. If you notice any of the following symptoms, see a doctor immediately.

➤ Rapid or difficult breathing
➤ Wheezing
➤ Chest pains when you breathe
➤ Feeling faint or lightheaded
➤ Spitting up blood
➤ Severe sore throat
➤ Extremely irritable or weak
➤ Earache
➤ Neck pain or stiffness

If you've had the flu once, you know you never want to have it again. Here's what you can do to avoid the flu the next time around.

☐ Get a flu shot. A flu shot is especially important for people who are 65 or older, have blood or immune disorders, diabetes, heart, lung or kidney disease, live in a nursing home or work in the medical profession. Get your shot between mid-October and mid-November, and you'll have the best protection between December and March, the peak flu season.

Since viruses A and B can mutate to create new virus strains, a vaccine won't always prevent you from coming down with the flu. However, a flu shot can reduce the length of your illness and the risk of complications or death. Don't get a flu shot if you are in the first three months of pregnancy or are allergic to eggs (the vaccine is egg-based).

☐ Stay away from people who have colds or the flu.

☐ Reduce your risk factors. You're more likely to come down with the flu if you are stressed, tired, overworked or don't eat a well-balanced diet.

Medical Sources ─────────────────
Mayo Clinic Health Letter (11,11:1)
The American Medical Association Encyclopedia of Medicine, Random House, Inc., New York, 1989
Complete Guide to Symptoms, Illness and Surgery, 2nd edition, The Body Press/Perigee Books, New York, 1989

Sinus sufferers alert

Ever have aching pains and pressure in your face? If so, you're not alone.

Sinus complaints are a common problem. They affect over 32 million people in the United States. In spite of these vast numbers, most people seem to think that sinus complaints are overexaggerated.

The problem is called sinusitis, and it's the result of inflammation of the hollow spaces in the bones of your face (sinuses). Normally your sinuses work to drain the mucus which filters the air we breathe.

But, some people have sinuses that are just too small to handle the flow. In other people, irritations such as cigarette smoke or allergies can create too much mucus for normal sinuses and they can get clogged. In any case, if you have clogged sinuses, they can become infected and hurt even more.

If you seem to get colds that go on and on, snore and have trouble sleeping because it's so hard to breathe, the area around your sinuses is tender and swollen, or even if you seem to get toothaches often, there is a good chance that you suffer from sinusitis.

What will help? you ask. The popular advice to drink eight glasses of water a day may help your sinuses as well as benefit the rest of your body. Vaporizers with added menthol may also help.

Other temporary home remedies include chewing horseradish or eating soup made with lots of garlic.

If your problem is an allergy, however, the remedy can be as simple as avoiding the allergy trigger. If it's cigarette smoke, for example, that bothers you, curing your sinusitis could be as simple as avoiding places where people are smoking.

Antihistamines may help reduce the swelling in your nose and dry up the mucus, but many of these have side effects such as sleepiness. Decongestants can also help reduce swelling. Be sure to check with your doctor or pharmacist before using any medications.

If your sinus problem goes on for a long time, a specific medication can stop working and you may have to switch to a medication with a different active ingredient.

If your sinusitis begins to interfere with your daily activities, or you have to take naps or miss work frequently, it may be time to see a physician for more extensive treatment.

Medical Source ————————————————
FDA Consumer (26,8:20)

How to tell if you have hay fever, a cold or a sinus infection

Suffering from sneezing, sniffling, coughing? You could have hay fever, a cold or a sinus infection.

The symptoms often overlap, sometimes making diagnosis difficult even for the family doctor.

For this reason, researchers undertook a study to determine the most reliable predictors of sinus infections.

The investigators found five consistently reliable indicators of infected sinuses. The last two will only be evident to a doctor.

- ☐ Ache in the upper jaws.
- ☐ Creamy yellow or greenish colored discharge from nose.
- ☐ Condition is not improved by taking antihistamines or decongestants.
- ☐ Pus and mucus are found in nose or sinus cavities.
- ☐ Abnormal transillumination. This means that the light from the flashlight the doctor uses to examine the nose will not pass through the cartilage that divides the nose into two passages.

Other possible symptoms are listed below. These are not generally as reliable as the ones previously mentioned.

> - ➤ Nasal speech
> - ➤ Difficulty sleeping
> - ➤ Sinus tenderness
> - ➤ Sore throat
> - ➤ Loss of sense of smell
> - ➤ Sneezing
> - ➤ Aching muscles
> - ➤ General ill feeling
> - ➤ Cough
> - ➤ Headache
> - ➤ Recent upper respiratory infection
> - ➤ Facial pain

If you suspect that you have a sinus infection, see your doctor immediately. A confirmed sinus infection should be quickly treated with antibiotics. If left untreated, it can lead to serious disorders, such as bacterial meningitis which can cause brain damage and death.

Your best bet is to avoid sinus infections completely, if possible. Here are a few suggestions for heading off sinus infections:

☐ Sleep with your head elevated, especially if you have allergies or a cold. This will help keep the infected mucus from draining back into your sinuses and infecting them.
☐ Avoid tobacco smoke.
☐ Consider taking decongestants. They will decrease the amount of mucus produced, making it less likely that mucus will drain into your sinuses and cause an infection.

Do not take decongestants for long periods of time or if you have high blood pressure, heart disease, irregular heartbeat or glaucoma.

These extra precautions will be well worth avoiding a sinus infection.

Medical Sources ————————————————————
Annals of Internal Medicine (117,9:705)
Postgraduate Medicine (91,5:281)

Body temperatures: the 98.6° fallacy

Feeling feverish? Don't get overheated if your temperature is not exactly 98.6° Fahrenheit.

Never a hot topic of debate, the average body temperature of healthy adults has been accepted as 98.6° since 1868 when Carl Wunderlich, a scientific investigator, examined 25,000 people, taking 1 million temperature readings. He determined average body temperature to be 98.6°.

Recently, researchers at the University of Maryland School of Medicine challenged Wunderlich's findings. They found 98.2° a more accurate description of the normal adult's average body temperature.

After taking 700 temperature readings from 148 participants, researchers found only 56 to have a temperature of 98.6°. Temperatures ranged from 96.0° to 100.8°.

Temperatures vary according to the individual and the time of day. Your temperature may change as much as 1.09 degrees. Between individuals, temperatures can differ as much as 4.8 degrees. Temperatures tend to be lowest at 6 a.m. and highest at 4 p.m.

Researchers recommend that you consider the time of day in determining the presence of fever. In the morning, 99° is the temperature level considered to constitute fever, while in the afternoon that level is 100° or more.

The researchers discovered that women's temperatures tend to be about .3 degrees higher than men's. For each degree that body temperature rises, your heartbeat rate increases 2.44 beats per minute. Neither age nor smoking seem to affect normal body temperatures.

Researchers believe that the equipment used for testing caused the difference in results.

While the Maryland researchers used digital thermometers, Wunderlich used awkward thermometers that had to be held under the armpit for 15 to 20 minutes. He also didn't have computers or statistical sources to help interpret his findings.

The difference between temperature norms is so small that researchers do not foresee any changes in medical practice.

Medical Source ————————————————
The Journal of the American Medical Association (268,12:1578)

DIGESTIVE DISORDERS

Conquering constipation

Constipation is one of those subjects that we just don't like to talk about, but it's a real problem for some of us — especially among the elderly.

But don't diagnose yourself with constipation too quickly. A decreasing number of bowel movements is normal as colon and rectal muscles weaken with age.

While most young people often have at least one bowel movement a day, it's not uncommon for older people to have only three bowel movements a week.

Actually, regular bowel habits that don't cause discomfort are more important than how many weekly bowel movements you have. If you have fewer bowel movements than you used to, but your stools are not hard and dry, you're probably not suffering from constipation.

If regularity really is a problem, making a few simple diet and lifestyle changes can relieve those constipation woes:

Eat more fiber. Many older people live alone or have difficulty getting around, so they don't prepare proper meals for themselves as they once did. This usually results in a lack of important foods in the diet, including fiber.

The loss of fiber in the diet usually leads to constipation. Some easy-to-find sources of fiber include whole-grain bread, leafy green vegetables and fresh fruit.

Drink plenty of liquids. Many elderly people have a diminished sense of thirst, so they don't drink as much water or other liquids as their bodies really need.

This can result in constipation as well. You should drink four eight-ounce glasses of water for every 1,000 calories you eat. If you consume about 2,000 calories a day, you need to drink eight eight-ounce glasses of water.

Stay active. Constipation is sometimes caused (and often aggravated) by too little activity. Spend at least 20 to 30 minutes three times a week walking or exercising in some other way. This helps keep your abdominal muscles healthy and toned, and it will relieve your constipation complaints.

Limit use of over-the-counter laxatives. Laxatives are the most commonly overused nonprescription drugs. Long-term use of laxatives can weaken colon muscles and actually contribute to constipation. Many other drugs, including sedatives and tranquilizers, can cause constipation as a side effect.

If you suspect you're taking medication that may be contributing to your constipation problems, talk with your doctor. He may be able to recommend a substitute drug that doesn't cause constipation.

If your constipation problem appears to be a simple combination of age and old habits, here's a natural laxative recipe for relief you may want to try.

Ingredients:
1 pound raisins
1 pound currants
1 pound prunes
1 pound figs
1 pound dates
1 container (28-ounce) of undiluted prune concentrate

Directions:
Place the fruit in a food grinder or food processor and grind thoroughly. Add the prune concentrate to the fruit mixture. Mix the ingredients well. The mixture will be very thick. Store in the refrigerator.

---

1) Drink one glass of prune juice each morning before breakfast.
2) Drink about 1/4 cup of the natural laxative mixture around 9 a.m. every morning for one week.
3) During that week, keep a record of how often you have a bowel movement and check for stool consistency (hard, soft, or loose and watery).
4) After one week, if your stools are very loose, only take the laxative mixture three mornings per week (Monday, Wednesday and

Friday). Try this for another week and keep track of bowel movements again. If your stools are still loose, take the laxative mixture only two days per week.

5) After the first week, if your stools are still dry, hard and infrequent, take 1/4 cup of the laxative mixture twice a day. Once constipation is relieved, cut back to one dose a day to maintain regular bowel movements.

Although natural laxatives are great for relieving constipation, and are much healthier than drug laxatives, it is important not to overuse the natural laxative mixture.

If your stools get too loose and watery or if bowel movements occur too often, you can begin to suffer from diarrhea and dehydration. This can result in hospitalization and serious complications.

Severe dehydration can even be fatal. If you are having at least three bowel movements a week and pass soft stools easily, don't use this natural laxative more than once or twice a week. You may not need to use it at all.

Occasionally, constipation can be a sign of a more serious disorder. If you're over 40 and you've had a recent unexplainable change in your bowel movement patterns, see your doctor.

Medical Source ———————————————————
Journal of Gerontological Nursing (18,10:5)
The American Medical Association Encyclopedia of Medicine, Random House, New York, 1989

When sweets turn sour

Sugar-free foods seem like the miracle answer for dieters, diabetics, and cavity-conscious folks. Artificial sweeteners are a great way to enjoy the taste of sugar while avoiding many problems associated with real sugar.

However, you can have too much of a good thing.

Sorbitol is a sugar alcohol found in many sugar-free foods and candies. As little as ten grams of sorbitol can cause bloating and gas. Twenty grams may lead to cramping and diarrhea.

Since some candies contain as much as three grams of sorbitol per piece, people susceptible to side effects from this artificial sweetener would have to eat only three pieces before experiencing discomfort.

Usually symptoms occur 30 to 90 minutes after consuming the sorbitol. Complications from sorbitol are especially likely to occur around holidays such as Halloween and Christmas when eating large amounts of sweets is common.

Besides sugar-free foods and candies, sorbitol is used to give many toothpastes their sweet taste. It is also used to sweeten vitamin C tablets, which have been known to cause diarrhea in children. Medications which contain sorbitol can cause chronic diarrhea.

Diabetics seem to suffer more side effects from sorbitol than non-diabetics. This is most likely due to diabetics' more frequent use of sugar-free products.

Cramps and diarrhea related to sorbitol are not usually accompanied by a fever and normally disappear after 24 hours if no more sorbitol is consumed during this time. Replace fluids lost during diarrhea by drinking plenty of clear liquids.

To avoid future problems with sorbitol, either eliminate or reduce consumption of sorbitol. Read product labels to help you reduce your risk.

If your symptoms persist after 24 hours, consult your doctor. Be sure to tell him about any sorbitol you may have ingested. Otherwise you may risk an incorrect diagnosis and have to pay for expensive tests when the only problem is a little overindulgence.

Medical Source ————————————————
Postgraduate Medicine (92,5:63)

Heartburn: Get it off your chest

Heartburn is not a pleasant, heartwarming sensation. You know what it's like. After a spicy meal or a too-quick lunch, you feel pain in your chest, back, neck and even jaw.

Constant heartburn often signals gastroesophageal reflux disease, a disorder in which acidic stomach contents come burning back up into your esophagus, the tube that connects your mouth and your stomach.

Gastroesophageal reflux commonly affects older adults. Forty-four percent of American adults report a heartburn attack once a month; seven percent suffer from daily heartburn.

Acid reflux occurs when the muscle between your stomach and your esophagus, the lower esophageal sphincter, relaxes at the wrong time. The sphincter should only relax when you swallow to allow food to pass from your esophagus to your stomach.

If there is too much pressure in your stomach or if the muscle between your stomach and esophagus becomes weak, stomach acids flow back up into your esophagus.

Although the lining of the stomach can handle the high acid content of the digestive juices, the lining of the esophagus is more sensitive to acid damage. The stomach acid irritates the lining of the esophagus, and you feel that burning sensation known as heartburn.

Another common cause of heartburn is poor esophageal clearance. This means the muscles of the esophagus that move food down the tube after you swallow don't work smoothly enough.

The swallowed food takes longer to travel down the esophagus than it should. The sphincter muscle has to stay open too long, and acid from the stomach can slosh back into the esophagus.

A third common culprit behind heartburn is a hiatal hernia. A hiatal hernia means part of your stomach pokes up through the hole in the diaphragm where the esophagus goes through.

Hiatal hernias can cause little pockets of acid that predispose you to gastroesophageal reflux.

The most common symptoms of gastroesophageal reflux are:

- ☐ Burning or discomfort in the center of your chest that is worse after eating.
- ☐ Painful, difficult or delayed swallowing when you eat or drink.
- ☐ Belching that brings food from your stomach back up into your mouth.
- ☐ Sudden filling of your mouth with salty-tasting fluid, known as water brash.

❏ A sour or unpleasant taste in your mouth after eating.

Other possible symptoms include hoarseness, postnasal drip, voice changes, persistent cough, excess salivation, bad breath, throat clearing, neck pain, sore throat, ear pain and choking spells.

Some people experience all these symptoms and never have burning chest pains.

Many people are sent home with some over-the-counter cough medicine or decongestant because the doctor thinks he's treating a common cold instead of gastroesophageal reflux.

Heartburn may occur when you lie down, bend forward, exercise, strain muscles and even when you sleep. Many pregnant women suffer from heartburn because the baby puts pressure on the stomach.

Heartburn resulting from pregnancy always disappears after childbirth and shouldn't be a cause for concern.

Although gastroesophageal reflux can be very uncomfortable, it's typically very easy to relieve. Lowering the amount of acid in the stomach is the simplest and quickest way to get relief from heartburn. The easiest way to do that is to take antacids.

Antacids are available as over-the-counter drugs in several different forms — pills, chewable tablets and liquids. Whatever the form or brand name of the drug (Rolaids, Tums, Mylanta, Phillips' Milk of Magnesia, etc.), they all seem to bring quick and soothing relief.

For people who experience only occasional cases of heartburn, antacids might be the best therapy.

But, for people who experience gastroesophageal reflux on a daily basis, making some simple lifestyle changes may be more helpful than buying stock in an antacid company.

❏ Cut down on fatty and spicy foods, alcoholic beverages, coffee (caffeinated and decaffeinated), other caffeinated drinks, chocolate, peppermint and citrus juices.

These foods cause the sphincter muscle to relax, and caffeine stimulates production of extra stomach acids. Fatty foods take longer to digest, so they stay in the stomach longer. That increases the likelihood that digestive juices will leak back up into the esophagus.

☐ Stop smoking cigarettes. Smoking also causes the sphincter to relax. Avoid other tobacco products, such as cigars, chewing tobacco and snuff.

☐ Lose excess weight. Fat around the abdomen increases the pressure on the stomach.

☐ Eat smaller meals. A full stomach can push stomach acid back into the esophagus and cause heartburn. Try eating four to six small meals per day instead of two to three large meals.

☐ Eat slowly, taking small bites and chewing completely. Many people suffer from heartburn because they "eat on the run."

☐ Don't eat for three hours before bedtime.

☐ Don't lie down immediately after meals. You may even want to take a walk. Lying down allows stomach contents to leak back into the esophagus more easily. Stay upright for at least two hours after every meal.

☐ If you have to "hit the hay" after a large meal, lie on your left side instead of your right. Lying on your left side causes only half the heartburn experienced when lying on your right. When you lie on your left side, your stomach is below your esophagus. In this position, gravity works to keep stomach acids from rising into the esophagus.

☐ Avoid bending over or stooping after meals.

☐ Avoid wearing tight clothing or belts around your waist (including girdles). This increases the pressure in the abdomen and literally pushes food into the esophagus from the stomach.

☐ Use lozenges to stimulate saliva production. Saliva helps neutralize the acid in the stomach. Remember to avoid peppermint lozenges.

☐ Avoid chewing gum. When you chew gum, you usually swallow mouthfuls of air. This causes heartburn. Swallowing air also causes stomach pain and bloating.

☐ Elevate the head of your bed six to eight inches. You can do this by placing blocks under your headboard, putting books or pillows between your mattress and box spring, or by using extra pillows to keep your head elevated. You can also buy wedge-shaped foam rubber pillows that keep your head and upper body slightly elevated.

This helps gravity "pull" the contents of the stomach away from the esophagus while you are asleep. It's harder for the stomach contents to travel "uphill."

☐ Ask your doctor or pharmacist about possible side effects of the medications you're taking. If they cause heartburn, ask your doctor about substituting a medicine that does not cause heartburn. Don't stop taking medication without your doctor's advice.

Drugs that can cause heartburn include:

➤ Alpha-adrenergic antagonists, such as phenoxybenzamine, phentolamine, prazosin, terazosin and labetalol

➤ Anticholinergics, such as atropine, scopalamine, pirenzepine and vecuronium

➤ Beta-adrenergic agonists, such as isoproterenol, metaproterenol, albuterol, bitolterol and terbutaline

➤ Calcium-channel blockers, such as verapamil, diltiazem, nifedipine (Procardia) and bepridil

➤ Diazepam

➤ Dopamine

➤ Narcotics

➤ Progesterone

➤ Theophylline

➤ Nitrates

These lifestyle changes are not short-term remedies. You'll only get relief from heartburn symptoms for as long as you follow them. When you switch back to old habits, the heartburn will return.

If you still suffer from gastroesophageal reflux after trying these tips, see your doctor. Continuous gastroesophageal reflux can cause asthma and bronchitis.

Swallowing may become extremely painful. It's also possible to mistake chest pains that signal potential heart problems for heartburn.

Medical Sources ————————————
The Journal of Family Practice (35,6:673)
American Family Physician (46,2:536)
Annals of Internal Medicine (117,12:977)
Geriatrics (48,3:60)
Emergency Medicine (23,20:98)
Modern Medicine (59,9:14 and 60,1:24)

Antacids: fighting the fire of heartburn

Over-the-counter antacids provide quick and easy relief for heartburn. They work by neutralizing stomach acids. But with so many to choose from, which antacid should you pick?

Use ingredient listings as a guide. Listed below are some common antacid ingredients and their possible side effects:

- ☐ **Aluminum hydroxide.** May cause constipation.
- ☐ **Magnesium salts.** May cause diarrhea.
  Tip: Choose an antacid that contains both these ingredients, and it will probably balance out the negative side effects of each.
- ☐ **Calcium carbonate.** Often the most effective antacid ingredient. Avoid these antacids if you are prone to kidney stones.
- ☐ **Alginic acid.** These antacids actually prevent acid reflux.

If you have high blood pressure, ask your doctor to recommend an antacid that is low in sodium. Antacids sometimes interfere with absorption of iron supplements or prescribed medicines such as tetracycline or ciprofloxacin. If you are taking these medications yet think you need an antacid, ask your doctor for suggestions.

Even though antacids provide relief, you should see your doctor if you have persistent heartburn.

Medical Sources ————————————
Geriatrics (48,3:60)
FDA Consumer (26,1:19)

'Coke is it' for digestive ills

Coca-Cola is normally a no-no for heartburn sufferers, but there is a reason to have a Coke and a smile when your digestive system is giving you trouble.

Everyday Coca-Cola can work even better than surgery to clear up a problem caused by heartburn. That problem is getting food stuck in your throat, and it can be more serious than it sounds.

Constant heartburn is more than just irritating. All that acid coming up from your stomach actually damages your esophagus, the canal that carries food from your mouth to your stomach.

You can develop ulcers and swelling in your esophagus, or even a buildup of scar tissue that narrows your esophagus.

When your esophagus narrows, food tends to get stuck on the way down. It's bad enough when you can feel the food going through your throat and esophagus, but it's worse when it really gets stuck. You can wind up needing surgery.

When food gets trapped in your damaged esophagus, doctors will remove the food with an endoscope and then dilate your narrow esophagus with a balloon dilator. Usually, the food breaks into pieces, and the doctor has to put the endoscope tube down your throat four or five times. It's a miserable experience.

Instead of rushing to the hospital and going through this painful surgery, all you have to do is grab a fizzy Coke to break up the lump of food in your esophagus.

Two British doctors studied eight people who came to the hospital a total of 13 times with food trapped in a damaged area. Every time the doctors gave Coca-Cola to the suffering people, the food disappeared before the next day. Seven times, the people didn't drink Coca-Cola, and they had to have the food removed surgically.

Fizzy drinks seem to work their way into the food and release carbon dioxide gas, disintegrating the trapped food. Some of the drink may seep through into the stomach and cause you to burp. Burping also helps get the stuck food moving.

At some point, the doctor may still have to look down your throat with an endoscope and then dilate your esophagus if it's too narrow. But if you've gotten rid of the lodged food with a Coca-Cola, the surgery will be much less difficult and painful.

When you get a piece of food stuck in your esophagus, try Coke — "it's the real thing" to make you feel better.

Medical Source —————————————————————
Annals of the Royal College of Surgeons of England (75,2:94)

Move over headache, here comes IBS

Doctors have a new medical puzzle on their hands. It ranks right up there with chronic lower back pain and headaches — two maladies which leave most doctors feeling hopeless, helpless and useless.

Irritable bowel syndrome (IBS) is a digestive disorder that affects one in four to five people, making life miserable for some. It equals the common cold as a major reason people are absent from work.

Everyone with irritable bowel syndrome has different symptoms, but there are four which most IBS sufferers have in common. They are called the Manning criteria:

- ❏ Your stomach hurts and cramps, bringing on loose stools (like diarrhea). You have an urgent need to go to the bathroom.
- ❏ Stomach pain or cramping brings on more frequent stools. In other words, you will defecate much more than normal.
- ❏ Stomach pain is eased after you defecate.
- ❏ Your stomach becomes bloated.

Other symptoms people frequently have include burning, cutting or strong stomach pain, gas, diarrhea (especially in the morning or after a meal), constipation, nausea, tenderness on the left side of the stomach, stools that are pellet-like or pencil-shaped or stools laced with mucus.

These symptoms come and go — you're likely to have a bad week or couple of days, then have no trouble at all for a week or two. The symptoms also vary: You may have diarrhea one week and constipation the next.

All IBS symptoms are probably caused by intense contractions or muscle spasms of the bowel.

Why your intestines don't work right remains a mystery. It could be a problem with your hormones, your nervous system or your biochemistry. It could be that your rectal area is more sensitive than other people's.

Many people with irritable bowel syndrome are depressed, anxious or stressed, especially right before a bout of stomach pain, diarrhea or constipation. But nobody knows which came first — the chicken (the IBS symptoms) or the egg (the depression or anxiety).

Is your mind affecting your stomach or your stomach your mind, or, more likely, does it go both ways?

Practicing relaxation techniques and working to remove the causes of your stress could relieve your bloating, diarrhea and stomach cramps. The most common causes of stress are marital problems, anxiety over your children, loss of a loved one and worrying obsessively over trivial, everyday problems.

Try to relax at mealtimes. Don't rush your lunch, eat during a stressful business meeting or talk with your spouse about finances over supper.

Getting to work late makes for an anxious day for many people. Try to wake up 30 minutes earlier and have a calm morning.

Some doctors recommend hypnotherapy, psychotherapy and anti-stress or anti-depressant medication as the only ways to ease the symptoms of IBS. However, you may be able to control many of your symptoms just by changing what and how you eat.

☐ If diarrhea is your main symptom, avoid sugar-free mints, gum and diet foods that contain sorbitol and limit lactose-rich dairy products. These sugars promote diarrhea because they are hard to digest. Also avoid beans, broccoli, apples, alcohol and fats. High-fiber foods, such as salads and bran, can worsen diarrhea and cause cramping if you eat too much.

You may want to try Imodium, an over-the-counter diarrhea medication, especially if your social life is limited by a fear of no nearby bathrooms. Consider taking Imodium before a special dinner out. But don't take any antidiarrheal medicine on a regular basis. You'll only make your IBS symptoms worse.

☐ Make sure you're getting enough fiber in your diet. Fiber promotes normal bowel function and relieves constipation. Most Americans only get half the 20 to 40 grams of daily fiber they need. Five servings a day of high-fiber foods such as fruits, vegetables and grains will help keep you regular. Fiber adds bulk to your stools and speeds their passage along your intestinal tract.
If you can't get enough fiber in your diet, use an over-the-counter fiber supplement such as Metamucil or Fiberall. Take the fiber with two glasses of water. Don't boost your fiber intake too quickly or your IBS symptoms may temporarily worsen.

☐ When you're troubled by gas and bloating, watch out for beans, cabbage, apple juice, grape juice, bananas, nuts and raisins.

☐ Limit the amount of caffeine and alcohol you drink. Both irritate the lining of your stomach. Nicotine from cigarette smoking and caffeine can worsen stomach cramps.

☐ Candy, gum and carbonated beverages can make you feel gassy and bloated. Candy and gum cause you to produce more saliva and swallow more often. Every time you swallow, you unintentionally gulp down air. The air and carbonation add to levels of gas in your stomach.

☐ Don't drink too much at mealtimes. Too much liquid will dilute your digestive juices and hinder digestion. Drinking plenty of water between meals is good for you.

☐ Get regular exercise. People who exercise have fewer stomach problems than couch potatoes. Exercise is a stress and tension reducer and promotes regular bowel movements.

Irritable bowel syndrome isn't harmful to your health, but make sure you see your doctor to ensure that your IBS symptoms aren't a sign of another disorder. IBS can be mistaken for something as easy to control as lactase deficiency, which means you lack the enzyme you need to digest milk properly. Your doctor also needs to check for cancer, gallbladder disease, ulcers or other problems with your digestive system.

Medical Source ――――――――――――――――――
   The Lancet (340,8833:1444 and 341,8836:36)

Fish oil for healthy intestines

It's no fish tale — fish oil might help improve your digestive problems.

Adding fish oil to the diet seems to help relieve the pain, discomfort and diarrhea associated with ulcerative colitis. Ulcerative colitis is a disease of the large intestines that causes inflammation, pain, fever, abdominal cramping and bloody diarrhea. It affects nearly 500,000 Americans.

Recent studies indicate that taking daily supplements of fish oil cuts the symptoms of ulcerative colitis by more than 50 percent.

About 72 percent of the people testing the effects of the fish oil cut down on the amount of anti-inflammatory medicine they were taking for the intestinal disorder.

Some encouraging news for those who aren't willing to risk the odor produced by taking 18 fish oil capsules a day: Drug companies are working on "designer drugs" that will mimic the action of the fish oil, providing the same relief without the fishy smell.

Fish-oil supplements appear to be effective in relieving ulcerative colitis without causing any negative side effects. Check with your doctor before adding large amounts of any dietary supplement to your daily diet.

Medical Sources ――――――――――――――――――
   Drug Therapy (22,76:83)
   Medical Tribune (33,9:13)

Say yes to yogurt

If milk and ice cream send your stomach into spasms and you running for the bathroom, you're probably lactose intolerant, a common disorder that affects millions of people. Common symptoms include stomach cramping and bloating, gas, diarrhea and nausea.

Nothing serious is wrong with you if you're lactose intolerant. Your small intestine simply doesn't produce lactase, the enzyme necessary to break down lactose, the sugar found in dairy products.

However, lactose intolerance can sometimes lead to other problems. Diarrhea can wash important nutrients from your intestines and eventually cause mild malnutrition. Also, many lactose-intolerant people avoid dairy products altogether and run the risk of calcium, protein and vitamin-D deficiencies.

This is especially dangerous in the elderly. Vitamin-D and calcium deficiencies can lead to osteoporosis (the brittle bone disease). Protein deficiency can cause muscle wasting and weaken your immune system, making your body less resistant to infections.

You know you need dairy products to stay healthy, but the thought of eating them still makes your stomach shudder.

What can you do? Try yogurt. Yogurt contains bacteria that help ease lactose intolerance.

Yogurt is plain milk that has been allowed to ferment. Yogurt manufacturers add the two bacteria *Lactobacillus bulgaricus* and *Streptococcus thermophilus* to milk and let it sit for several hours.

The bacteria grow in the milk and turn the milk into a tart, acidic gel that everyone now knows as yogurt. (Most manufacturers sweeten their yogurt with fruit and flavorings.) Apparently these bacteria help break down lactose so that lactose-intolerant people can actually absorb sugars from the yogurt.

Many kinds of yogurt still contain live bacteria when you eat them. However, some manufacturers "heat-treat" their yogurt to make it last longer on the shelf. This heat-treating process kills the bacteria.

If a manufacturer heat-treats the yogurt, the label must say "heat-treated after culturing." If the yogurt has not been heat-treated and still contains live bacteria, the label must say "active yogurt cultures" or "living yogurt cultures."

If you're lactose-intolerant, try adding yogurt to your diet. Yogurt provides a good supply of vitamin D, calcium and protein that people need in their diets, and it helps them to avoid the nausea, diarrhea and cramping that lactose normally causes.

Remember to read the yogurt labels and find the brands that contain live bacteria to get the best results.

Medical Sources ————————————————

Journal of the American College of Nutrition (11,2:168)

FDA Consumer (26,5:27)

Put the brakes on peptic ulcer pain

It started out as mild discomfort after you ate. But lately you've noticed that the former dull aching has turned into a sharp, knife-like pain after meals. Sometimes it even strikes in the middle of the night.

You may be suffering from peptic ulcer disease. And you're not alone. Up to 10 percent of all male Americans and up to 5 percent of all female Americans suffer from peptic ulcer disease at some point.

Peptic ulcer disease occurs when you develop ulcers (small, open sores) on the lining of your stomach or intestines. This can happen because something damages the lining of the digestive system or because the stomach acid has "eaten away" part of the lining.

Often peptic ulcers follow an intestinal infection caused by the bacteria *H. pylori*. Scientists report that *H. pylori* is present in up to 95 percent of people with intestinal ulcers and in 75 percent of the people with stomach ulcers.

You can avoid some of the other causes of peptic ulcers:

Try not to use nonsteroidal anti-inflammatory drugs (NSAIDs). These painkillers significantly increase your risk of digestive ulcers. Aspirin, ibuprofen and naproxen are some of the more well-known NSAIDs. These substances disturb the sensitive lining in the stomach and intestines. Using them frequently increases your risk of ulcer by about 50 percent.

Avoid caffeine, alcohol, tobacco and spicy foods. These substances can cause irritation of the stomach and intestinal lining. That leads to bleeding and the development of ulcers. Surprisingly, milk can also lead to ulcers. Although milk is bland and would seem to soothe the digestive tract, the calcium in milk actually increases the amount of acid in the stomach, which can lead to ulcers.

Be happy. One risk factor for peptic ulcer disease is stress. Stress may lead to higher levels of acid in the digestive tract, and it can also lead to high-risk behaviors like drinking alcohol and smoking.

If you do develop an ulcer, try these tips for relief:

Stop smoking, stop drinking alcohol and cut down on NSAID use. Changing these habits will prevent your ulcer from getting worse and will also help your ulcer heal and protect you from getting another one.

Ask your pharmacist to recommend a good over-the-counter antacid. An antacid will lower the amount of acid in your digestive tract. This will create a better environment for the ulcer to heal. In many cases, the ulcer will heal within six to eight weeks.

If your ulcer doesn't seem to be improving, see your doctor. Ulcers caused by the *H. pylori* bacteria often need to be treated with antibiotics.

Medical Source ————————————————
American Family Physician (46,1:217)

Dizziness

Dealing with dizziness

"I'm so dizzy; my head is spinning." If you have the same sensations Tommy Roe sang about in 1969, you may be worried that something besides love is making you dizzy.

Although some 8 million of us visit doctors for dizziness each year, it may be comforting to know that most of the time those spinning sensations don't signal a serious disorder.

In fact, dizziness in middle-aged and elderly people is commonly caused by ear infections or psychological problems.

The balance mechanism of the inner ear is a factor in about half of all dizziness complaints. A disruption in this balance mechanism causes feelings of spinning or moving.

Usually these dizzy spells, also called vertigo, last less than a minute. The most common type of vertigo occurs with a change in head position. Simply rolling over in bed can make you feel as if the world's turned upside down.

Vertigo can be almost completely cured with exercise. Rehabilitation therapists can show you how they are done. Regular walking for exercise can restore balance upset by vertigo.

Other conditions that can affect the balance mechanisms of the inner ear and cause dizziness include shingles of the ear and Meniere's disease.

Shingles of the ear is characterized by a rash inside the ear canal, severe vertigo, and problems controlling face muscles. Rest is the best treatment. In some cases, prescribed medicines can help.

Meniere's disease is characterized by dizziness, periods of hearing loss, ringing in the ears and a feeling of fullness in the ears. The dizziness may persist for hours or even days. Hearing loss usually worsens. In addition to medical treatment, a low-salt diet may help.

Dizziness may accompany a migraine headache or occur if you get up too fast. If your doctor can find no physical cause of dizziness, it may be related to depression, anxiety or panic.

One study found psychological problems to be the primary cause of dizziness in 16 percent of the people studied and a contributory cause in another 40 percent of people complaining of dizziness.

This type of dizziness may be accompanied by feelings of sadness or hopelessness, memory loss, sleep and appetite changes and suicidal thoughts. Counseling or short-term medication can help.

Often dizziness has more than one cause. It is usually brief, often disappearing in two weeks or less, and rarely signals a life-threatening disease. However, you should consult your doctor if you have long-term or recurrent dizziness.

Medical Sources ————————————————————

Annals of Internal Medicine (117,11:898)
Medical Tribune (33,24:2)

Headaches

Help for your aching head

Often headaches are only mildly irritating and can be explained by changes in the weather, irregular eating or stress. Some headaches, however, are considerably more painful.

About 11 million people suffer from extremely severe headaches, including migraines. The number of sufferers seems to be increasing, having risen about 60 percent in the last 10 years.

Often incapacitating, migraines cost American employers about $17.2 billion yearly due to missed workdays and decreased productivity.

The best way to treat a headache is to prevent it from developing. Know the most common causes of your headaches and avoid them. If you aren't sure what these triggers are, keep a headache diary. Record each headache and the factors that could have led to its development.

Common headache triggers include:

☐ Alcohol

☐ Weather or altitude changes

☐ Hormone changes, especially during menstruation

☐ Bright light or glare

☐ Missed meals

☐ Odors, such as:
  ➤ Perfume
  ➤ Flowers
  ➤ Natural gas

☐ Loud noises

☐ Too little or too much sleep

☐ Vigorous exercise

❐ Stress

❐ Certain foods or food additives, such as:
  ➤ Ripened cheese
  ➤ Chicken liver
  ➤ Citrus fruits
  ➤ Chocolate
  ➤ Red wine
  ➤ Caffeinated beverages
  ➤ Monosodium glutamate (MSG)
  ➤ Preservatives found in smoked and processed meats

If your teen or preteen has recently started to complain of headaches, check for these common headache culprits:

❐ Chewing gum. Big gum balls can be especially troublesome. The strain on the jaw caused by chewing big wads of gum can lead to tension headaches. To stop the headache, stop the gum chewing.

❐ Eyestrain caused by overuse. Long periods of time spent at the computer either working or playing games can cause headaches or make them worse.

❐ Foods and drinks. Many of teens' favorite foods and drinks (chocolate, colas, etc.) may contain ingredients that cause headaches. Headaches are a common symptom of caffeine withdrawal. Artificial sweeteners may also be at fault.

Another good way to prevent headaches is to start on a wellness program when you're feeling good. Get enough sleep, exercise regularly and eat balanced meals. Avoid food or food additives that seem to give you headaches.

You may want to explore various ways to relax, especially if you feel stress plays a big role in your headaches. Some researchers have speculated that there is a "migraine personality." They say that people who get migraines are perfectionists and driven to succeed.

Other researchers say that's not true, but everyone agrees that how you deal with anger, anxiety and tension can lead to a migraine.

If you feel a headache coming on, try the following techniques to help reduce its severity or duration:

- ☐ Avoid a lot of activity.
- ☐ Rest in a quiet, dark room if possible.
- ☐ Apply an ice pack to your forehead or the base of your neck.
- ☐ Take an over-the-counter painkiller, such as aspirin or acetaminophen. Use acetaminophen for children younger than age 19 to lower the risk of Reye's syndrome.

If you continue to have recurring or extremely severe headaches that neither preventive measures nor over-the-counter medicines seem to help, see your doctor.

He will either give you "abortive" medicine, which will relieve pain once you're hit with a migraine, or "prophylactic" medicine, which will prevent the headache completely. You may need preventative medicine if you suffer from more than two migraines a month.

Medical Sources ——————————————
American Family Physician (47,1:21)
Postgraduate Medicine (93,1:51 and 223)
National Headache Foundation, 5252 N. Western Ave., Chicago, IL 60625

Headband eases headache

Have a hard time getting headache relief from medications? You may want to try this simple headache remedy.

An elastic headband designed to apply continuous pressure on the temples, forehead and back of the head effectively relieves migraine headaches. One study found that the headband relieved headaches in over half the volunteers.

Medical Source ——————————————
American Family Physician (47,1:22)

Headache? Check your drinking water

Your drinking water could be the culprit behind your headaches! Unsafe levels of trichloroethylene (TCE), a chemical solvent used in a variety of industries, may cause severe, chronic headaches. Polluted wells of a western Illinois community contained TCE levels ranging from 10 to 2,441 parts per billion. Only five parts per billion of TCE is safe to drink, according to the Environmental Protection Agency.

Severe or frequent headaches were reported by 62 percent of the 106 Illinois residents questioned about their symptoms. As a precaution, you may want to have your drinking water tested to ensure it's not harmful to your health.

Medical Source ———————————————————
Medical Tribune (33,20:1)

Stress goes straight to your head

Proposal due tomorrow. Briefcase. Laptop computer. Pencil. Paper clip. — Am I forgetting anything? Oh yes, the headache.

Of all the items people bring home from the office at the end of the day, by far the most common is a headache.

Some people suffer from the crippling, one-sided migraine accompanied by nausea, the sinus headache which can be treated with nasal decongestants and antibiotics, or the intensely painful "cluster headache" which develops around the eyes and often hits in the middle of the night.

However, nine out of every 10 headaches are the "tension-type," says the National Headache Foundation, the kind you get during a stressful or tiring day at the office, after a confrontation that left you biting back words on the tip of your tongue or after serving a Thanksgiving feast to 20 of your loudest relatives.

Everyone knows the signs of a tension headache — a dull, constant ache slowly grows on both sides of your head. You may feel as though a headband is squeezing tighter and tighter around your temples and the back of your skull.

Your shoulders, neck and head muscles often feel tight and tense. Extreme tiredness and sensitivity to light and sound may accompany your headache. There's no doubt about it — a tension headache can hurt worse than a migraine.

The most important step in fighting a tension headache is to stop the pain before it gets out of your control. As soon as you notice a headache coming on, immediately take aspirin, acetaminophen or ibuprofen.

Keep an ice pack or a hot pack at the office so you can place it on your head or neck at the first sign of pain. A long, hot shower will help ease tension and an aching head.

Other ways to prevent tension headaches are:

- ☐ Get plenty of sleep on a regular schedule.
- ☐ Exercise at least three times a week.
- ☐ Take breaks to stretch, walk or just relax during stressful situations.
- ☐ Take a vacation or a day off work when headaches become a daily trial.
- ☐ Reduce stress with deep breathing, gentle music or other relaxation techniques.

A caffeine-withdrawal headache feels just like a tension headache. If you normally drink several cups of coffee, tea and soda a day, your head will probably ache dully when you miss your regular dose of caffeine. Too much caffeine can give you a headache, too, so try to wean yourself off slowly.

Depression may be the cause of a daily tension headache that hits the moment you wake up or early in the morning.

If your headache falls into this pattern, you may have a chemical imbalance that may be improved with medication or you may need to work with friends, family members, a local support group or a counselor to pull yourself out of the dumps.

For chronic headaches that occur more than 15 times a month, don't keep taking over-the-counter pain relievers without visiting your doctor.

Pain relievers that you can buy without a prescription are generally less harmful than prescription medications, but they do have their side effects.

Aspirin, ibuprofen and acetaminophen, especially those products that contain caffeine, can lead to a "rebound effect." Your body adapts to the pain reliever being in your system, and you become extra-sensitive to pain when the medicine starts to wear off.

You need to see your doctor if you're taking a large number of pain relievers, if frequent headaches are interfering with your daily life, or if a severe or constant headache is accompanied by weakness, dizziness, numbness or other strange physical sensations.

Medical Sources ─────────────────────

American Family Physician (47,4:799)

National Headache Foundation, 5252 N. Western Ave., Chicago, IL 60625

HEMORRHOIDS

At-home remedies for hemorrhoids

If you're at the end of your rope with hemorrhoids, you're not alone. Half of all people over the age of 50 live with the painful nuisance of hemorrhoids — swollen veins in the rectum caused by too much pressure. Yet most cases of hemorrhoids don't need surgery, and many of us can find relief by changing a few habits.

People develop hemorrhoids for a variety of reasons, including constipation, diarrhea, pregnancy, obesity and liver disease. When pressure causes the veins inside the rectum to swell and stretch, internal hemorrhoids develop.

Usually the only sign of these internal hemorrhoids is bright red blood on the surface of your stool, in the toilet bowl or on the toilet paper.

Internal hemorrhoids may not be painful even if they are bleeding because internal vein walls don't have pain-sensitive nerves.

It's possible for these hemorrhoids to swell so much that they fall out of the rectum. They normally pull back inside the rectum without any help. Occasionally, you may need to push them up with a lubricated finger.

External hemorrhoids develop in the veins around the anus. You can feel these with your finger. External hemorrhoids bleed easily from straining or rubbing, and they may itch and be extremely painful.

You may experience especially severe pain if a blood clot forms in an external hemorrhoid. But Dr. Lee Smith of the George Washington University Medical Center says that these blood clots are like a black eye and will eventually disappear.

To prevent and treat hemorrhoids, relieve the pressure and strain that causes them to develop:

☐ Eat a high-fiber diet and drink several glasses of water daily. This will help prevent constipation, a major cause of hemorrhoids. Excellent sources of fiber include bran cereals, fruits, potatoes, beans (kidney, navy, lima and pinto) and vegetables, especially asparagus, brussels sprouts, cabbage, carrots, cauliflower, corn, peas, kale and parsnips. Limit low-fiber foods, such as ice cream, soft drinks, cheese, white bread and meat. You can also increase your fiber intake with a fiber pill, powder or liquid drink from the local pharmacy.

❏ Avoid all laxatives except stool softeners. Other laxatives can cause diarrhea, which will just make your hemorrhoids worse.

❏ Don't linger on the toilet to catch up on your reading. This habit puts too much pressure on the anal region, making hemorrhoids worse and bleeding more likely. Never push long or hard for a bowel movement.

❏ Try to avoid lifting heavy objects, which puts pressure on the anal area. If a heavy lifting situation can't be avoided, be careful not to hold your breath while you lift. Grunting is a sure sign that you're holding your breath. Concentrate on breathing in and out steadily during physical labor or weight-lifting.

❏ Take three to four warm baths in plain water daily. Don't make the bathwater too hot, and don't add any bubble baths, Epsom salts or soaps. They may irritate hemorrhoids.

❏ Use cold packs to relieve swelling. You can also relieve irritation by applying a thin coat of petroleum jelly to the anal area. Petroleum jelly works as well as over-the-counter hemorrhoid medication and is a lot cheaper.

❏ Clean yourself with a soft, moist pad or even rinse in the shower instead of wiping with plain toilet paper. Baby wipes also work well.

Continuous hemorrhoid pain usually means that you have a break in the skin called a fissure or an external hemorrhoid with a blood clot. If you have continuous pain or bleeding from the rectum, see your doctor.

Hemorrhoids don't cause cancer, but bleeding from the anal area can be a sign of cancer.

Medical Sources ———————————————————
FDA Consumer (26,2:31)
Postgraduate Medicine (92,2:141)

Hiccups

Hiccups: home remedies and why they work

Your grandmother may have told you that if you drink a glass of water without stopping for air that it would stop your hiccups.

If that didn't work, she may have moved on to one of the other popular home remedies such as holding your breath, blowing into a paper bag, swallowing several times while holding your nose, or maybe swallowing a spoonful of dry, granulated sugar. Were these effective treatments for hiccups or merely old wives' tales?

Excluding hiccups caused by underlying medical problems, you probably get hiccups most often after eating too fast, experiencing sudden changes in temperature, dealing with emotional stress, drinking alcohol, or some other irritation to the nerves that control the diaphragm.

When you hiccup, your diaphragm contracts involuntarily. As you inhale, the space between the vocal cords closes quickly, interfering with the flow of air and causing the hiccup sound.

Your grandmother might not have known that all this was happening inside your body, but somehow she learned that by controlling breathing or soothing the diaphragm, she could control the hiccups.

Raising carbon dioxide levels helps reduce hiccup frequency. This may explain why holding your breath and other techniques designed to interrupt your respiratory rhythm work wonders.

Remedies that soothe your diaphragm, such as swallowing a spoonful of dry sugar, somehow interfere with the nerve signal that tells the diaphragm to behave like a nervous jumping bean.

Although most hiccup attacks only last a few minutes, they make it difficult to concentrate on anything, much less sit still.

Here are a few remedies to try the next time you need hiccup relief. Keep in mind that not all cures work for everybody. By the time you've run through the entire list, you'll have either stopped your hiccups or they will have gone away naturally.

- ❏ Hold your breath for as long as you can and swallow each time you feel the urge to hiccup.
- ❏ Try the old paper-bag remedy. Breathe for about a minute into a paper bag gathered tightly to your lips. The buildup of carbon dioxide might shut down the hiccups. Don't try this for more than a minute at most.
- ❏ Chug-a-lug a glass of water.
- ❏ Eat some dry bread.
- ❏ Swallow some crushed ice.
- ❏ Tickle the top of your mouth with a cotton swab.

Helping your baby cope with hiccups can be a ticklish experience. Tickling your baby's tummy causes him to hold his breath, temporarily raising carbon dioxide levels and putting the lid on a pesky case of hiccups.

If your hiccups persist for more than a day or two, see your doctor. Occasionally, hiccups can signal a serious medical problem.

Medical Source ——————————————————
British Medical Journal (305,6964:1237)

Some hiccup remedies not always safe

Some people try to put a stop to their hiccups by touching the back of their throat with a fingertip or cotton swab. This interferes with the nerve impulse that tells your diaphragm to contract and stops your hiccups. However, gagging as a method of relieving hiccups may not be as safe as originally thought.

A 39-year-old man with a history of medical problems entered an emergency unit after hiccuping constantly for three days. The gagging technique was used several times in the emergency room as a means of stopping his persistent hiccups.

He was also given a prescription for controlling hiccups and one to control stomach acid which was believed to be the cause of his hiccups.

After leaving the hospital, his hiccups resumed but ceased after self-induced gagging. The man did not have his prescriptions filled and continued to gag himself. The frequent retching caused internal bleeding resulting in further emergency treatment, including a transfusion of several pints of blood.

It seems that gagging may be an effective, temporary means of controlling hiccups, but you should be aware of possible side effects. Don't use this method of treatment on a regular basis without medical supervision. Pulling on your tongue works just as effectively, but won't cause any harm. Just remember to pull gently!

Medical Source ─────────────────────────
Emergency Medicine (24,15:82)

Preventing and treating major illnesses

Cancer
Diabetes
Heart and blood
 vessel disease
Kidney problems
Thyroid problems

CANCER

Improving your odds

Chemo. Mammogram. Biopsy. Surgery. Tumor. Bone marrow transplants. Cancer. These words ring round and round prayer groups, bridge clubs and gatherings of friends. Everybody knows somebody with cancer these days.

How likely is it that you'll become a statistic in the cancer "epidemic"? Your chances of developing cancer aren't completely out of your control.

In fact, scientists believe that the food we eat is directly linked to about 40 percent of all cancers in men and 60 percent of all cancers in women.

The American Institute for Cancer Research says that 80 percent of cancer cases can be prevented by making changes in your lifestyle: eating a healthy, low-fat diet rich in vegetables, fruits and whole grains, quitting smoking and limiting your exposure to the sun.

Take these steps to prevent cancer, then stop worrying about it. One reason we are so fearful of cancer is that the media has led us to believe that everything causes cancer. That isn't so.

Less than 10 percent of all cancer cases are caused by smaller risk factors such as occupational exposure, radon, pollution, manufactured chemicals, medical X-rays, electromagnetic fields and fluoride.

Scientists are still investigating whether strong electromagnetic fields have any effect on cancer risk, and they've found no evidence that fluoride causes cancer.

What is cancer?

There are more than 100 different types of cancer, but they all are a disease of the body's cells. To keep the body in good repair, healthy cells grow, divide and replace themselves.

Sometimes cells lose control, begin to divide too quickly and grow without any order. They form tumors. Tumors that are malignant, not benign, are cancer. They can move into and destroy tissue and organs and spread to other parts of the body.

The most common signs and symptoms of cancer are:

> ➤ Changes in bowel or bladder habits
> ➤ A sore that doesn't heal
> ➤ Unusual bleeding or discharge
> ➤ A lump or thickening in the breast or elsewhere
> ➤ Indigestion or difficulty swallowing
> ➤ Changes in a wart or a mole
> ➤ A nagging cough or hoarseness

Of course, all these symptoms can be caused by many other less serious health problems. But if a problem lasts for more than two weeks, be sure to see your doctor.

Take care of your body by paying attention to it and by making healthy lifestyle changes. That's the surest way to improve your odds in the fight against cancer.

Medical Sources ————————————————

American Institute for Cancer Research, 1759 R Street N.W., Washington, D.C. 20069

National Cancer Institute, Building 31, Room 10A24, Bethesda, MD 20892

Take the best anti-cancer 'pill' available

The best anti-cancer "pill" now known is not a vitamin supplement or a prescription medicine. The prescription you need against cancer is to eat your fruits and vegetables every day.

Such simple advice seems too good to be true, but a group of scientists who closely analyzed 156 dietary studies says to believe it:

People who eat little or no fruits and vegetables on a daily basis experience about twice the risk of cancer as people who eat fruits and vegetables regularly.

The nutrients found in fruits and vegetables — especially vitamin C, vitamin E and carotenoids — are on the front line in the battle against cancer.

Cancer is frequently caused by highly unstable chemicals in our body known as free radicals. These free radicals are missing an electron, and so they run around in our bloodstream trying to steal electrons from other cells.

They cause other cells to become unstable, a process called oxidation. While they're bouncing around, the free radicals damage cells, even altering their DNA coding, and create a ripe environment for cancer.

Vitamin C, vitamin E and carotenoids can neutralize these free radicals, prevent the oxidation process and even repair much of the damage they do. That's why these anti-cancer nutrients are often referred to as "antioxidants."

Folate and ascorbic acid are two additional cancer-fighting nutrients found in fruits and vegetables. These nutrients seem to act as scavengers — they pick up and get rid of dangerous poisons in the body that can cause cancer.

The individual nutrients do help to prevent cancer, but the natural combination of vitamins and nutrients found in fruits and vegetables seems to be the best recipe for cancer prevention.

Apparently, the anti-cancer effects of natural fruits and vegetables cannot be matched or duplicated in vitamin supplements. Eating the real thing is the best way to reduce your risk of cancer.

Medical Source ————————————————
   Nutrition and Cancer (18,1:1)

Organic produce not always best

Think home-grown produce is safer for you and your children than commercially grown fruits and vegetables? Think again.

Some parents are concerned that pesticide residues on produce increase their children's risk of cancer in later years. As a result, several have started to grow their own produce or to buy only organically grown fruits and vegetables.

However, it's not necessary to switch to home or organically grown produce. It's more important to make sure that you and your child eat enough fruits and vegetables.

As a matter of fact, your family could be at greater risk from unwashed organically grown produce than from exposure to pesticide residues. One child died after eating unwashed produce grown in soil that had been fertilized with manure contaminated with bacteria.

Either commercially or organically grown produce is safe to eat as long as it is thoroughly washed with water, says John Hotchkiss, associate professor of food chemistry and toxicology at Cornell University.

Medical Sources ——————————————

Medical Tribune (34,17:31)
Tufts University Diet & Nutrition Letter (11,8:3)

Garlic may do more than spice up your life ... it could prolong it

If you are like most Americans, you probably have some garlic on hand to spice up anything from chicken to potato salad.

The potent herb does more than spice up your favorite dishes, though. It also has medicinal capabilities that include preventing and treating illnesses ranging from colds to cancer.

Eating garlic appears to slow down the first stages of skin cancer and reduce the risk of lung cancer. In animal studies at the American Health Foundation in Valhalla, N.Y., garlic prevented almost 80 percent of colon cancer tumors.

And good news for people with cancer already: Garlic seems to reduce the toxicity of certain cancer-therapy drugs without interfering with the drugs' effectiveness. It tends to lessen damage to organs and tissues from toxic chemotherapy drugs and radiation treatments.

Garlic (*Allium sativum*) is a member of the allium family. Onions, scallions, chives, leeks and shallots are also members of the allium group and have garlic's healing and preventative characteristics.

While it is probably not feasible to eat a pound of garlic and onions each week and still maintain a social life, include as many members of the allium family in your diet as possible.

You may want to talk to your doctor about taking garlic tablets as a supplement to your daily diet. Many tablets are odorless and have no aftertaste.

Medical Sources ——————————————

Nutrition and Cancer (17,3:279)
Medical Tribune (33,18:33)

Another spice of life: cancer-fighting turmeric

If you and your family are fans of spicy foods, you might be getting more than just a tasty meal. Studies suggest that the main ingredient of the spice turmeric helps fight against cancer.

Turmeric is one of the most commonly used spices in India, but in the United States you're more likely to find it in cosmetics and food colorings.

Scientists report that eating turmeric stopped the growth of stomach cancer and skin cancer in laboratory mice. It also prevented the growth of cancer cells in humans with myeloid leukemia.

For people who smoke, turmeric might help fight against lung cancer.

The spice seems to change the makeup of a chemical in the body that promotes cancer growth.

So, treat your family to a spicy meal. Adding a little spice to your life just might help you lower your risk of cancer.

Medical Source ———————————————
The Journal of the American College of Nutrition (11,2:192)

Want more lycopene? Try tomato juice

You might say tomay-to, or you might say tomah-to, but you should definitely drink processed tomato juice more often.

Tomatoes in any form are a super source of lycopene, which helps defend your body against cancer. But nutritionists have learned that processing tomatoes and other foods can actually make lycopene more available to your body.

Researchers compared how people absorbed lycopene from unprocessed tomato juice and from tomato juice that had been processed (cooked slowly with 1 percent corn oil for one hour). People were able to absorb more lycopene from the cooked tomato juice.

Red berries, fruits and vegetables also contain lycopene, but tomatoes are one of the best sources of this cancer fighter.

Choose a low-sodium tomato juice if you are on a salt-restricted diet.

Medical Source ———————————————
The Journal of Nutrition (122,11:2161)

Detecting breast cancer before it's too late

About one out of every nine American women will develop breast cancer in her lifetime. Fortunately, only about one in 30 will die from it.

The best way to sway those odds in your favor is to make sure that your breast cancer is detected in its earliest stages through regular mammograms and regular self-exams. More than 80 percent of breast cancers are discovered as a lump found by the woman herself.

Early detection is particularly important for you if you have a mother or other close relative with breast cancer, if you're older, if you began menstruation early, if your first pregnancy was at a late age or if you began menopause late.

Unfortunately, early detection in women who have no symptoms has been difficult up to this point. But a new test that pulls fluid from the nipple with a device similar to a breast pump could help doctors spot future breast cancer victims before the disease strikes.

When researchers pulled breast fluid from almost 3,000 women in the late 1970s, they were able to fairly accurately predict who would have breast cancer more than 10 years later. The breast fluid of some women had abnormal or "precancerous" cells years before they were diagnosed with breast cancer.

The women who did not produce any fluid at all had a lower risk of developing breast cancer. However, even women who have never been pregnant or given birth have some fluid secretion and reabsorption going on in their breasts all the time. The presence of fluid is not an accurate indicator of breast cancer risk.

If you are experiencing any abnormal secretions from your breasts (secretions that contain pus or are discolored), contact your doctor right away.

Medical Source ————————————————————
Science News (141,11:165)

More news on mammograms

Staying abreast of the latest theories concerning mammogram screening can be a real challenge. New studies keep the matter on the front burner of discussion.

A hot debate started in 1992 when the Canadian National Breast Screening Study suggested that women in their 40s receive no benefits from these breast X-rays that detect possibly cancerous tumors.

Mammograms can detect smaller tumors than those found in a regular physical exam and pick up malignant tumors before any other symptoms are apparent.

Even though the screenings turn up almost twice as many tumors in women ages 40 to 49 than just a physical exam, mammograms don't seem to help women in this age group survive the cancer.

After menopause, breast tissue becomes less dense. Many women in their 40s have not yet undergone menopause, and their thick breast tissue prevents mammograms from revealing as many potentially cancerous tumors as the procedure can in older women.

Cancer may grow so fast in women in their 40s that mammogram's earlier detection of the tumors doesn't help.

Some specialists recommend that only those women in their 40s who have a family history of breast cancer or another cancer risk factor should receive regular mammograms.

However, researchers agree that women in their 50s and 60s do get significant benefits from mammograms. Women ages 50 to 69 who receive regular mammograms have an average 30 percent reduction in deaths caused by breast cancer.

Some specialists recommend that women over age 65 only have mammograms every other year instead of yearly. The U.S. Health Care Financing Administration, the unit that directs Medicare and Medicaid, will only pay women 65 and older for a mammogram screening done once every two years.

Other researchers say that since age is associated with a higher incidence of breast cancer, older women should be screened more, not less.

The American Cancer Society and the National Cancer Institute may review their current recommendations for receiving mammograms.

For now, however, women in their 40s are still encouraged to have mammograms every year or at least every other year. Women over 50 should get a mammogram every year.

All women should have a yearly physical exam and continue monthly breast examinations at home.

Medical Sources ——————————————————
Science News (143,10:149)
Journal of the National Cancer Institute (84,24:1860)

The anti-breast-cancer diet

Does eating too many fats put you at risk for breast cancer or not?

For 15 years, we've heard that we can lower our risk of breast cancer by eating a diet low in fat and keeping our weight down. Now, for the past two years, reports have surfaced stating that breast cancer isn't linked to how much fat you eat at all.

Controversy rages, but most doctors and researchers agree that a low-fat diet will help reduce your risk of breast cancer. The new studies showing no link between diet and breast cancer have some obvious flaws, such as studying a small slice of the population whose diets are so similar that you can't draw any solid conclusions from the results.

When researchers look at the international picture, the role of fats in breast cancer risk seems obvious. For instance, Japanese women with their low-fat diets have a 20 percent lower annual risk of breast cancer recurrence than Americans.

The low-fat traditional Hispanic diet may help lower the risk of breast cancer in American women. The high intake of beans in the Hispanic diet could be one of the keys to Hispanic women's low rate of breast cancer.

Hispanic women typically eat twice as many beans as Caucasian women. The beans seem to contain anti-cancer properties due to their low-fat, high-nutrient makeup.

Hispanic women also use large amounts of olive oil, which is high in monounsaturated fat (a "good" kind of fat). This also seems to reduce the risk of breast cancer.

Research by the American Health Foundation found that fruits and vegetables in the diet reduce the risk of breast cancer in women.

Women who don't suffer from breast cancer eat more fruits and vegetables than women who do suffer from the disease. In other words, the fruits and vegetables seem to help protect women from developing breast cancer.

Scientists are still conducting tests, but a diet high in fruits and vegetables and low in fat shows promise for reducing the risk of breast cancer in women.

Medical Source ────────────────────
Medical Tribune (33,13:14)

No link between stress and breast cancer

Stress is inconvenient, worrisome and irritating, but it won't increase your risk of breast cancer recurrence.

Women who suffer from severe stress are no more likely to suffer from breast cancer relapses than women who are not under severe stress.

Scientists recently studied women who had been diagnosed with breast cancer.

During the four-year study, over half of the women experienced a severely stressful event, such as the loss of a loved one, divorce or their home burning down.

The researchers found no link between stress and breast cancer relapse. However, it's still important to cope with stress and reduce anxiety and depression to maintain a healthy outlook on life.

Medical Source ────────────────────
American Medical News (35,18:33)

Age at last pregnancy: important cancer risk factor

You've probably heard that the earlier you have your first child, the lower your risk of breast cancer. Well, new research indicates that your age at your last pregnancy is more important than age at your first.

Two recent studies conducted in Norway and Brazil suggest that women may want to complete their families by age 35 in order to reduce their risk of breast cancer. Later pregnancies may cause unnecessary breast tissue growth and increase the risk of developing a malignant cancer.

Giving birth to large numbers of children does seem to protect you from breast cancer.

Birth rates are decreasing worldwide, and that may cause a rise in the number of breast cancer cases. You may be able to counter the rising risk of breast cancer by having your children before the age of 35.

Medical Source ─────────────────────────────
The Lancet (341,8836:33)

Battling prostate cancer

One out of every 10 men in the United States develops prostate cancer. It's the second leading cancer killer among men, following closely behind lung cancer.

The prostate is a walnut-sized gland that surrounds the neck of a man's bladder and the upper part of the urethra (the tube that drains urine through the penis). The prostate produces the fluid that helps nurture and transport sperm.

Risk factors for prostate cancer are:

- ☐ Race. African-Americans have a higher risk for prostate cancer than other races in the United States. Their increased risk may be due to their slightly higher levels of testosterone.
- ☐ History of prostate cancer in your family. The more relatives you have with prostate cancer, the greater your risk.
- ☐ High-fat diet. The more animal fat you eat, the more likely you are to die of prostate cancer. Greek men eat about half the fat that American men do and are half as likely to die of prostate cancer.
- ☐ Exposure to cadmium. People working in the welding or electroplating industries are often exposed to high levels of cadmium, a mineral commonly found in cigarette smoke and alkaline batteries.
- ☐ Age. By age 80, 60 to 70 percent of all men will have developed cancer cells in their prostate, no matter what their nationality. Nearly 100 percent of 90-year-old men have prostate cancer.

Researchers still haven't been able to pin down one specific cause of prostate cancer, but they expect the cancer rates to continue to rise. With advances in medicine that effectively treat and control the common killers of older men, including infection, pneumonia, heart disease and lung cancer, men are living long enough to develop prostate cancer.

Many prostate cancer cases are not found until the cancer has spread beyond the prostate gland, becoming almost impossible to cure.

The digital rectal exam, in which a doctor uses his finger to feel the prostate gland, is the most common prostate cancer test. This is not a particularly popular exam and may not detect prostate cancer in its early stages.

While this is an uncomfortable procedure, it's definitely worth the embarrassment. Less than half of all American men who should be having a yearly rectal exam do so, says Gerald P. Murphy, chief medical officer of the American Cancer Society.

You should also have your prostate specific antigen (PSA) levels tested at the same time you have your rectal exam. PSA is a protein produced by the prostate gland and found in increased levels in men with prostate cancer. A simple blood test can tell your doctor if your PSA level is normal.

Some doctors have been hesitant to do the two exams together, believing that the digital rectal exam actually causes the prostate gland to release more protein specific antigen than normal, causing the test of PSA levels to be inaccurate.

Researchers stress that this is not the case and that the two tests are most effective at detecting prostate cancer when performed together. Done during the same exam session, these two tests catch up to 70 percent of all prostate cancers before they've had time to spread.

If the cancer doesn't spread beyond the prostate, either because it's a slow-growing cancer or because you receive treatment, your chances for survival are excellent.

Don't hastily assume you're prostate cancer positive if you have high PSA levels. An enlarged, irritated or infected prostate can also elevate PSA levels. If either your yearly digital rectal exam or your PSA levels are irregular, your next step should possibly be a prostate ultrasound. This test produces a photograph of your prostate.

All men over 40 should have regular screenings for prostate cancer. If you have a history of prostate cancer in your family, talk with your doctor about beginning these screenings earlier.

Your family doctor or a urologist (a specialist in problems of the prostate and other urinary disorders) can give you an examination. Also, many hospitals and community health centers offer prostate cancer screening during Prostate Cancer Awareness Week, held at the end of September every year.

If your high PSA levels do indicate cancer growth, you may be eligible to try 4HPR. 4HPR is a new drug, similar to vitamin A, that may halt prostate cancer growth in men who have mildly elevated PSA levels. Researchers are currently testing the drug for effectiveness and side effects.

If you have any of these symptoms of prostate cancer, see a doctor immediately:

> Painful or frequent urination
> Sudden decrease in size and force of urinary stream
> Pain in lower back, pelvis or thighs

There are several options for treating prostate cancer.

☐ Radiation. Radiation may involve the use of an external beam or implanted pellets. Radiation may cause incontinence or impotence.

☐ Hormone therapy. It sometimes helps to reduce the level of testosterone in men with prostate cancer. This may be done through drugs called hormone blockers or castration. However, once the cancer has spread beyond the prostate, odds of survival drop dramatically.

☐ Chemotherapy

☐ Surgical removal of the prostate gland. Many men think this cure is worse than the disease as surgery can cause impotence and urinary incontinence (loss of bladder control).

However, a new surgical technique (anatomic radical retropubic prostatectomy) may make incontinence and impotence from prostate cancer operations problems of the past.

Commonly known as nerve sparing, this surgery spares the nerve bundles that are usually cut during conventional prostate cancer surgery. Two-thirds of some 1,200 men who underwent the nerve-sparing operation were able to continue their normal sexual activities.

In a study of 955 men who had undergone a nerve-sparing operation, more than 80 percent were free from cancer four to five years later.

Support groups are available to help men and their families cope with prostate cancer. For more information contact:

> American Cancer Society, 1-800-ACS-2345
> American Foundation for Urologic Disease, 1-800-828-7866. They provide information on the latest developments in the diagnosis and treatment of prostate cancer and can refer you to local chapters of the support group, Us Too.
> National Cancer Institute, 1-800-4-CANCER

Medical Sources
Science News (139,17:261)
The New England Journal of Medicine (324,17:1156)
Geriatrics (48,8:15)
Pharmacy Times (59,12:29)
Nutrition Action (20,2:5)
Annals of Internal Medicine (118,10:793)
Medical Tribune (34,22:4)
The Wall Street Journal (April 22, 1992, B1)

Treating prostate cancer: Is waiting wiser?

Once you're diagnosed with prostate cancer, should you have prostate surgery or should you wait? Opinions are so conflicting, you may think it's easier to decide by coin toss than logic.

Many researchers believe that too many men with prostate cancer undergo treatment, while too little is known about the surgery's effectiveness.

Some doctors are even reluctant to perform the PSA test because of its ability to detect small cancers.

These doctors believe that men, especially men over 65, would be better off not knowing about a small prostate cancer which may not spread. They say that treatment may be worse than the disease and have more fatal consequences.

One study actually found that older men who underwent aggressive treatment, such as surgery or radiation therapy, for prostate cancer lived an average of one year less than those men who did not have treatment. Many men will die of other causes before a slow-growing cancer has time to spread.

"Watchful waiting" (simply having your doctor monitor the progress of the cancer) may be more beneficial for older men than aggressive treatment, some researchers say.

So, what should you do if you've been diagnosed with prostate cancer?

A new test being developed may help you decide. This test would help doctors predict which men diagnosed with prostate cancer have fast-growing tumors. Men with slow-growing tumors would not have to undergo unnecessary surgery or other painful treatments.

Developed by Dr. Judah Folkman, director of the Surgical Research Laboratory at Children's Hospital in Boston, this test measures the number of blood vessels present in a tumor. The more vessels that are present, the greater the chance the cancer will spread rapidly.

If you are diagnosed with prostate cancer, discuss your treatment options with your doctor. He will be able to best help you decide which treatment route is right for you.

Medical Sources ————————————————
Medical Tribune (34,21:8)
Pharmacy Times (59,12:29 Hospital Edition)
The Atlanta Journal/Constitution (May 26, 1993, A1)
The Wall Street Journal (April 22, 1992, B1)

Prostate and breast cancers linked

Did your mother have breast cancer? If so, you may be at an increased risk of prostate cancer. If you're diagnosed with prostate cancer, your daughter may have an increased risk of breast cancer.

Researchers discovered this surprising link while studying men who had been diagnosed with breast cancer. (Yes, it is possible for men to develop breast cancer although less than one in every 100 breast cancers are found in men.)

The investigators discovered that female relatives of men who had breast cancer had a doubled risk of developing breast cancer themselves. Then, they found that a family history of prostate cancer also doubled a woman's risk of developing breast cancer.

The researchers now speculate that there is some type of genetic link between prostate cancer and breast cancer. It appears that the relationship between prostate and breast cancer is a two-way street. A study done in Iceland found that the male relatives of women diagnosed with breast cancer had a 40 to 50 percent increase in prostate cancer risk.

A high-fat intake is associated with an increased risk of both breast and prostate cancers.

Medical Sources ————————————————
> *Journal of the National Cancer Institute* (85,10:776)
> *Annals of Internal Medicine* (118,10:793)

Good news about colon cancer

The best news about colon cancer, one of the most common cancers and one of the major killers in America, is that it can be detected and stopped early.

A very simple and most important warning sign of colon cancer is blood in your stools. Bloody stools are usually caused by hemorrhoids, but never just assume that cancer is not the cause.

Other signs and symptoms are:

> ➤ A change in bowel habits
> ➤ Recurrent abdominal pain or cramps
> ➤ Unexplained weight loss
> ➤ Unexplained anemia (low red blood cell level —
>   pale skin and fatigue are two common signs)

More good news is that you can do much to reduce your risk of getting colon cancer in the first place:

- ❏ Eat a healthy diet rich in the mineral selenium. Good sources include liver, seafood, eggs, cereals, dairy products and vegetables.
- ❏ Get plenty of exercise. Walking for 30 minutes three days a week is a good anti-cancer exercise program to start with.
- ❏ If you are overweight, begin a healthy diet and exercise plan to shed your increased risk of cancer along with your extra pounds.
- ❏ Talk to your doctor about the benefits of taking a weekly aspirin to reduce your risk of colon cancer.
- ❏ Cut down on the amount of cancer-causing fatty foods in your diet. Only 30 percent of your calories should come from fat.
- ❏ Cut down on the amount of beef in your diet. Red meat contains large amounts of fat. Leaner meat, such as chicken, turkey and fish, are healthier for you and your family.
- ❏ Increase the amount of fruits and vegetables you eat daily. Fruits and vegetables contain cancer-fighting vitamins and minerals and provide natural fiber. Fiber helps food travel through the intestines more quickly, reducing your risk of colon cancer.
  Other ways to up your fiber intake are:
  - ➤ Eat whole-grain breads and cereals.
  - ➤ Add dried beans to soups, casseroles and salads.
  - ➤ Substitute brown rice for regular white rice.
  - ➤ Substitute whole-wheat or spinach pasta for regular pasta.
- ❏ Drink eight to 10 glasses of water each day. This also helps move food (and wastes) through the intestines more quickly. (It prevents constipation, too.)
- ❏ Make sure you are getting the recommended daily allowances (RDAs) of important vitamins and minerals. Vitamins A, C and E are especially helpful "anti-cancer" vitamins. Some important sources of these vitamins include the following:

Vitamin A — fish liver oils, eggs, vitamin A-fortified

breads, vegetable-based soups, milk, carrots, peaches, spinach, squash and sweet potatoes

Vitamin C — tomatoes, red and green peppers, strawberries, apricots, potatoes, citrus fruits, collard greens, broccoli, spinach and other leafy vegetables

Vitamin E — soybeans, nuts, whole grains, vegetable oils (such as soybean, corn and safflower oils, margarine), and green, leafy vegetables

Medical Sources

Cancer, Epidemiology, Biomarkers and Prevention (2,1:41)
Medical World News (34,4:16)
Medical Tribune (34,7:1)
Nutrition Research Newsletter (12,1:7)

A natural colon cancer fighter

It's what is known as a "trace element" — your body needs only a trace of this dietary mineral to function properly.

But that little bit is crucial to your good health. In fact, a deficiency of this trace element could increase your risk of developing deadly colon cancer.

This vital mineral is selenium. Two recent studies indicate that getting the proper amount of selenium can prevent the development of colon polyps.

A colon polyp is a small growth on the wall of the large intestine that can easily turn into colon cancer. If removed before turning into cancer, the polyp is harmless.

Selenium helps the body produce a substance known as glutathione peroxidase. The body needs this substance to prevent damage to cells that could lead to cancer.

Getting the right amount of selenium is tricky. A deficiency of selenium can be dangerous, but getting too much can cause negative side effects such as hair loss, nail loss, joint inflammation and garlic-smelling breath.

The recommended daily allowance for selenium in men over the age of 25 is 70 micrograms per day. For women over the age of 24, the RDA is 55 micrograms per day.

Seafood, kidney and liver are good dietary sources of selenium that will help you avoid selenium deficiency and reduce your risk of colon cancer.

Be sure not to overeat foods that are rich in selenium. If you develop symptoms of selenium overdose (hair or nail loss, joint pains or garlic breath), call your doctor right away.

Medical Sources ————————————————
Medical World News (34,4:16)
Cancer, Epidemiology, Biomarkers and Prevention (2,1:41)

Cholesterol can cause colon cancer, too

We know cholesterol is a risk factor for heart disease. Now researchers say it may put you at risk for cancer, too.

Colorectal adenomas are not exactly cancer — not yet, anyway. They are growths that can turn into cancer of the colon and rectum. And they seem to be related to the amount of cholesterol in your blood.

High levels of HDL cholesterol (the "good" cholesterol) decrease your risk of developing colorectal adenoma.

High levels of LDL cholesterol (the "bad" cholesterol) and VLDL cholesterol (very low-density lipoproteins — very bad cholesterol) increase your risk of colorectal adenoma.

Your cholesterol levels may directly impact the amount of various enzymes your intestines produce to help digest food. Making too much of some of the enzymes might have cancerous effects on the walls of the intestines.

Medical Source ————————————————
Annals of Internal Medicine (118,7:481)

An aspirin a week for colon cancer

You have taken aspirin for years to relieve all kinds of aches and pains. It has been called the "most common of all medicines" and the "wonder drug."

And by now you have probably heard that aspirin can help prevent heart disease and strokes. Studies now show that aspirin may have a third benefit

— it may help protect you from colon cancer.

Some researchers say that taking just one aspirin a week can slash by half your risk of developing this deadly disease. An aspirin a day seems to work even better, cutting your risk by about 60 percent.

People with rheumatoid arthritis seem to have a 30 to 40 percent decreased risk of digestive cancers such as cancers of the stomach, colon, rectum, liver and bladder. Arthritic women even have reduced risks of breast, gallbladder and pancreas cancers.

After a 20-year study of over 1,000 people with rheumatoid arthritis, researchers believe that aspirin and nonsteroidal anti-inflammatory drugs (NSAIDs) such as ibuprofen are responsible for the decreased cancer rates. Many people with rheumatoid arthritis take these medications to relieve pain and improve mobility.

Aspirin and NSAIDs inhibit the production of prostaglandins, a chemical produced naturally by the body which may promote tumor growth.

Some people who have been diagnosed with rheumatoid arthritis modify their diets to include more vegetables, which may also reduce their risk of colon cancer.

Scientists may have only begun to discover what ailments aspirin can relieve and what diseases it may prevent. But aspirin can also have potentially harmful side effects.

Most doctors believe that further research is needed before they recommend widespread aspirin use in the prevention of digestive cancers. Be sure to consult your doctor before taking aspirin on a regular basis.

Medical Sources ————————————————
American Journal of Gastroenterology (87,9:346)
The New England Journal of Medicine (325,23:1593)
Journal of the National Cancer Institute (84,19:1491 and 85,4:258, 307)

How to detect colon cancer early: the screening test

A "sigmoidoscopy" is a test commonly used to detect colorectal cancer.

It's a visual examination of the lower part of the colon and the rectum using a lighted tube. This test appears to be the most effective way to detect colon cancer early, especially when you've had no warning signs of the cancer.

Colon cancer is fairly uncommon in people under age 40, but your risk almost doubles every seven years after you reach age 50.

There's some good news and some bad news concerning a sigmoidoscopy. First, the bad news: The test can be uncomfortable, not to mention embarrassing. You lie on your side with your knees to your chest draped in a hospital gown while the tube is inserted into your rectum.

The good news is that you may only have to have the test done every 10 years rather than every three or five years as previously thought.

According to a new study, having the test done every 10 years is about as effective as having the test done more often.

You do need to have the test done more often if you are at high risk for developing colon cancer.

Possible risk factors for colon cancer include:

> A family history of colon cancer
> A close relative with multiple colon polyps
> A history of colon polyps
> Inflammatory bowel disease
> Diet high in fat and low in fiber
> Lack of physical activity
> Excess weight

Medical Source ───────────────────
The New England Journal of Medicine (326,10:654)

Skin cancer: Pale is in, tan is out

Let's face it. You know you're not going to call off your vacation or stop playing golf because you're afraid of skin cancer.

So if you're Caucasian, get ready to invest in the protection that sunscreens can provide. Whites get skin cancer more than any other form of cancer.

In fact, the most common forms of skin cancer, basal and squamous cell carcinomas, account for more than one-third of all cancers. Fortunately, basal and squamous cell cancers rarely lead to death, although their removal can leave disfiguring scars.

The most important cause of these cancers is exposure to ultraviolet B radiation from the sun, and the majority of basal and squamous cell cancers show up on the head, neck and arms, where skin meets sun most often.

Unfortunately, as we spend more leisure time in the sun and the protective ozone layer depletes, the incidence of skin cancer is increasing.

Tanning booths are not a good alternative to sun exposure. Ultraviolet A radiation from tanning booths is not safe either. In fact, the law requires all tanning salons to post a warning about the danger of skin cancer from ultraviolet A.

If several of the following characteristics describe you, you are particularly vulnerable to skin cancer:

> Older
> Don't tan
> Stay red after sunning
> Scottish or Irish ancestors
> Cigarette smoker
> Red, blond, or light brown hair
> Male
> Easily sunburned
> Freckled
> Blue eyes
> Fair skin

Some medical conditions that predispose you to basal and squamous cell cancers are burn scars, sinus drainage, chronic ulcers and lowered immunity.

The most important thing you can do to prevent skin cancer is avoid the sun. Wear hats and clothes that shield your skin, and stay out of the sun from 10 a.m. until 2 p.m. When you are in the sun, use a sunscreen with a sun protection factor (SPF) of at least 15.

If you do notice a new or unusual place on your skin, ask your doctor to evaluate it. The most common skin cancer, basal cell carcinoma, can look like a little pink nodule, a crusted scaly patch, or a sore that refuses to heal. Squamous cell cancers might resemble eczema or psoriasis, a red and scaly nodule, or a flat, pink, scaly place.

Regardless of the type of skin cancer you have, the sooner you find it, the cheaper it is to treat, and the better your chance of avoiding scarring from extensive surgery.

Although surgery usually stops these skin cancers, about half of the people who have a squamous or basal cell carcinoma will have another skin cancer within 5 years. So watch carefully for telltale signs, and remember your sunscreen.

Medical Source ——————————————————
The New England Journal of Medicine (327,23:1649)

The ABCD's of skin cancers

Malignant melanoma is the most serious of all skin cancers and is now the eighth most common cancer in the United States. Growing faster than any other cancer, rates of malignant melanoma have risen 500 percent since the 1980s. The largest increase is in men over 50.

Melanoma often grows from an existing mole. Sometimes, however, the tumor will simply appear on normal skin. A malignant melanoma can appear anywhere on the body, including under the nails or in the eye.

A family history of melanoma or unusual moles, fair skin and a large number of moles on the body increase the risk of developing this skin cancer. Repeated sunburns or even just one massive burn can also raise your risk.

At this time, the only way to screen for skin cancer is visually. Even if you're not at high risk, it's important to examine your skin regularly. Watch for changes in existing moles.

The American Academy of Dermatology developed the ABCD guidelines to help identify possibly cancerous moles:

☐ Asymmetry — Mole is not exactly round or oval.
☐ Border Irregularity — Mole's outside edge appears notched or scalloped. It may be difficult to tell where mole ends.
☐ Color Variation — Mole has shades of brown/tan, red, white, blue/black or some combination of these colors. Cancerous moles tend to develop dark-black areas.
☐ Diameter — Mole is 6 millimeters (about 1/4 inch) or larger in size.

Some moles do not develop any ABCD features. The only indication of cancer in these moles is their extremely rapid growth.

When checking your moles, be sure to do a total body exam. Check the bottoms of your feet, between your toes and personal areas. You may want to have someone help you check difficult areas such as your back, back of legs and scalp. Some cancers are mistaken for birthmarks and are not diagnosed until they have already started to spread.

Although the face is the area most regularly exposed to the sun's ultraviolet rays, many malignant melanomas appear on the chest, stomach, back, legs and feet. Doctors speculate that recreational tanning, which is the most damaging type of ultraviolet radiation exposure, is responsible for the large numbers of malignant melanomas that appear in these areas.

The U.S. population has an estimated total of 6.1 billion moles. Each person probably has between 10 and 40 moles.

Checking all those moles may seem troublesome, but it's worth the effort when you consider that early detection of malignant melanoma can mean a 100 percent cure.

The important factor is how far the cancer has invaded the skin. There is a 99 percent disease-free survival rate for cancers that have not progressed beyond the skin's surface.

The earlier you have a suspicious mole examined, the better.

Medical Sources —————————————————————
Medical World News (33,2:19)
Journal of the National Cancer Institute (85,2:87)

Dietary changes cut lung cancer risk in half

Lung cancer heads the pack as the leading cause of cancer deaths for both men and women in the United States.

Millions of people across the nation are being diagnosed with lung cancer these days, including people who never smoked a single cigarette. Only 13 percent of women diagnosed with lung cancer will survive for five years or more. It's a deadly disease with little hope of survival for those who develop it.

So, scientists have been focusing on ways to prevent the disease from ever occurring. Recent research indicates that diet is one of the best weapons in the fight against lung cancer.

One medical study of 41,000 women suggests that making a few dietary changes can cut a woman's risk of lung cancer in half.

Women who reported the highest intakes of fruits and vegetables, especially green, leafy vegetables, had only 50 percent of the risk of developing lung cancer compared with the women who reported the lowest intakes of the same foods.

Fruits, vegetables and vitamins can do wonders to reduce your risk of lung cancer, but the best way to prevent lung cancer is to quit smoking. Smoking is the largest and most dangerous risk factor for lung cancer, and huge quantities of healthy foods cannot completely overcome it.

Talk with your doctor about a stop-smoking program to reduce your (and your family's) risk of developing lung cancer.

Medical Source ———————————————
Cancer Research (53,3:536)

Stop beta-carotene from going up in puff of smoke

Beta-carotene can help prevent the development of cancer. Study after study has proven it. But can the anti-cancer vitamin even help protect smokers from lung cancer?

Most smokers have abnormally low levels of beta-carotene in their blood due to the harmful effects of cigarette smoke on some vitamins in the body.

In a recent study, men who smoked more than 15 cigarettes per day took a 20-milligram beta-carotene supplement every day for 14 weeks. They were able to boost their blood levels of beta-carotene by more than 13-fold.

The increased levels of beta-carotene strengthened certain cells in the blood that help prevent the development of cancer. More beta-carotene in the blood means stronger and more effective cancer-fighting immune cells. And that means a lower risk of developing lung cancer.

Beta-carotene is a natural precursor of vitamin A.

To maximize your body's defense against developing cancer, get your vitamin A the natural way instead of in supplement form. Taking a supplement just won't give you the same cancer-fighting protection that vitamin A-rich fruits and vegetables can provide.

The combination of nutrients and protective chemicals in fresh food can't be duplicated. Broccoli, for instance, contains beta carotene, but it also contains sulforaphane, a natural cancer-fighter.

People who eat plenty of vegetables and have high levels of beta carotene in their blood consistently have a low risk of lung cancer.

Here are a few of the best vegetable and fruit sources of vitamin A:

broccoli	carrots	spinach
squash	zucchini	romaine lettuce
peaches	sweet potatoes	apricots

Some good natural sources of beta carotene include mangoes, tomatoes, yellow squash, kale and cantaloupe.

Vitamin A also seems to work against mouth cancer for people who smoke or use smokeless tobacco.

The cancer-causing part of tobacco damages the genetic material in the cells of your mouth. If the cells don't have a chance to repair themselves, the damaged cells can duplicate themselves and develop into cancer.

Vitamin A gels that you could apply directly to your mouth are only in the testing phase now. Until their worth is fully established, eating foods rich in beta carotene could be your best protection against mouth cancer.

Medical Sources ─────────────────────

The American Journal of Clinical Nutrition (57,3:402)
Nutrition Research Newsletter (12,4:41)
Medical Tribune (33,16:24)
Nutrition and Cancer (17,3:263)
The Lancet (339,8809:1562)
Drug Therapy (22,7:55)

Pet birds linked to lung cancer

Cigarette smoking accounts for about 80 percent of lung cancer cases.

The remaining 20 percent of lung cancer deaths have not been completely explained. Recently, researchers have begun to investigate a new possible contributor to mysterious cases of lung cancer — the keeping of pet birds.

Past studies have shown that pet birds can cause lung problems — coughing, difficulty breathing and even permanent lung damage.

Birds carry parasites and other foreign particles which you may inhale into your lungs. Your body will then begin to produce antibodies to protect itself against the foreign matter. The longer you're exposed to birds, the more antibodies you produce.

When too many antibodies build up, they start to destroy lung cells. Changes in the cells brought about by the parasites or the antibodies may lead to the development of cancerous cells.

A general practitioner in the Netherlands was the first to suspect a connection. He noticed that people who had kept pet birds for five to 14 years were more prone to malignant lung tumors. His studies led him to conclude that bird keepers are 6.7 times more likely to develop lung cancer than people who don't keep birds.

A later study done in Berlin found lower, yet still significant, increases in the risk of lung cancer among bird keepers. Those investigators found people exposed to pet birds to be twice as likely to develop cancer as those not exposed. If you had kept a bird for 10 years or more, you were three times more likely to develop lung cancer.

Scottish researchers found only pigeon keepers to be four times more likely to develop lung cancer.

Although further research needs to be done to measure the risk levels accurately, researchers agree that prolonged exposure to pet birds may increase your chances of developing lung cancer.

If you are a smoker, are regularly exposed to cancer-causing agents, if your family has a history of lung cancer, or you consider yourself a high risk for lung cancer, you may want to minimize your exposure to pet birds.

If you keep pet birds in your home, keep them in well-ventilated areas — preferably not a bedroom, and keep their cages and surrounding space extra clean.

Medical Source ————————————————————
British Medical Journal (305,6860:970, 986, 989)

Warning: Applying powder here can cause cancer

Most women have experienced that "less than fresh" feeling at one time or another. But if you use talcum powder to help you feel fresh, you could be setting yourself up for ovarian cancer.

Long-term use of talc in the genital area greatly increases your chances of developing ovarian cancer, according to a recent study from Harvard Medical School. Long-term use of talcum powder is not a major cause of ovarian cancer, but it might account for nearly one out of every 10 ovarian-cancer cases.

Women who applied the talc directly onto the genital area were at the greatest risk of developing ovarian cancer, especially if they used the powder every day for over 10 years. Women who used talcum powder before 1960 when it might have contained asbestos are also at high risk for ovarian cancer.

In many cases, ovarian cancer can be difficult to detect early because there are no definite symptoms. According to the National Cancer Institute, some symptoms are swelling, bloating and discomfort in the lower abdomen, a feeling of fullness even after light meals, gas and indigestion.

Sometimes menstrual periods can remain normal, misleading some women into neglecting their routine pelvic examinations.

If you don't catch ovarian cancer before it spreads, your chances of survival are bleak — only 10 to 20 percent. Catching it early raises your survival chances to 60 to 70 percent.

Medical Sources —————————————————————
Obstetrics and Gynecology (47,9:81)
The American Medical Association, Random House, New York, 1989

Drinking water linked to bladder cancer

"Drink more water" are words you're sure to hear if you're plagued by a urinary tract infection, kidney stones, a weight problem, the flu or even the common cold.

The more water you drink the better, right? Not where bladder cancer is concerned, says a new study. Drinking a lot of beverages, especially chlorinated tap water, appears to increase men's risk of developing bladder cancer.

Researchers questioned 351 white males with bladder cancer and 855 healthy white males about their intake of milk, coffee, tea, juices, bottled drinks, tap water and alcohol.

Men who drank over 14 cups of fluids a day had more than four times the risk of bladder cancer than men who drank less than seven cups a day. Most of the fluids came from the local tap water, including glasses of water taken directly from the tap, plus coffee, tea and frozen juices.

The risk of bladder cancer appeared to be associated more with these tap-water sources than with the non-tap-water sources.

Several other studies agree that the more you drink, especially chlorinated water, the greater your risk of bladder cancer. Researchers have several different theories.

When you drink beverages all day, and particularly when you don't urinate often enough, your bladder has to stretch. The stretched bladder lining increases the contact between your body tissues and cancer-causing substances in your urine.

Also, compounds formed from chlorine, which public water systems often use as a disinfectant, have been shown to increase the risk of cancer in laboratory rats. And, the pollution levels in some public water supplies exceed safety standards, according to some studies.

What can you do to protect yourself? You may want to support measures to control pollution into rivers and other water areas to reduce the need for chlorine in the water supply.

Using a water filter may help decrease your risk of bladder cancer.

Also, be sure to urinate often so that your bladder doesn't have to stretch too much.

While there does appear to be a link between increased beverage intake and bladder cancer, the benefits of drinking adequate amounts of water probably outweigh any bad side effects.

Medical Source ─────────────────────────
Archives of Environmental Health (48,3:191)

DIABETES

What causes diabetes?

Diabetes is a disease that affects the way your body uses food. It comes in two types — noninsulin-dependent (or Type II) diabetes mellitus and insulin-dependent (or Type I) diabetes mellitus.

If you have diabetes, an organ in your abdomen, known as the pancreas, doesn't make enough of the chemical insulin.

Your body needs insulin to convert sugar from the food you eat into energy for all the cells in your body.

People with Type I diabetes would die if they didn't give themselves at least one shot of insulin every day. With Type II diabetes, sometimes your pancreas does make enough insulin, but your body can't use it for some reason.

By far the most common type of diabetes (nine out of 10 of all cases) is Type II, or noninsulin-dependent diabetes. It used to be called maturity-onset diabetes because it usually develops later in life — after age 40.

Medical experts don't know what causes Type II diabetes. It does seem to run in families, so you can inherit the tendency to be diabetic. However, it usually takes a factor like obesity to bring on the disease.

Type II diabetes often develops slowly. Common signs and symptoms are:

> ➤ Excessive thirst
> ➤ Frequent urination
> ➤ Extreme fatigue
> ➤ Nausea
> ➤ Unexplained weight loss
> ➤ Blurred vision
> ➤ Hard-to-heal infections of the skin, gums, vagina or bladder
> ➤ Tingling or loss of feeling in hands or feet
> ➤ Dry, itchy skin

Most people with Type II diabetes can control their blood-sugar levels with a special diet, exercise program and weight loss and quitting smoking.

If diabetes isn't controlled, it can cause problems with your kidneys, legs and feet, eyes, heart, nerves and blood flow. You can have kidney failure, blindness, stroke, gangrene and amputation. Because diabetes can be such a serious, even life-threatening illness, the best way to deal with it is to avoid it.

Medical Source ────────────────────────

American Diabetes Association Inc., 1660 Duke Street, Alexandria, VA 22314

Health risk weight chart

Most people who have noninsulin-dependent diabetes are overweight. Some people can avoid Type II diabetes completely by simply losing weight.

When does your weight put you at risk for diabetes? When you are 20 percent over your ideal weight, your health is affected. The chart below shows 20 percent over ideal weights for people of average bone size:

Women	Men
4'9" — 127	5'1" — 146
4'10" — 131	5'2" — 151
4'11" — 134	5'3" — 155
5'0" — 138	5'4" — 158
5'1" — 142	5'5" — 163
5'2" — 146	5'6" — 168
5'3" — 151	5'7" — 174
5'4" — 157	5'8" — 179
5'5" — 162	5'9" — 184
5'6" — 167	5'10" — 190
5'7" — 172	5'11" — 196
5'8" — 176	6'0" — 202
5'9" — 181	6'1" — 208
5'10" — 186	6'2" — 214
	6'3" — 220

Medical Source ────────────────────────

American Diabetes Association Inc., 1660 Duke Street, Alexandria, VA 22314

Sweating away a 'sweet' disease — diabetes

Sweat. Some think it's sexy. Others think it's disgusting. But it could help prevent life-threatening, noninsulin-dependent diabetes. If you work up a sweat at least once each week, that is.

Harvard University researchers studied the effects of vigorous exercise on 22,000 male doctors to see if exercise reduced their risk of developing diabetes.

They found that the men who exercised vigorously enough to work up a sweat at least once a week reduced their risk of developing Type II diabetes by 23 percent.

The men who exercised vigorously between two and four times each week enjoyed a 38 percent lower risk of developing diabetes. Exercising five or more times a week gave men a huge 42-percent drop in their diabetes risk.

Fortunately, the benefits of vigorous exercise seemed to be the greatest in overweight men. Overweight men who vigorously exercised at least once a week had a 40 percent lower risk of diabetes than overweight men who exercised less than once a week.

Although the Harvard study was conducted with male volunteers, the effect of exercise on diabetes seems to hold true for women, too. An earlier study showed that exercising at least once a week decreased women's diabetes risk by 33 percent.

A healthy lifestyle that includes regular exercise is the only practical way to prevent Type II diabetes.

Medical Sources ————————————————

The Journal of the American Medical Association (268,1:63)
Medical World News (33,7:16)

An aspirin a day to prevent heart disease

The age-old doctor's line "Take two aspirin . . ." might turn out to be a bit of heartwarming advice for people suffering from diabetes.

Diabetics who take two 325-milligram aspirin tablets a day could reduce their risk of having a heart attack by as much as 17 percent.

Apparently, men who have diabetes have about twice the risk of getting heart disease as other men. Diabetic women are in even greater danger — they have three to five times the risk of developing heart disease compared with nondiabetic women.

Aspirin therapy isn't for everyone, but since diabetic people already have an increased risk of heart disease, taking daily aspirin to reduce their risk of heart attack could be wise.

Always talk to your doctor before taking any medications. Taking too much aspirin can cause dangerous side effects. Your doctor can help determine a safe and effective dosage for you.

Medical Source ————————————————
> *The Journal of the American Medical Association* (268,10:1292)
> *Medical Tribune* (33,18:3)

Foot-care tips for diabetics

If you suffer from diabetes, you might have poor circulation in your legs and feet. The skin on your feet can sometimes be very thin and can break easily, and things might take a little longer to heal.

Some diabetics can injure themselves because they have nerve damage that causes their legs and feet to feel numb.

Injuries can sometimes go unnoticed and can lead to more serious problems like gangrene (when the tissue dies). That could result in amputation of the foot or leg.

Here are some simple, natural tips to help keep your legs and feet healthy:

- ❒ Be sure your shoes fit properly and you have plenty of cushioning.
- ❒ Break in new shoes gradually — wear them for short periods of time at first.
- ❒ Do not go barefoot. Shoes protect your feet from injury.
- ❒ Check your feet every day for cuts, blisters and redness. Make sure the doctor checks them each time you go for a visit or checkup.
- ❒ Trim your toenails straight across instead of curved, or file them very carefully.
- ❒ Don't dig under your toenails or around your cuticles with a sharp instrument.

❏ Wash your feet with warm water and use a mild soap.
❏ Change your socks or stockings every day. Make sure they aren't too tight.

Medical Source ———————————————————
Postgraduate Medicine (92,2:289)

Pain relief for diabetes sufferers

If you have pain from diabetes, arthritis or shingles, we've got hot news for you. Researchers have found that the active ingredient in red peppers, capsaicin, is effective in relieving discomfort caused by these disorders.

Does this mean you should start a red pepper roundup? No, ready-made relief is as close as your nearest pharmacy. Made from dried cayenne peppers, capsaicin is available as an over-the-counter cream. It is absorbed through your skin and works by deadening local nerves.

Capsaicin works especially well in relieving pain from diabetic neuropathy, a complication of diabetes that results in damaged nerves.

Eight percent of all diabetics are diagnosed with diabetic neuropathy at the same time they are diagnosed with diabetes. After 25 years of diabetes, one-half of all diabetics have nerve damage.

Improvement sometimes occurs spontaneously after six to 10 months, or symptoms may last for many years.

If you suffer from diabetic neuropathy, simply touching your skin can cause a painful burning sensation. Symptoms depend on which muscles are affected and are often worse at night. They may interfere with your sleep and work.

Symptoms include:

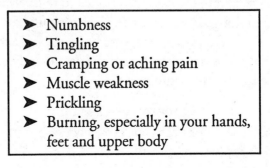

> Numbness
> Tingling
> Cramping or aching pain
> Muscle weakness
> Prickling
> Burning, especially in your hands, feet and upper body

In one eight-week study, more than 70 percent of the people who used capsaicin to treat the symptoms of diabetic neuropathy relieved their discomfort. They walked and slept better and were able to work comfortably and participate in recreational activities.

Using capsaicin can also make exercise less painful and enable you to follow a regular exercise schedule.

Capsaicin cream is applied directly to your skin and it shouldn't interact with any medications you take by mouth.

Distributed under the name of Zostrix, the cream comes in two strengths, regular and high potency (HP). High potency is three times as strong as regular strength. Although capsaicin cream is available over the counter, you have to ask for it in most pharmacies.

When purchasing capsaicin, be careful not to confuse it with capsicum, capsicum oleoresin, capsaicin oleoresin or nonivamide (pelargonic acid vanillylamide), which is sometimes incorrectly referred to as synthetic capsaicin.

Products that contain capsicum or capsicum oleoresin often are not as effective as products that contain capsaicin.

When you first begin using capsaicin, you may experience burning, stinging or redness. These effects normally disappear after you have used capsaicin for one to two weeks.

If the burning persists, try treating the area with a local skin anesthetic, such as 5 percent Xylocaine, or applying capsaicin to a smaller area.

You can also take a simple painkiller, such as aspirin or ibuprofen, for the first few days. It may take two weeks or longer, especially if your pain is due to nerve damage, before the capsaicin begins to relieve your discomfort.

Even after prolonged use, researchers haven't found capsaicin to have any adverse side effects. Capsaicin appears to be just as safe and effective now as it was centuries ago when the Mayan and Incan Indians used it to treat arthritis, epilepsy and the common cold.

How to use capsaicin

☐ Don't use on or near your eyes, nose or mouth.
☐ Don't apply to broken or irritated skin.

- ❏ Don't use on children younger than two years of age except under a doctor's supervision.
- ❏ If you have shingles, don't apply Zostrix until the skin blisters have healed. Don't tightly bandage the affected area after you apply the cream.
- ❏ Massage a small amount of the cream onto all sides of the painful area.
- ❏ Apply the product three or four times a day. As pain is relieved, you may gradually reduce the number of times you use capsaicin to once or twice a day or as the directions recommend.
- ❏ Wash your hands thoroughly after applying the cream.
- ❏ Stop using the product if your symptoms get worse or persist after 28 days or if your condition is relieved yet recurs in a couple of days.

Medical Source ————————————————
U.S. Pharmacist (18,8:20)

HEART AND BLOOD VESSEL DISEASE

Cough to survive a heart attack

Most people have read enough or heard enough about heart attacks to know the symptoms: the crushing pain in the chest, left arm or jaw. Some people begin to sweat or feel queasy before the pain begins. Others remember their heart feeling "funny" or racing just before the other symptoms started.

In many cases, the heart stops beating altogether. When your heart stops, you begin to feel as if you're about to faint.

In this situation, you have only about 10 seconds before you lose consciousness. What happens during those 10 seconds can be the difference between life and death.

You could save your life with a new method called "cough resuscitation." Cough resuscitation is a crude alternative to CPR (cardiopulmonary resuscitation) — the more traditional form of resuscitation that involves another person performing chest compressions and mouth-to-mouth breathing for the unconscious person.

Coughing repeatedly and very vigorously can help keep you conscious until help arrives. In some cases, the coughing can actually force the heart back into a semi-normal rhythm.

Cough resuscitation involves taking a deep breath and expanding your lungs and chest as much as possible. Then, the cough should be deep and prolonged, like you're trying to cough up sputum from deep inside your chest. A deep breath and a deep cough must be repeated every two to three seconds until help arrives or until the heart feels like it has a normal rhythm again.

The deep breaths fill the lungs with air and help oxygenate the blood so that the heart, brain and other organs in the body will suffer as little damage from oxygen-loss as possible.

The deep, vigorous coughs squeeze the heart and keep the blood circulating. Coughing also creates a certain amount of "electricity" in the heart muscle that sometimes will shock the heart back into a normal or semi-normal rhythm.

Using cough resuscitation, heart attack victims can stay conscious, get to a phone and call for help in between breaths and coughs.

Talk to your doctor if you have questions about cough resuscitation or other questions about your risk of heart attacks. And contact your local American Heart Association about taking a course in CPR, so that you'll be prepared to help others when needed.

Medical Sources ────────────────────────

Emergency Medicine (24,12:170)

U.S. Pharmacist (18,1:98)

The dangers of borderline high blood pressure

Just when you thought you were safe, they lowered the blood pressure standards again. The National High Blood Pressure Education Program has changed the normal blood pressure level to 130/85 mm Hg. Anything over that can damage you heart and put you at risk for a stroke or heart attack.

What hypertension, or high blood pressure, really means is that flow of blood from the heart is literally under high pressure. Usually the increased pressure is due to a narrowing of the blood vessels in the body — when the same amount of blood has to travel through a narrower space, the pressure goes up.

One problem with high blood pressure is that the heart muscle has to work harder to force the blood through those narrowed vessels. The heart muscle is like any other muscle in the body: The harder it works, the thicker it gets.

However, unlike a thickened biceps muscle, a thickened heart muscle is not such a great thing. In fact, it can predispose you to heart trouble in the future.

The good news is, if you do lose weight, exercise, cut back on salt and alcohol and quit smoking, you can dramatically improve the condition of your heart.

Dr. Paul Whelton, a professor of medicine and epidemiology at Johns

Hopkins University, says that if everyone in the United States lowered his systolic blood pressure (the higher number in the blood pressure reading) by 3 mm Hg, we'd have 8 percent fewer deaths from stroke every year and 5 percent fewer heart-attack deaths.

You may be willing to get your blood pressure checked, but what should your next step be? Here's a chart to help you know what to do:

Systolic (higher number)	Diastolic (lower number)	What to do*
Less than 130	Less than 85	You're safe. Get your blood pressure checked again in 2 years.
130-139	85-89	Have blood pressure checked again in one year; modify lifestyle
140-159	90-99	Have blood pressure checked again within two months
160-179	100-109	Have medical evaluation or treatment within one month
180-209	110-119	Have medical evaluation or treatment within one week
210 or higher	120 or higher	Have medical evaluation or treatment immediately

* This advice may not be the best for you. For instance, you may need more regular checkups if you have a family history of heart disease, poor health or other risk factors. Check with your doctor.

Even mildly elevated blood pressure is nothing to fool around with. Talk to your doctor about your blood pressure. If it is elevated — even mildly — ask your doctor about a plan to help lower it to reduce your risk of heart disease.

Medical Sources —————————————————
Circulation (87,2:476)
Hypertension (18,5:4)

How to reduce your risk of high blood pressure

☐ Keep your weight within 10 pounds of your "ideal" weight. Ask your doctor what your ideal weight is, based on your height and body build.

☐ Get regular exercise. Walking for 30 to 45 minutes at a time three to five times each week will help reduce your risk of high blood pressure.

☐ Cut by at least half the amount of alcohol you drink each week. You shouldn't drink more than two ounces of 100-proof whiskey, eight ounces of wine or 24 ounces of beer each day.

☐ Restrict your intake of salt to six grams of table salt per day.

☐ Increase the amount of fiber in your diet, especially natural fruit fiber.

☐ Make sure you get the recommended daily allowances of potassium, calcium and magnesium.

☐ Reduce the amount of fatty foods and cholesterol in your diet.

☐ Stop smoking.

☐ If you have diabetes, keep your blood sugar under tight control.

☐ If you are using oral contraceptives, corticosteroids, decongestants, or appetite suppressants, talk to your doctor about your increased risk of high blood pressure.

Medical Sources ────────────────

U.S. Pharmacist (18.3:13 Cardiovascular Disease Supplement)
Postgraduate Medicine (93,4:193)

A vitamin that lowers blood pressure

Good news for the millions of Americans with high blood pressure who worry about the possibility of stroke or heart attack: Doctors have found another natural remedy for hypertension.

Increase the amount of the mineral potassium in your diet.

To prove this theory, a team of Italian researchers tested the effects of increased potassium on a group of people who were already taking medicine for hypertension.

The test group upped the amount of potassium-rich foods they ate by more than 60 percent for a year. As a result, these people were able to cut by more than half the amount of medicine they took for high blood pressure. This is good news since blood pressure drugs often cause unpleasant side effects.

The test group consumed about 4,460 milligrams of potassium daily by including three to six servings of peas, beans, fruits and vegetables in their meals every day. They also cut back slightly on fats.

Potassium appears to prevent thickening of artery walls that slows down blood flow and can trigger strokes or heart attacks.

A 12-year California study reaches a similar conclusion about potassium. The report indicates that men in the lower third of the population in potassium consumption are more than 2 1/2 times more likely to have a stroke than men who consume more of this valuable mineral.

Medical Sources ————————————————
The Johns Hopkins Medical Letter (4,3:1)
Annals of Internal Medicine (115,10:753)
Hypertension (19,6:749)
Harvard Health Letter (17,7:1)

Potassium do's and don'ts

The recommended dietary allowance for potassium is from 1,600 to 2,000 milligrams.

But you might need to raise your potassium intake to about 3,500 milligrams a day for it to work to lower high blood pressure.

For the best results, follow these potassium do's and don'ts:

Do's:
  ✔ Check with your doctor before increasing potassium intake if you have kidney disease.
  ✔ Steam or microwave vegetables to preserve potassium.
  ✔ Check the list below of high-potassium foods for a wide range of tasty suggestions. Skim milk is also high in potassium.

Don'ts:
  ✗ Don't rely on meat, poultry or fish for your potassium. Although they are good sources of potassium, they are also higher in calories

and fat than vegetables, fruits, and peas and beans.

✗ Never stop taking your high blood pressure medicine without asking your doctor first.

Potassium Sources

Vegetables	Fruits	Peas and beans
asparagus	apples	pinto beans
artichoke	apricots	kidney beans
broccoli	bananas	chickpeas
carrots	cherries	broad beans
cauliflower	grapefruit	lentils
eggplant	grapes	string beans
romaine lettuce	oranges	peas
mushrooms	peaches	
peppers	pears	
baked potato	plums	
spinach		
turnips		

Medical Sources ——————————————

The Johns Hopkins Medical Letter (4,3:12)

Recommended Dietary Allowances, 10th Edition, National Academy Press, Washington, D.C., 1989

The truth about fish oil

Fish oil does work to lower blood pressure, but don't get too excited about it. A little rush of adrenaline may undo all the good your weeks of popping fish oil supplements have done.

Fish oil can lower blood pressure, but the effects aren't nearly as breathtaking as some scientists have claimed. Whether or not fish oil benefits you at all depends on your health.

☐ If you're healthy with normal blood pressure, fish oil supplements will do nothing for you. Don't take them as a "preventative," or in an attempt to keep from developing high blood pressure later. You won't get anything out of it except, possibly, an upset stomach.

❏ If you have high blood pressure but don't have any heart or artery damage, fish oil supplements may or may not help you lower your blood pressure. You have to take a lot of fish oil to get any effect at all.

On average, people with high blood pressure can lower their systolic blood pressure (the upper number) by 4 mm Hg and their diastolic blood pressure (the lower number) by 3 mm Hg by taking 7.7 grams of omega-3 fatty acids a day. That's about 15 fish-oil capsules every day.

❏ If you have hardening of the arteries because of heart disease or high cholesterol, you may really benefit from fish oil. Three of four small studies on the effect of fish oil on blood pressure in people with heart disease showed systolic decreases of 10 to 17 mm Hg and diastolic decreases of 3 to 10 mm Hg.

The higher your cholesterol levels and the worse your heart disease, the better fish oil works. People with heart disease and high cholesterol levels have high levels of thromboxane in their bodies. Thromboxane is a "vasoconstrictor," which means it raises blood pressure by narrowing your blood vessels.

Fish oil contains the omega-3 fatty acid eicosapentaenoic acid (EPA), which seems to lower blood pressure by stopping your body from making thromboxane. EPA also seems to help lower your blood pressure by stimulating your body to make a certain type of "vasodilator," which causes the blood vessels to relax and dilate.

If you have high blood pressure and you're ready to try fish oil, don't let us discourage you. One thing is certain: Fish oil works better for some people than for others. It may be your miracle cure.

Just don't pin all your hopes on it. Your best bet for preventing and lowering high blood pressure and heart disease is to lose weight, exercise, stop smoking, cut down on alcohol and salt, avoid stress and eat a healthy diet.

Instead of taking fish oil supplements, consider eating cold water fish that contains omega-3 fatty acids, such as cod, tuna, salmon, halibut, shark and mackerel, three times a week. You'll get the fish oil benefits without the unpleasant side effects, such as diarrhea, gas and upset stomach.

Medical Source ——————————————————
Circulation (88,2:523)

Good HDL sweeps up bad LDL in the cholesterol wars

Ever since your heart attack last year, your doctor has been telling you to keep your cholesterol level under 200 to reduce your risk of another heart attack.

So you had your cholesterol level checked at a health fair, and it was under 200, the magic number. You're safe.

Unfortunately, you might not be as safe as you think.

People who have a low level of HDL cholesterol (the good kind of cholesterol) have an increased risk of heart attack and sudden death even if their total cholesterol levels are normal, or below 200.

In one study, people who had suffered from heart problems in the past managed to keep their cholesterol levels to an average of 175. However, 60 percent of them experienced a serious heart problem over the next 13 years, mainly because their HDL levels were too low.

The HDL cholesterol serves as a kind of cleaning crew in the body. The HDL molecules "sweep up" extra cholesterol in the blood and transport it to safe locations, away from the walls of the coronary arteries. When there are low levels of HDL in the body, the extra cholesterol does not get "swept" away.

When a lot of that extra cholesterol builds up on the artery walls — a condition known as atherosclerosis — blood can no longer get through the vessels. When blood flow to the heart is blocked, a heart attack occurs. Atherosclerosis also increases the risk of strokes.

Average HDL levels for men are 45 to 50, and 55 to 60 for women. People with HDL levels below 35 are in danger of suffering from future heart problems, warns the American Heart Association.

Two important ways to raise HDL levels are regular exercise and quitting smoking. For obese people, losing weight can help raise HDL levels by as much as 10 percent.

During your next checkup, ask your doctor to check your HDL levels in addition to your total cholesterol level. If your HDL levels are below 35, talk to your doctor about a safe way to keep your total cholesterol level below 200 while raising your HDL to a safe level.

Medical Source ─────────────────────
Circulation (86,4:1165)

Coffee gets the O.K. for the heart

Worried about coffee elevating your risk of heart disease? Well, you can now show your face, proudly, at the coffee shop again.

The final word on coffee and heart disease is that the two are not related. Drinking coffee does not increase your risk of heart disease, indicates an analysis of 11 major coffee-and-cholesterol studies done in the past 25 years.

Dr. Martin B. Myers of the University of Toronto and his colleagues concluded that the risk of heart disease is the same for people who drink no coffee as it is for people who drink six cups a day.

Coffee has also been standing "trial" on the charge that filtered coffee is a health hazard. Some researchers believe that filtered coffee can raise cholesterol levels and therefore increase your risk of heart disease.

A team of researchers at the Johns Hopkins Medical Institute did a study to settle the issue, and their results turned out to be in favor of coffee.

The investigators recruited 100 volunteers for the strict, scientific, 16-week study.

The first half of the study was an eight-week "washout" period in which the volunteers had no coffee or other caffeine-containing foods, medications or drinks to "clean out" their systems.

Then, some volunteers drank 24 ounces of coffee a day, some drank 12 ounces, some drank decaffeinated coffee, and other had no coffee at all.

The final study results showed a slight increase in the amount of blood cholesterol in the volunteers who drank 24 ounces of regular caffeinated coffee each day. None of the other volunteers experienced a rise in blood cholesterol levels.

The researchers concluded that even though the volunteers who drank the most coffee experienced a slight increase in blood cholesterol, the increase was so small that it shouldn't have any effect on the risk of heart disease.

In other words, although you may suffer from side effects of caffeine, you can drink coffee to your *heart's* content.

Medical Sources ————————————————————
Archives of Internal Medicine (152,9:1767)
The Journal of the American Medical Association (267,6:811)

Nutty way to lower cholesterol

Your family and friends might think you're a little ... eh, nutty, but you could help lower your risk of heart disease by eating more of a tasty snack food — walnuts.

A recent study indicates that increasing your daily intake of walnuts could help lower your blood-cholesterol level and reduce your risk of heart disease.

Researchers recruited 18 men with blood-cholesterol levels ranging from 137 to 250. The men were divided into two groups, and each group was placed on a special healthy diet.

Both diet plans contained identical foods and nutrients, except that 20 percent of the calories of one diet came from walnuts instead of other foods. The walnuts were served as snacks and mixed into entrées, breakfast cereals and salads.

After the eight-week test period, the researchers came up with some promising results: Replacing a portion of fatty foods in your diet with walnuts can lower cholesterol levels by more than 10 percent.

Substituting the walnuts into the diet also seems to improve the ratio of LDL cholesterol (the bad stuff) to HDL cholesterol (the good stuff).

Walnuts have a very high ratio of polyunsaturated fat to saturated fat, and scientists think this might be the key to the health benefits of eating more walnuts.

Walnuts are also an excellent source of an important dietary fatty acid (n-3 linolenic acid).

Researchers report that people who eat nuts fewer than four times a week have a 78 percent relative risk of suffering a heart attack, whereas people who eat nuts more than five times a week cut their risk down to 49 percent.

Americans eat an average of four grams of walnuts a week. Increasing your walnut intake to 28 grams a day could significantly lower your blood-cholesterol levels and lower your risk of heart disease. Almonds and hazelnuts might have the same cholesterol-lowering effect as walnuts.

Do cut down on other fatty foods in your diet to avoid gaining weight from the extra calories in the nuts.

Medical Source ─────────────────────────
The New England Journal of Medicine (328,9:603)

Margarine-butter battle, 'Round 2'

You switched from butter to margarine a few years ago to try to lower your cholesterol levels.

Well, it might be time to switch again. But, this time, you may be switching from margarine to corn oil.

In a recent study, 14 volunteers received meals approximating the current U.S. diet for four weeks. These meals contained 36 percent of calories from fat.

For another four weeks, the volunteers ate meals with 30 percent of calories from fat, which is what the American Heart Association recommends. These meals were cooked with both corn oil and margarine, and were much better at reducing blood cholesterol levels than the butter-enriched standard American diet. The corn oil/margarine meals also lowered LDL levels by an average of 10 percent.

But for another portion of the study, the volunteers ate meals that contained 30 percent of calories from fat and completely substituted liquid corn oil for butter and margarine.

When the volunteers ate these meals, they enjoyed significantly lower blood cholesterol levels than when they ate the meals cooked with both corn oil and margarine. And, the meals cooked with liquid corn oil alone lowered

LDL cholesterol by 17 percent.

The study indicates that switching from butter to margarine is a great way to lower your cholesterol levels. But, switching to liquid corn oil is even better.

Only liquid vegetable oils will help lower cholesterol levels. Solid shortenings are just as bad as butter.

Apparently, the process of converting a vegetable oil into a solid or semi-solid form (a process known as hydrogenation) is what makes the difference between good and bad shortening. The thicker (or the more solid) the shortening, the more hydrogenated it is. And the more hydrogenated it is, the worse it is for you.

If you must use margarine, use liquid margarine spreads instead of margarine sticks.

Even though the researchers used liquid corn oil in the study, other liquid vegetable oils such as olive, soybean, sunflower, safflower and canola oils are as good or better for lowering blood cholesterol levels, too.

Medical Source ————————————————
Arteriosclerosis and Thrombosis (13,2:154)

Change when you eat, not what, to cut cholesterol

Millions of Americans have given up some of their favorite foods in a valiant attempt to lower their cholesterol levels and reduce their risk of heart disease.

A recent study suggests that combining a low-fat diet with a simple dietary trick could help lower cholesterol levels even more.

"Oh, no!" most people groan. "What else am I going to have to give up?"

The answer is nothing. The number of meals you eat each day is the magic behind this new trick.

The volunteers for the cholesterol study received a diet plan that contained balanced meals with only 30 percent of the calories from fat. Half the group was instructed to eat their food in three meals per day. The other half was instructed to divide the food into nine meals per day.

The three-meals-a-day group received 25 percent of their energy allowance at breakfast, 25 percent at lunch, and about 50 percent at dinner, with a small snack during the day.

The other group divided their energy allowances into smaller meals: early morning, 8.3 percent; breakfast, 8.3 percent; late morning, 8.3 percent; lunch, 8.3 percent; mid afternoon, 8.3 percent; late afternoon, 8.3 percent; dinner, 16.6 percent; mid evening, 16.6 percent; and late evening, 16.6 percent.

Compared with the three-meal diet plan, the nine-meal plan helped lower total blood cholesterol by 6.5 percent and LDL cholesterol (the bad cholesterol) by 8.1 percent.

Every 1 percent drop in total cholesterol can cause a 2 percent drop in the risk of heart disease. So, eating nine meals a day can lower the risk of heart disease by a good 12 percent.

Remember that the volunteers eating nine meals a day did not eat more food (total calories) than the volunteers eating three meals a day. They just had more, smaller meals.

Talk to your doctor about changing the number of meals you eat a day to help lower your cholesterol and reduce your risk of heart disease.

Medical Source ——————————————————————
The American Journal of Clinical Nutrition (57,3:446)

Good news about garlic

It's an old superstition that you can keep vampires away with a clove of garlic around your neck, but it's no superstition that garlic is good for your blood.

Yet another study shows that eating garlic can lower the amount of fat in your blood. This study suggests that you can lower your total cholesterol by 6 percent (average drop in the study volunteers was 262 to 247) and your LDL cholesterol by 11 percent if you take three 300-milligram garlic tablets every day for 12 weeks.

Garlic also works against heart disease by making the blood less sticky and less likely to clot, by dilating the blood vessels and by lowering blood pressure.

The part of garlic that smells so strong, allicin, is what seems to work so well against heart disease. Formed from alliin (which doesn't smell), allicin is produced by a chemical reaction that occurs when you break open a garlic clove.

Natural garlic can vary in how much allicin it contains, but a dried garlic powder tablet always provides the same amount of the anti-heart-disease compound.

The tablets used in this study, which was supported by a grant from a manufacturer of garlic tablets, provide 1.3-percent alliin, which releases 0.6-percent allicin. Look for information about alliin or allicin content on your garlic-tablet label.

Garlic tablets are a good option if you're concerned about bad breath. The tablets don't give off the odor natural garlic does.

However, eating natural garlic with your meals is probably the safest way to go.

Medical Source ——————————————————————
American Journal of Medicine (94,6:623)

Grape beverage gives heart disease protection

By now you may have heard results of studies that say drinking small amounts of alcohol is associated with a reduced risk of coronary heart disease.

In France, where a typical meal has an abundance of fatty sauces and creams, they have a relatively low death rate from heart disease. Researchers believe this may be partly due to the French habit of drinking wine with meals.

But did you know that you can get some of the same protective benefits from drinking a natural, nonalcoholic beverage? Purple, concord grape juice also contains the cholesterol-lowering chemical naturally produced in grapes.

Levels of this chemical, resveratrol, differ from wine to wine but are usually higher in red wines made from grapes fermented in their skins. (Resveratrol is concentrated in the skins of grapes.)

Purple grape juice actually contains more of the protective chemical than many wines.

White wine and white grape juice contain very little resveratrol. Just eating grapes themselves won't work because the actual fruit contains only slight amounts of the cholesterol-lowering chemical.

Medical Source ————————————————————
  Science News (142,3:47)

Building up iron supply could be tearing down heart

The government requires some food manufacturers to fortify the foods they produce with iron. This extra iron is supposed to improve your health. But it could be doing the exact opposite.

High levels of iron stored in the body could more than double your risk of heart attack, claims a study of almost 2,000 men by Finnish researcher Dr. Jukka T. Salonen.

Iron is an essential part of red blood cells, which carry oxygen through the body. When the body has more iron than it needs to produce red blood cells, it puts it into storage. Too much stored iron may promote the formation of dangerous free radicals in the blood, which can lead to a heart attack.

Scientist Jerome L. Sullivan of the Medical University of South Carolina in Charleston also thinks that lowering the amount of stored iron in the blood can help reduce the risk of heart attacks.

In fact, he believes that one reason premenopausal women have such a low rate of heart attacks is that the blood loss of monthly menstruation helps keep the amount of stored iron at low levels.

Aspirin and fish oil may help protect people from heart attacks partly because they lower the amount of stored iron in the body, Sullivan believes.

Scientists have not been able to prove absolutely that high levels of stored iron cause heart attacks, but there does seem to be a strong link.

Because iron is an important nutrient that is essential for the production of red blood cells, don't try to avoid iron or iron-fortified foods.

However, some scientists suggest that adults should avoid iron-supplement pills unless your doctor recommends them or you are suffering from iron deficiency.

Medical Sources ─────────────────────
   Circulation (86,3:803)
   Science News (142,12:180)

Folate and B6 fight silent killer

It's a dangerous condition that damages the arteries and heart of about one out of every 10 people. The worst of it is, you don't know whether or not you are that one person in 10 until it's too late.

You see, the condition is "silent" — it doesn't cause any bad symptoms.

The good news is that getting enough vitamin B6 and folate can head off the problem.

Here's the story: Your body produces an amino acid known as homocysteine when it breaks down proteins from your diet. Normally, your body processes the homocysteine so that it is not hazardous to you.

However, sometimes your body cannot process the homocysteine well enough, and you get a buildup of the amino acid. That's when things get dangerous.

High levels of homocysteine can more than triple your risk of a heart attack. Scientists are not sure how the homocysteine might trigger a heart attack. But, they suspect that the amino acid damages the cells that line the arteries and heart.

Fortunately, getting enough of the vitamins B6 and folate should help keep your homocysteine levels low.

The recommended daily allowance (RDA) of folate is 200 micrograms for men and 180 micrograms for women. The RDA of vitamin B6 is 2 milligrams for men and 1.6 milligrams for women.

Some natural sources of folate are liver, broccoli, leafy green vegetables and citrus fruits. Some natural sources of vitamin B6 are chicken, fish, liver, pork, eggs, whole-wheat products, peanuts and walnuts.

Medical Source ─────────────────────
   The Journal of the American Medical Association (268,7:877)

Slash heart disease risk the 'E'asy way

Ward off heart disease with a pill that you can buy over-the-counter? Give yourself an "E," say researchers at Brigham and Women's Hospital and the Harvard School of Public Health.

Taking a vitamin E supplement each day dramatically reduces the risk of developing the number one killer in the United States — heart disease — in middle-aged men and women, two new studies report.

Researchers found that men and women who took vitamin E supplements for at least two years had about a 40-percent lower risk of developing heart disease.

And, they found that the benefits of vitamin E supplements are stronger the longer you take them.

How does vitamin E work to fight heart disease?

We have highly unstable chemicals in our blood known as free radicals. These free radicals are missing an electron, and so they run around in our bloodstream trying to steal electrons from other cells. They cause other cells to become unstable, a process called oxidation.

The free radicals also change the surface of LDL cholesterol molecules. The cholesterol becomes "stickier" and more likely to clog arteries. This ultimately leads to the development of atherosclerosis, or hardening of the arteries.

Vitamin E helps to lower the risk of heart disease by neutralizing the free radicals before they can attack the LDL molecules. Vitamin E is a strong "antioxidant" that can block the whole process of atherosclerosis before it even begins.

The researchers did find that taking vitamin E supplements was better than getting vitamin E through diet only.

Normally, getting vitamins and minerals from your diet is recommended over taking supplements. But, in this case, many foods high in vitamin E are also high in fat — such as oils, nuts and seeds — and since we've been told to avoid fatty foods, it's difficult to get large quantities of vitamin E from food only. Other natural dietary sources of vitamin E include whole grains, soybeans, corn and wheat germ.

The Recommended Dietary Allowance for vitamin E is 10 milligrams (15 international units) for men and 8 milligrams (12 international units) for women.

The volunteers in the studies took vitamin E supplements containing 100 international units or more.

Most vitamin E pills contain this much, but multivitamins usually contain less — about 30 international units.

While study results suggest a strong association between vitamin E supplements and a reduced risk of heart disease, most doctors aren't ready to recommend the widespread use of vitamin E. The long-term effect of large doses of vitamin E hasn't been tested yet.

Remember that taking vitamin supplements is no substitution for getting plenty of fresh vegetables and fruits in your diet.

Medical Source ————————————————————
The New England Journal of Medicine (328,20:1444, 1450)

Beta-carotene may work against vitamin E

Beta-carotene, that important vitamin found in orange and yellow vegetables, could be defeating you in your battle to reduce your risk of heart disease.

Vitamin E can dramatically reduce your risk of heart disease, but taking beta-carotene supplements on a long-term basis decreases the amount of vitamin E in the blood.

After nine months of taking beta-carotene supplements, the volunteers in one study had lost 40 percent of the vitamin E in their bloodstream. They took supplements ranging from 15 to 60 milligrams of beta-carotene.

The relationship between vitamin E and beta-carotene is just another thing you have to worry about when you take vitamin supplements. Most doctors and nutritionists discourage the regular use of vitamin supplements unless you have a vitamin deficiency or are unable to eat a well-balanced diet.

Beta-carotene is a natural precursor of vitamin A.

Medical Source ————————————————————
Journal of the National Cancer Institute (84,20:1559)

Less hair, more heart disease risk

Going bald? Don't worry about your looks; worry about your heart.

Male pattern baldness might be a significant warning sign of heart disease, including heart attacks.

It's not only how much hair you lose, but where you lose it. A receding hairline is not nearly so risky as losing hair on the top and crown of your head.

To test the relationship between male pattern baldness and heart disease, a team of scientists collected information from 1,437 men under age 55 who were admitted to various hospitals in eastern Massachusetts and Rhode Island.

About half of the men had been admitted to the hospitals for a first heart attack. The rest of the men had been admitted for non-heart-related problems.

Hospital nurses recorded information about the men's extent of baldness using a five-point scale in which a score of one (1) indicated no hair loss and a score of five (5) meant extreme baldness.

The nurses also used the Hamilton Baldness Scale as modified by Norwood (see the accompanying chart) to record the type of baldness each man in the study had. The Hamilton Scale shows different patterns of baldness. All the study data indicated that the degree of risk for cardiovascular disease depended on the different baldness patterns.

Men with frontal baldness had only a slightly greater risk of heart disease than men with no hair loss.

However, men with baldness involving the vertex scalp (see Hamilton scale) experienced a greater risk of heart disease — these men were 1.4 times more likely to develop heart disease than those without hair loss.

The men with severe vertex baldness had 3.4 times the risk of developing heart disease compared with those with no hair loss.

The results suggested that the greater the amount of hair loss on the vertex scalp, the greater the relationship to heart disease.

Men who suffer from male pattern baldness (especially involving the vertex) should talk to their doctors about taking steps to reduce their risks of developing heart disease.

Medical Source ————————————————————
The Journal of the American Medical Association (269,8:998)

The Hamilton Baldness Scale as modified by Norwood

Men with frontal baldness had only a slightly greater risk of heart disease than men with no hair loss.

Men with receding hairlines (even if it is extreme) but no baldness on top had no increased risk.

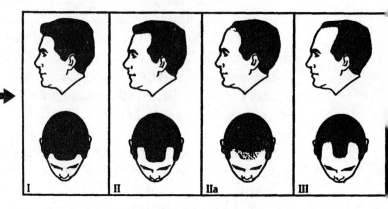

However, men with baldness involving the vertex scalp — on top of the head (III) — experienced a greater risk of heart disease. These men were 1.4 times more likely to develop heart disease than those with frontal baldness or no baldness.

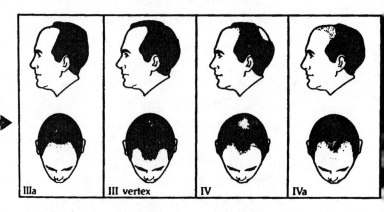

Men with severe vertex baldness (VII) had 3.4 times the risk of developing heart disease compared with those with no hair loss.

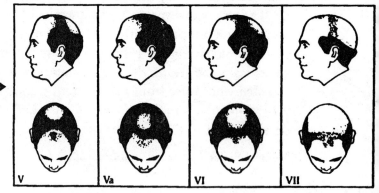

Children can be a heartache

If your heart can barely handle your two or three children, imagine having six. Women who've had six or more pregnancies have one and a half times greater risk of heart disease than women who've had no children, says a not-so-surprising recent report.

Insulin resistance might play a role in the effect of pregnancy on your heart. Your body needs insulin to keep your blood sugar at its proper level.

The more children women have, the more resistant to insulin they become, perhaps because of changes in how their body fat is distributed. Insulin resistance is a major heart-disease risk factor.

The heart disease risk was slightly higher for women with six or more pregnancies who didn't work outside the home than for women with six or more pregnancies who did work outside the home.

Cardiovascular disease is the leading cause of death for women in the United States. If you've had six or more pregnancies, get regular medical checkups for high cholesterol, high blood pressure and diabetes.

Take care of your heart. Don't smoke. Lose weight if you need to (without yo-yo dieting). Eat low-fat foods, exercise regularly and keep your stress level as low as possible.

Medical Source ————————————————
The New England Journal of Medicine (328,21:1528)

Belly fat is a safety hazard

When you think of the spare tire that you always carry with you in your car, you usually think of it as a safety precaution.

But the other spare tire that you carry with you — the one around your belly — is a safety hazard. In fact, it could mean the difference between life and death for some people.

That extra stomach fat increases your risk of heart and blood vessel disease much more than extra fat about the hips or rear end.

People with more stomach fat have greater amounts of triglycerides in the blood after eating the same high-fat meal that other people eat. Somehow the extra stomach fat influences how the body processes the fats from the meal.

People with more stomach fat also have unfavorable levels of cholesterol, insulin and saturated fats in the blood compared with people with less stomach fat.

High levels of blood triglycerides can lead to hardening of the arteries and result in strokes and heart attacks. Unfavorable levels of cholesterol, fats and insulin in the blood can add to heart and blood vessel risks, as well as increase the risk of getting diabetes and other dangerous health conditions.

Apple-shaped people (those with fat stomachs) have significantly greater risks of heart and blood vessel disease than pear-shaped people (those with fat around the hips and thighs).

People with a lot of stomach fat should begin a safe weight loss program to reduce their risk of heart and blood vessel diseases.

Medical Source ————————————————————
American Heart Association news release (Nov. 17, 1992)

Heart disease sufferers: Got the hots for hot tubs?

Relaxing in hot tubs traditionally has been one of the big "no-nos" for people with coronary artery disease. Up until now, anyone with heart disease who even mentioned the word *hot tub* to his doctor received a quick lecture on how dangerous that evil thing could be.

Now, however, doctors are beginning to realize that the hot tub might not be as dangerous for people with coronary artery disease as they once thought.

The old school of thought behind the hot tub taboo was very logical: Sitting in a hot tub causes the blood vessels in the body to relax and expand, which can result in low blood pressure.

In response to this low blood pressure, the heart starts beating faster to try to maintain the correct blood pressure. Doctors thought that this extra work could put too much stress on an already-damaged heart.

However, a new study comparing 15 minutes of pedaling a stationary bike with 15 minutes of sitting in a hot tub found that the exercise placed more strain on the heart than sitting in the hot tub did.

Using the hot tub seems to be safe for people with stable coronary artery disease. But it's only safe if you follow these important guidelines:

☐ Limit the amount of time you spend in the hot tub to 15 minutes. If you want to spend more time in the hot tub, get out and cool off for 30 minutes to an hour before getting back in.

☐ Never allow the temperature of the water in the hot tub to rise above 104° F (40° C).

☐ If you have low blood pressure, avoid using the hot tub. The hot water will cause your blood pressure to drop even more — possibly to dangerous, or even life-threatening, levels.

☐ If you experience light-headedness or dizziness when you stand up to get out of the hot tub, you should avoid using the hot tub in the future. Your blood pressure could be getting too low.

☐ Do not use a hot tub if you are pregnant — even early in the pregnancy.

☐ Do not use a hot tub if you are taking several medications to help lower your blood pressure.

☐ Do not get in a hot tub if you have been drinking alcoholic beverages.

☐ After a vigorous physical workout, be sure to cool down completely before getting in a hot tub. Never go straight from a hard workout into the hot tub.

☐ Avoid using the hot tub if you have severe coronary artery disease or other types of serious heart disorders. (The men in the study had stable heart disease.)

☐ Always follow your doctor's advice. If he recommends that you avoid hot tubs, please do so. He knows your individual health status and can make the best recommendation for your continued good health.

Medical Source ——————————————————
Mayo Clinic Proceedings (68,1:19)

Aspirin therapy not for everyone

Maybe you've been taking an aspirin a day for years to reduce your risk of a heart attack.

But it might not be such a good idea anymore.

Up until now, many doctors have recommended that all adults should consider taking an aspirin a day to prevent the development of heart disease.

Now, the American Heart Association is cautioning doctors about that liberal advice.

The benefits of aspirin in preventing a first heart attack might be limited to men who are middle-aged and older and who have significantly high risk factors for coronary heart disease. And even then, you should begin aspirin therapy only with your doctor's recommendation.

The underlying problem that leads to many heart attacks is hardening of the arteries, also known as atherosclerosis.

The hardening of the blood vessels that supply the heart occurs when cholesterol and other sticky substances build up on the vessel walls. That buildup narrows the vessel openings, and smaller and smaller amounts of blood can flow through.

A heart attack occurs when a blood clot clogs up one of those narrowed vessels. This stops all the blood from flowing to a part of the heart, and that portion of the heart muscle stops working.

Aspirin helps prevent heart attacks by preventing platelets in the blood from clumping together and forming blood clots that can block the vessels. However, aspirin will not prevent or reverse the fatty buildup on the linings of the arteries.

The major risk factors for atherosclerosis that people should avoid are tobacco smoke, high cholesterol, lack of regular exercise, obesity, stress and high blood pressure.

The problem is that aspirin has many side effects that could be very dangerous for some people. For example, people with kidney disease, liver problems, peptic ulcers, gastrointestinal problems and bleeding disorders may not be able to take aspirin without suffering serious — even deadly — side effects.

Since negative side effects can come with taking aspirin on a long-term basis, the American Heart Association cautions that only middle-aged or older men whose arteries are already narrowed with fatty deposits should use aspirin. All others who are taking aspirin daily should reconsider doing so.

If you are taking an aspirin a day to reduce your risk of heart attack, talk with your doctor about the benefits and possible dangers of the aspirin therapy. You might need to change your routine.

Medical Sources ──────────────────────────
> American Heart Association news release (Feb. 9, 1993)
> *The Lancet* (340,8812:143)

Low dose of aspirin is effective

For people on aspirin therapy who have advanced heart disease or who have already suffered from a stroke, studies show that low doses of daily aspirin are as good or even better at preventing another stroke or heart attack as high doses.

The low-dose aspirin helps keep the clotting factors (platelets) from getting sticky and forming "clumps" in the blood vessels.

Low doses of aspirin also prevent the release of enzymes from other cells that can damage vessel walls and lead to clots — an event that sometimes occurs with high doses of aspirin.

Another benefit of low doses of aspirin is that low doses cause fewer stomach problems than higher doses.

Do not start taking aspirin daily without your doctor's advice — she can make sure daily aspirin is safe and effective for you.

Medical Source ──────────────────────────
> *Emergency Medicine* (24,14:26)

A night on the town turns deadly

Ever heard of someone walking out of a smoky bar and dropping dead on the spot? This strange and all-too-common incident may not be just a coincidence.

Smoking and recent heavy alcohol drinking seem to increase your risk of a life-threatening form of stroke.

Both smoking cigarettes and drinking alcohol can temporarily send your blood pressure skyrocketing, causing a sudden increase in the flow of blood to your brain. The blood vessels in the brain burst because they can't handle the extra blood flow.

Finnish researchers studied the smoking and drinking habits of people 15 to 60 years old who suffered an aneurysmal subarachnoid hemorrhage (SAH).

SAH is a type of stroke caused by a damaged blood vessel on the surface of the brain ballooning out and bleeding into the space between the brain and skull. About a third of the people in the study died from the bleeding.

The risk of stroke went up more than fourfold for men who had drunk more than 120 grams of alcohol (that's about six mixed drinks or nine 12-ounce beers) within 24 hours of the stroke.

Women who had drunk more than 40 grams of alcohol (that's about two mixed drinks or four glasses of wine) on the day of the stroke were more than six times as likely to have an SAH than women who had nothing to drink.

Most of these alcohol-related strokes occurred during the hangover period. Your blood pressure can be dangerously high when you're withdrawing from alcohol.

Men who smoked at least 20 cigarettes a day were seven times more likely to have the brain hemorrhage than men who had never smoked. Women who were smokers, no matter how many cigarettes they smoked, doubled their risk of SAH.

Smoking is probably at the root of almost half of all SAHs. Over the long term, smoking weakens the walls of blood vessels in the brain, leaving you at risk for stroke.

Even smoking just one cigarette may have the short-term effect of increasing your blood pressure for two to three hours.

Thousands of Americans die of stroke every year, making it the third largest cause of death in the United States. Reduce the chances of it happening to you — don't drink heavily and don't smoke.

Medical Source ————————————————
Stroke (24,5:639)

KIDNEY PROBLEMS

Calcium helps, not hurts, kidney stones

They affect over 350,000 Americans every year, and they cause some of the most excruciating pain known to man.

"They" are kidney stones, and they are more common than you think.

The odds of getting a kidney stone are about one in seven for men and one in 10 for women. And, to add insult to injury, all the people who've ever experienced kidney stones before have a 50 to 60 percent likelihood of experiencing them again some time in the next 10 years.

Kidney stones usually are made up of calcium and a substance known as oxalate. They start off as tiny, unnoticeable crystals in the kidney.

Over time, however, the crystals grow into large stones that can lodge in the ureter — the tube that connects the kidney with the urinary bladder. Once the stones lodge in the ureter, that's when the pain begins.

How can I avoid these painful stones? you ask. Well, up until now, many doctors have recommended cutting down on the amount of calcium in the diet (since the stones are made up largely of calcium).

However, researchers from the Harvard School of Public Health are now suggesting that a diet low in calcium actually increases your risk of getting kidney stones.

In fact, a recent study indicates that men who eat a diet rich in calcium might reduce their risk of getting kidney stones by 34 percent.

Apparently, kidney stones form when calcium binds with oxalate in the kidneys, forming crystals that grow into stones. (Oxalate is present in many foods.) A diet high in calcium may help bind, or tie up, the oxalate in the intestines.

So, the oxalate-calcium complexes pass right through the intestines without ever reaching the kidneys.

However, a diet low in calcium leaves some "unbound" oxalate that can be absorbed into the bloodstream instead of passing out through the intestines.

That oxalate in the blood travels to the kidneys, where it can form crystals that might lead to kidney stones.

Don't go calcium-crazy, however.

Unless your doctor recommends it, you shouldn't eat more than the recommended daily allowance (RDA) of calcium, which is 800 milligrams per day.

Medical Source ————————————————
Science News (143,13:196)

Coke is out for people with kidney stones

If you've ever suffered from kidney stones, you might want to think twice before guzzling down that soft drink. You may be setting yourself up for your next bout with those painful stones.

Cutting down on soft drinks may help reduce your risk of recurrent kidney stones.

In a recent study, men who normally drank at least 1.1 liters of soft drinks each week were able to reduce their risk of developing recurrent kidney stones by reducing their soft drink consumption.

Medical Source ————————————————
ACP Journal Club (118,1:15)

THYROID PROBLEMS

Hypothyroidism: Are you at risk?

Have you felt tired lately? Are you constipated? Has your weight crept up even though you've lost your appetite?

Symptoms like these might indicate that you have hypothyroidism, a common condition that mostly affects the elderly and women between the ages of 35 and 60.

Of the 6 to 7 million Americans who suffer from hypothyroidism, about half don't seek medical treatment because they don't know they have a problem. Many of those affected think that their symptoms are signs of aging.

Here are some questions and answers to help you identify and prevent hypothyroidism:

Q. What is hypothyroidism?

A. Hypothyroidism is a condition that develops when your thyroid, a butterfly-shaped gland surrounding the Adam's apple at the base of your neck, slows down or stops producing a hormone called thyroxine or T4. T4 is very important because it controls your metabolism: how fast your body uses the food you eat, how fast your heart beats, your body temperature and all the other chemical reactions in your body.

Once it begins to develop, hypothyroidism continues to get worse the longer you have the condition. A lack of T4 can affect every organ in the body.

Q. What are the warning signs of hypothyroidism?

A. The symptoms of hypothyroidism develop slowly over months or years, and you might not notice the changes in your body at first. If several of these characteristics apply to you, ask your doctor to check you for hypothyroidism:

- ❏ Fatigue, a feeling of being worn out
- ❏ General aches and pains, muscle weakness

- ❏ Slow heart rate
- ❏ Constipation
- ❏ Depression
- ❏ Weight gain in spite of smaller appetite
- ❏ Sensitive to cold
- ❏ Thin, dry and lifeless hair
- ❏ Dry, thick and puffy skin
- ❏ Tingling hands
- ❏ Heavy menstrual periods
- ❏ Brittle nails
- ❏ In rare cases, you become cold, drowsy and even comatose.

Q. What causes hypothyroidism?

A. Most often, hypothyroidism develops because the thyroid gland degenerates for some reason and can no longer produce the amount of the hormone T4 your body needs.

It can develop because of a lack of iodine in your diet. The thyroid gland requires a certain amount of iodine to produce and release T4. Iodine deficiency is rare in the United States because most Americans get plenty of iodized salt in their diets.

Occasionally, treatment for hyperthyroidism (an overactive thyroid) might encourage the shutdown of the thyroid gland, causing hypothyroidism.

Another possible cause for hypothyroidism is Hashimoto's disease. This is a disorder in which your body's natural defense system starts to work abnormally, and your own antibodies attack the thyroid and keep it from producing T4.

Hypothyroidism also develops because of a breakdown in normal interactions with other hormone-producing glands, the pituitary and the hypothalamus. When these glands fail to contribute their hormones, the thyroid gland can no longer produce T4.

Q. What should I do if I think I have hypothyroidism?

A. See your doctor. Even doctors often don't recognize the signs of hypothyroidism, dismissing your forgetfulness and depression as normal in a person growing older. However, blood tests will reveal whether or not hypothyroidism is your trouble.

If you recognize the symptoms and react as soon as possible, you can add quality to your life. This potentially dangerous condition is easy to control with proper treatment.

Medical Source ———————————————————
    U.S. Pharmacist (17,3:H3)

Recognizing an overactive thyroid

Graves' disease, the most common form of hyperthyroidism, is a disorder that drew national attention several years ago when President Bush, the first lady and their dog all came down with it.

Hyperthyroidism occurs when the thyroid gland produces too much of the thyroid hormone. This extra hormone causes symptoms such as:

- ❑ Irritability
- ❑ Nervousness
- ❑ Increased sweating
- ❑ Weight loss despite increased food intake
- ❑ Heart fluttering
- ❑ Tremors in the hands and tongue
- ❑ Light menstrual periods
- ❑ Warm, moist skin
- ❑ Muscle weakness
- ❑ Frequent bowel movements
- ❑ Insomnia
- ❑ Fatigue
- ❑ Heat intolerance (feel hot when everyone else is cool or comfortable)

Another noticeable symptom of hyperthyroidism affects your eyes. High levels of the thyroid hormone can cause your upper eyelids to swell — giving you a constant staring appearance and causing your eyelids to droop.

Graves' disease can also inflame the muscles and fat around and behind your eyes, causing your eyes to bulge out of their sockets.

Graves' disease is much more common in women than in men, and frequently appears after hormonal changes, such as pregnancy. Stressful situations also appear to trigger the condition.

Doctors can treat Graves' disease by using medications or surgery to prevent the over-production of the thyroid hormone. If not treated, the disease can become life-threatening.

Medical Source ————————————————
FDA Consumer (26,10:34)

Cigarette smoke triggers Graves' disease

Scientists were not able to discover what triggered the first family's outbreak of Graves' disease, but they did find another possible trigger that's found in countless numbers of houses around the nation — cigarette smoking.

Although doctors are not absolutely sure what causes Graves' disease, they think that some people are genetically predisposed to developing the disorder. In other words, something in their genetic material makes them an easy target for getting the disease.

An environmental factor can trigger the disease in these people, and that's where cigarette smoking comes in.

Cigarette smoking weakens the immune system until it is no longer able to prevent Graves' disease from attacking the body.

Since Graves' disease seems to be passed down in families, relatives of people with Graves' disease need to avoid cigarette smoking and perhaps reduce their risk of triggering the disease.

If someone in your family has thyroid problems (including Graves' disease), talk to your doctor about your risk of getting a similar disorder. And, if you smoke, talk with your doctor about a stop-smoking plan to help protect you from Graves' disease.

Medical Source ————————————————
The Journal of the American Medical Association (269,4:479)

Working with your doctor

Alternative medicine
Surgery survival
Medications

ALTERNATIVE MEDICINE

The new alternative: when 'conventional' medicine lets you down

If the National Institute of Health awards medical research grants to an organization, the organization must be involved in answering important scientific questions like: "Is there a genetic factor involved in Alzheimer's?" "Can we develop a vaccine to stop HIV?"

Right?

Not always.

How about, "Can hypnosis heal broken bones?" "Can yoga help heroin addiction?" "Does prayer affect health?"

The Office of Alternative Medicine was recently established and funded to address just such unconventional medical issues.

Alternative medicine is a term that describes a myriad of unconventional approaches to healing and improving mental and physical health.

Although ridiculed in the past, alternative medical therapies are gaining greater acceptance.

One out of every three people in the United States today uses some form of "alternative" or "unconventional" medical therapies. In fact, Americans made 37 million more visits to unconventional health-care providers than primary care doctors in 1990.

Apparently, traditional health care does not satisfy all of our needs and these therapies provide some assistance.

Some of the most popular "alternatives" are:

- ☐ **Chiropractic:** This form of alternative medicine involves manipulation or adjustment of your spinal column (backbone) to relieve back problems and other complaints.

- ☐ **Acupuncture:** This natural healing approach makes use of needles to stimulate spots in your body that are supposed to have "nerve" connections with other places in your body.

☐ **Hypnosis:** Specialists trained in hypnosis try to produce hypnotic states in people to relieve pain or fight cravings through the subconscious mind.

☐ **Biofeedback:** This "unconventional" form of therapy involves monitoring skin temperature and electrical impulses to help you learn to control muscle tension, heart rate and other bodily functions.

☐ **Guided imagery, visualization and relaxation training:** These techniques involve the use of relaxation and meditation to change normal body responses.

☐ **Herbalism:** A practice which includes combinations of natural plant substances to treat illnesses, based on folk medicine and modern research.

☐ **Homeopathy:** This form of unconventional medicine is based on the practice of giving the body tiny doses of various substances to help your immune system fight off diseases (similar to how vaccines work).

Admittedly, the safety and medical benefits of some of the unconventional medical treatments are still in question. However, many Americans seem willing try the alternative forms.

Most Americans who use alternative treatments don't give up on conventional modern medicine altogether. Most people use a combination of the two.

Most people with serious or life-threatening illnesses (cancer, heart disease, diabetes, etc.) stick with their regular medical doctor for long-term treatment.

For more information on some of the alternative forms of medical treatment, talk with your doctor or contact the following agencies:

American Chiropractic Association
1701 Clarendon Boulevard
Arlington, VA 22209
(703) 276-8800

Committee for Freedom of Choice in Medicine
1180 Walnut Avenue
Chula Vista, CA 92011
(619) 429-8200

National Center for Homeopathy
801 North Fairfax Street, Suite 306
Alexandria, VA 22314
(703) 548-7790

Medical Sources ———————————————————
Consumer Reports (59,1:51)
Medical World News (34,4:48)
The New England Journal of Medicine (328,4:246)

Another alternative: Midwives deliver health and savings

Having a baby?

New research suggests you can save money and have a healthier delivery if you ask for a nurse-midwife instead of a physician. The one-to-one care a trained midwife provides may help you have fewer problems during childbirth and may lower your chances of having a risky Caesarean section.

Researchers studied 3,551 low-risk deliveries handled by a physician and 1,056 deliveries handled by a certified nurse-midwife. Midwives cut in half the diagnosis of fetal distress and the need for epidural anesthesia, painkiller placed into the membrane covering the spinal cord.

The women who were cared for by a nurse-midwife were 25 percent less likely to be diagnosed with a labor abnormality.

Most important to the researchers, though, was that nurse-midwives reduced the need for C-sections by 21 percent. Only slightly less than one in 10 of the women cared for by a nurse-midwife needed C-sections in contrast to around one in eight of the women cared for by a resident physician.

Many health-care professionals are concerned that too many unnecessary C-sections are being performed. In the last 25 years, Caesarean childbirth, which increases the mother's risk of infection and death, has shot up from 4.5 percent of all deliveries to a whopping 23.8 percent.

The babies and mothers under the midwives' care did not have more problems as a result of having fewer C-sections. The babies were, in fact, less likely to be admitted to the intensive care nursery.

When fetal distress or abnormal labor arose, the midwives consulted with the doctor in charge of labor and delivery.

The major difference between care by a nurse-midwife and care by a physician is that the midwives stay with you from the minute you're admitted into the hospital until after the birth of your baby.

Physicians are usually responsible for several labors going on at the same time and for any problems the newborn babies may have.

You are the midwife's only responsibility, and that continuous care can reduce your natural stress, fear and anxiety. Midwives also tend to keep expecting mothers walking around more, which can relieve pain and may shorten labor.

If you've had problems during pregnancy or have any health problem such as diabetes, thyroid, liver or kidney trouble, you should be under a physician's care in case you have complications during delivery.

Medical Source —————————————————
American Journal of Obstetrics and Gynecology (168,5:1407)

SURGERY SURVIVAL

When it comes to hospitals, is bigger better?

Bigger may not always be better, particularly if you're talking about mortgages or credit card balances. However, there seems to be growing support for "big" when you are selecting a hospital for emergency or planned care.

Large urban hospitals involved in teaching activities had better quality care than nonteaching, small and rural hospitals. This conclusion came from a study of 14,000 elderly Medicare patients in hospitals in five states.

Researchers found that death rates in rural or suburban hospitals with fewer than 100 beds were 25 percent higher than in large urban teaching hospitals.

The study also served to dispel one of the phobias people may have about public hospitals — even big city and county hospitals that serve poor patient populations scored high.

The people surveyed had been hospitalized for five diseases: congestive heart failure, heart attack, pneumonia, stroke and hip fracture.

The patients participating in the survey were cared for in about 300 different hospitals in various regions around the country.

To ensure the validity of the survey, the researchers used many criteria, including asking the question, "Would you send your mother to ... this hospital?"

Study results show that care given by nurses was about the same in big and small hospitals. The overall difference in the quality of care was attributed to the difference in the training of doctors at large, urban facilities and those at smaller hospitals.

The challenge is to get this type of information into the hands of the people who need it most — hospitals and the patients they serve.

Hospitals need to use this data to improve their own performance records. Consumers need to know this information so they can make wise choices about where they receive medical treatment.

Whether you decide to go with a small or large facility, you need to know that each has its good and bad points. The small, local hospital may be more friendly and the care more personal, but the larger hospital may be apt to provide you with better care.

Medical Source ————————————————
   The Journal of the American Medical Association (268,13:1709)

Concentrate your pain away during surgery

You close your mind to the pain. You think about sun-bleached beaches, chocolate sundaes and lazy Sunday afternoons. You tell yourself to do anything but concentrate on the pain you're about to experience in the dental chair.

However, suppression or escape tactics may not be the most effective way of coping with pain.

Recent studies recommend concentrating on the location, quality and intensity of painful sensations. To suppress or stop thinking about these sensations might actually prolong your discomfort.

Studies done on 63 college students appear to support this theory. The students immersed their hands in cold water for up to four minutes. Pain disappeared most quickly in students who were told to concentrate on the sensations and most slowly in students who were told to suppress all awareness of the painful feelings.

Researchers speculate that monitoring painful sensations makes it easier to notice lessening of the pain. Suppression seems to weaken feelings of control and even decreases a person's ability to enjoy pleasant sensations immediately after a painful experience. Distraction doesn't seem to work as well as monitoring painful feelings, but it is better than suppressing them altogether.

Try concentrating on the painful sensations the next time you find yourself in an uncomfortable situation. You may be pleasantly surprised.

Medical Source ————————————————
   Science News (143,10:156)

Donating blood for yourself

Donating blood for your own use during surgery was once rare.

But autologous transfusion (use of your own blood rather than blood from a donor) is becoming more and more common, even routine for those of us who must have elective surgery.

If the prospect of giving blood in the weeks before an operation scares you, you're not alone.

Many believe that donating blood can make you weak or anemic, or lower your immunity to infection. These popular myths just aren't true, according to a recent report.

People who are facing major surgery should plan ahead to have a supply of their own blood ready in case a transfusion becomes necessary. By using your own blood you can avoid the risks of using donated blood.

Young, healthy people who must have minor surgery need not donate blood for their own use, because it is unlikely they will require a transfusion.

Ask your doctor about giving your own blood back to yourself if you are anticipating major elective surgery.

If autologous transfusion is right for you, your doctor will carefully schedule your donations before your operation.

And don't worry about anemia; it takes only three days for your body to replace the amount of blood you give each time.

Although donated blood is now generally very safe, using your own blood can help you:

- ☐ Avoid viruses like AIDS, cytomegalovirus, hepatitis and T-Cell leukemia Type I.
- ☐ Stockpile your blood if you have a rare type.
- ☐ Avoid the possibility of an allergic reaction to donated blood.
- ☐ Be sure of an adequate supply if you live in a remote area.
- ☐ Use your own blood if you have religious objections to using donated blood.

You should not donate blood for your own use if any of these characteristics apply to you:

- ☐ You weigh less than 90 pounds.

❑ You are anemic.

❑ You have active epilepsy.

❑ You have an acute infection or a serious chronic disease.

❑ You have cardiovascular (heart and blood vessels) or cerebrovascular (blood vessels of the brain) disease or any of these symptoms: chest pain, irregular heartbeat or dizziness.

Medical Source —————————————————

Emergency Medicine (24,14:73)

Do you really need that surgery?

Suffering from appendicitis? Did your doctor recommend immediate, emergency surgery? You might want to check your wristwatch before agreeing to the surgery.

According to a recent medical report, many "emergency appendectomies" are actually unnecessary, and the time of day seems to have a lot to do with it.

Researchers obtained this information after carefully reviewing the case notes of 578 patients who underwent emergency surgery for suspected appendicitis during a four-year period at a hospital in England.

According to the researchers' review of the hospital records, 144 of the patients actually received unnecessary surgery, and the people that arrived at the hospital between the hours of midnight and 6 a.m. had the highest rate of unnecessary surgery. ("Unnecessary" means that there was no evidence that the situation could only be remedied by surgery.)

The rate of unnecessary operations in patients who arrived during that time period was highest in those who underwent surgery within three hours, without an extended period of medical observation.

Although no one disputes that some cases of appendicitis need immediate surgery to avoid life-threatening consequences, the researchers suggest that the early morning hours in the hospital might call for a second opinion before surgery is performed unnecessarily.

Medical Source —————————————————

British Medical Journal (306,6873:307)

MEDICATIONS

Ace inhibitor side effect: chronic cough

If you are currently taking ACE inhibitors, a commonly prescribed blood pressure medication, the side effects might leave you coughing.

According to a recent study, the use of ACE inhibitors for the treatment of high blood pressure results in fewer side effects than other medications, but might induce a chronic cough.

As many as one of every four people taking ACE inhibitors for several months came down with a persistent cough. That's a lot more coughing than doctors might expect. The researchers looked at side effects from only three of the most-used ACE inhibitors: captopril, enalapril and lisinopril.

Talk to your doctor if you experience a cough from ACE inhibitors and ask if she has heard about the new findings on ACE inhibitors.

In another development, a recent five-year study of 2,231 heart attack victims showed that ACE inhibitors reduced the risk of dying from a heart attack by 19 percent.

The risk of a second heart attack was reduced by 25 percent, and the risk of heart failure was reduced by 22 percent. Each participant had experienced heart damage to the left ventricle that reduced the heart's pumping efficiency.

Heart attack victims have an increased risk of a second heart attack, and they are also at risk for enlargement of the heart and heart failure. ACE inhibitors reduced the risks of heart attacks for the people who began taking this medication several days after heart attacks.

For people with persistently high blood pressure, the benefits of ACE inhibitors outweigh the coughing side effect, and new research shows that this medication reduces the risks of future heart attacks.

Do not discontinue medication to control your blood pressure without talking to your doctor.

Medical Sources ————————————————
Archives of Internal Medicine (152,8:1698)
The New England Journal of Medicine (327,10:669)

Beware of long-term use of this common drug

If you use nonsteroidal anti-inflammatory drugs (NSAIDs) to combat the pain and inflammation of rheumatic diseases (including osteoarthritis; rheumatoid arthritis; or other disorders of muscles, tendons, joints, bones, or nerves), you may be at risk of damaging your digestive tract.

This damage can occur in your mouth, esophagus, stomach or intestines. A whopping 66 percent of people with rheumatic diseases taking these pain relievers have ulcers in their small intestines. Taking aspirin to improve circulation may also put you at risk.

Ulcers may develop within weeks after beginning treatment. In addition, the risk of these problems rises as the dosage increases.

They may also cause serious complications and increase risks in people who already have a peptic ulcer, which can occur in the esophagus, stomach, or duodenum (part of the small intestine).

Furthermore, recent studies indicate that the pain relievers can cause perforation (holes) and hemorrhage (abnormal discharge of blood) in the small intestine.

People who use nonsteroidal anti-inflammatory drugs continually for six months or more have a greater chance of injuring the small intestine in contrast to aspirin users or people who continually use NSAIDs for less than six months or use only occasionally.

Ulcers in the digestive tract in the long-term-user group were single or multiple and ranged from tiny holes to deep masses of ulcers. An estimated two-thirds of the people using NSAIDs for at least six months experience damage to the digestive tract.

This damage is usually accompanied by intestinal inflammation, protein loss and inapparent blood loss.

However, consequences from gastrointestinal damage can be worse. Death can occur from perforated ulcer.

Unexplained weight loss and development of iron-deficiency anemia may signal gastrointestinal problems. If you have abdominal pain while taking these mild pain relievers, consult your doctor immediately.

If you must take NSAIDs, short-term use (less than six months regularly) or occasional use appears to cause the least amount of gastrointestinal damage.

Some NSAIDs may also put you at greater risk than others. Discuss potential risks and alternative solutions with your doctor.

Some common NSAIDs include the following:

> Acetaminophen   > Aspirin
> Naproxen   > Ibuprofen

Medical Source
The New England Journal of Medicine (327,11:749)

Aspirin vs. ibuprofen

Is ibuprofen better than aspirin? With ibuprofen sales up 13.6 percent and aspirin sales down 2 percent in 1992, you might think so. Experts, however, caution that this is not necessarily the case.

People tend to think ibuprofen is more effective because it has only recently become available as an over-the-counter drug and because it is still available as a prescription.

Ibuprofen sales may also be up because it is often advertised as an effective treatment for arthritis pain. However, aspirin may be just as effective as ibuprofen in relieving the painful inflammation associated with arthritis, studies report.

A plus for aspirin: studies have indicated that aspirin use reduces the risk of heart disease. However, the FDA prevents aspirin makers from advertising aspirin as being beneficial for the heart.

If you and your doctor decide that aspirin is a better choice than ibuprofen for your use, watch for these warning signs of excessive aspirin use:

❑ Stomach irritation, bleeding
❑ Problems with excretion of salt and water from the body
❑ Decreased absorption of glucose and amino acids
❑ Depletion of folic acid, vitamin C, vitamin K, thiamin and potassium
❑ Tinnitus (ringing in the ears), dizziness
❑ Hives, rashes
❑ Bronchospasm (constriction of the air passages of the lung by contraction of the bronchial muscles) in people with asthma

❏   Interference with blood clotting (talk to your doctor about discontinuing aspirin seven days before having any kind of surgery)

Medical Sources ─────────────────────

Drug Therapy (23,3:77)

1992 Drug Handbook, Springhouse Corporation, Springhouse, Pennsylvania, 1992

Nutrition And Diet Therapy Dictionary, Van Nostrand Reinhold, New York, 1991

Can't take aspirin? Here's how to use acetaminophen safely

If you're like most of us, you might be a little confused about acetaminophen. How does it differ from aspirin? When should you use acetaminophen instead of aspirin or ibuprofen? And why do we hear so much about it now?

Acetaminophen has been available over the counter since 1955. It appears to be a good remedy for fever and minor pain and has gained popularity since researchers found a link between aspirin and Reye's syndrome in children.

Ordinarily, you can count on acetaminophen to reduce a fever by 2 to 3 degrees within three to four hours.

Acetaminophen has these advantages over aspirin or ibuprofen:

> ➤ Less likely to upset your stomach
> ➤ Usually acceptable for people who are allergic to ibuprofen and aspirin or who have a bleeding disorder, such as hemophilia

Apparently, acetaminophen doesn't relieve inflammation (sore joints and muscles) like aspirin and ibuprofen do, and a few people are allergic to acetaminophen.

While an excess of aspirin will cause an early warning signal of ringing ears, there is no warning sign of overdose if a person has taken too much acetaminophen.

Acetaminophen poisoning has three stages. For the first 24 hours, you will feel bad, have stomach pain and upset, and might feel sleepy and/or sweaty.

For the next 24-48 hours, you will feel better, but liver damage is beginning. In the final stage, the liver and kidneys fail, and you can go into a fatal coma.

If you suspect that someone has taken too much acetaminophen, give the person syrup of ipecac to help void the drug from the stomach and take them to the hospital immediately.

Suggested guidelines for safe use of acetaminophen:

- ❑ Read the label and ask your pharmacist or doctor if you are confused about usage.
- ❑ Tell your pharmacist and doctor about any allergies you have. If you develop a new problem while using acetaminophen, check with your doctor because you could be allergic to acetaminophen.
- ❑ Don't use it for more than three days for fever or 10 days for pain.
- ❑ Avoid acetaminophen if you use alcohol heavily, or if you have liver or kidney disease.
- ❑ Don't use acetaminophen within four days prior to any lab tests. It can affect blood-glucose tests.

Be sure to follow these special safety tips if you give your children acetaminophen:

- ❑ Don't give it to children under age 3 unless advised by your doctor.
- ❑ Check to see if your liquid form of acetaminophen contains aspartame. If it does, be aware that it is dangerous for children with phenylketonuria.
- ❑ Don't substitute children's syrup for infant drops. Read the label carefully and rely on your doctor's or your pharmacist's advice for dosage.
- ❑ Don't use it as a pain reliever for more than five days.
- ❑ Never refer to acetaminophen or any other medicine as candy.
- ❑ Store acetaminophen and other drugs away from children.

By following the advice of your doctor or pharmacist, you can use acetaminophen as an effective and safe alternative to aspirin and ibuprofen for pain and fever relief.

Common over-the-counter forms of acetaminophen are:

➤ Acetaminophen Uniserts	➤ Neopap
➤ Anacin- 3	➤ Panadol, Infants' Drops
➤ Arthritis Pain Formula	➤ Phenaphen
➤ Bromo Seltzer	➤ St. Joseph's Aspirin-Free
➤ Datril Extra Strength	➤ Tempra
➤ Liquiprin	➤ Feverall
➤ Tylenol	➤ Dorcol Children's Fever and
➤ Valadol	Pain Reducer

Medical Source ————————————————
U.S. Pharmacist (18,3:26)

Two drugs never to take at the same time

Terfenadine is one of the most commonly prescribed drugs to help clear up congestion from allergies, colds and infections.

Terfenadine (also known by the trade name Seldane) was approved by the Food and Drug Administration (FDA) in 1985 as a safe and effective antihistimine. Over 16 million prescriptions for Seldane were issued in 1991 alone.

Seldane is popular because it doesn't make you sleepy. Many older antihistamines list drowsiness as a side effect. In fact, some over-the-counter sleeping pills actually are antihistamines.

Since the FDA approved the drug, the "safe and effective" terfenadine has run into some serious problems.

The problem comes when someone who is taking terfenadine for congestion also has some type of fungal infection and receives a prescription for ketoconazole, a commonly prescribed anti-fungal medication.

Taking both medications at the same time spells "danger" with a capital "D."

Taking terfenadine and ketoconazole together can cause a rare type of heartbeat abnormality that could lead to a heart attack, even in young, healthy people.

Apparently, ketoconazole fights against fungal infections by interfering with some metabolic pathway in the fungus. Ketoconazole can also interfere with some similar metabolic pathways in the human body. Normally, this is no problem.

However, when a person is also taking terfenadine, the ketoconazole interferes with the metabolic pathway that breaks down the terfenadine. This leads to a buildup of the terfenadine in the body.

When too much terfenadine gathers in the bloodstream (instead of being broken down and disposed of), it begins to bother the heart's electrical activity. This can lead to irregular heartbeats, which can increase the risk of a deadly heart attack.

Scientists warn that people who are taking terfenadine for congestion problems should avoid taking ketoconazole (also known by the trade name Nizoral) for fungal infections.

Scientists also suggest that people who have liver damage could have an increased risk of side effects from Seldane because the damaged liver is unable to filter and clear the drug out of the body as it should. When that happens, too much of the drug builds up in the bloodstream. The resulting "overdose" can cause the life-threatening heart problems.

Always check with your doctor or pharmacist about the side effects of the medications you are taking.

And be sure to tell your doctor about the medications (both prescription and over-the-counter drugs) you are taking when he prescribes a new medication for you.

The doctor can check to make sure your old medications don't interfere with the new ones he is prescribing for you.

Medical Sources ————————————————————
   Science News (142,3:46 and 143,14:220)
   The Journal of the American Medical Association (269,12:1513)

A tasteless drug reaction

It all began with what seemed like an innocent form of therapy for a common illness, but it ended up in a tasteless mess.

A 48-year-old woman was suffering from a condition known as onycho-mycosis, which is a fungal infection of the fingernails that causes the nails to be abnormally brittle and breakable.

Her doctor tried an anti-fungal cream that was applied directly to the fingernails, but the woman experienced no relief from the aggravating problem. So her doctor switched her to an anti-fungal pill called terbinafine, and that's where the trouble started.

After taking the medication every day for about six weeks, the lady noticed a loss of taste. She could no longer taste salty, sweet, sour or bitter foods, and the other things she ate tasted "mildewy."

Her doctor took her off the terbinafine right away, but even four weeks later, she still had no sense of taste.

If you are taking terbinafine or any other type of medication and notice a change in your sense of taste, talk to your doctor immediately. Catching a problem early might help prevent long-term or irreversible damage.

Medical Source ———————————————————
   The Lancet (340,8821:728)

Birth defect from common decongestant?

Just because a medicine is available over-the-counter doesn't mean you shouldn't check with your physician before taking it, if you are pregnant, that is. You should be especially cautious, if pregnant, because any medicine you take also affects your unborn child.

Studies show that women in their first trimester of pregnancy who take over-the-counter drugs containing pseudoephedrine, a common deconges-tant, for hay fever, colds or the flu, have given birth to babies with gastroschisis.

Gastroschisis is a hole in the baby's abdominal wall that allows the baby's intestine to protrude outside the body. Surgery is required immediately to close the hole. Research has shown that babies who were exposed to pseudoephedrine while in the womb have a three times greater risk of developing gastroschisis.

Further research is being done to prove the link between this over-the-counter drug and the abdominal defect.

In the mean time, if you need to use a nasal decongestant while you're pregnant or if you are trying to become pregnant, try using saline nasal drops, or ask your doctor about a safe alternative. Check with your doctor before taking any medication.

Medical Source ───────────────────────
Science News (141,17:262)

Using 'smart drugs' is stupid

They seem to be one of the latest trends among young professionals trying to sharpen their edge in the business world. Instead of working harder or studying more, they pop a magic pill known as a "smart pill."

Yes, "smart drugs." Taking these pills is supposed to make you smarter. But, "smart drugs" might be one of the most stupid trends to hit the public lately.

The original class of drugs that first received the nickname "smart drugs" were designed and approved to treat severe mental disorders such as dementia and Parkinson's disease among the elderly. People began to think that if those kinds of drugs could help improve mental disorders, then they could do even better things for people without mental disorders.

So, the latest trend involves creating and selling counterfeit "smart drugs" to people as a way to increase energy, improve memory and increase intelligence.

Unfortunately, these new counterfeit "smart drugs" do little to boost intelligence but have a lot of undesirable side effects. There has been no scientific evidence to suggest that smart drugs actually improve intelligence.

The lack of this supporting evidence and the presence of the negative side effects have lead the Food and Drug Administration to withhold approving the "smart drugs" for the purpose of increasing intelligence.

Even though people who take "smart pills" are still waiting for their surges of intelligence, they are not having to wait for side effects — they've already shown up.

The "smart drugs" Pracetam and Hydergine can cause insomnia, nausea and other stomach or intestinal problems.

Diapid is another type of "smart drug" that causes side effects such as runny nose, ulcers in the nose, abdominal cramps and increased bowel movements.

The "smart drug" Vincamine causes stomach and intestinal problems, especially in children and pregnant women.

One of the most alarming aspects of the "smart drugs" is that huge doses are required to achieve the so-called desired effects. Another dangerous aspect is that many "smart drug" users claim that you need to take various combinations of the different kinds of "smart drugs" to get the "best" effect.

And, to add insult to injury, "smart drug" supporters recommend taking the drugs for long periods of time to get the best effects.

All three of those factors spell "danger" to doctors, pharmacists and scientists from the Food and Drug Administration. Taking large doses, mixing different drugs and taking drugs for long periods of time can cause serious health problems and possibly serious long-term side effects.

A special report from the Federation of American Societies for Experimental Biology warns that the ingredients in these "smart drugs" can be dangerous and potentially harmful for healthy men. The report also cautions that if healthy men are at risk, other less healthy groups of people are at even greater risk for bad results.

The ingredients in the "smart drugs" have been blamed for side effects such as insomnia, irritability, gastroenteritis, pancreatitis and even birth defects.

The Food and Drug Administration suggests that since "smart drugs" have not been subject to proper scientific studies to prove their effectiveness and to document their safety, people should avoid using them under any circumstances.

If you are using "smart drugs" and have developed questionable side effects, stop taking the drugs immediately and contact your doctor right away. Getting rid of your "smart drugs" might turn out to be the smartest thing you could do.

Medical Source _____

FDA Consumer (27,3:24)

Taking medicine? Important but often neglected advice

If you are taking prescription or over-the-counter drugs, you might want to think about taking a simple but special precaution. Tell someone close to you exactly which medications you're taking.

Consider this real life experience. An older woman visited the emergency room at a hospital because of stomach pain, upset stomach and dizziness.

As part of the treatment for her dizziness, she was given a scopolamine patch, with the instructions that she should remove it if she had any bad side effects. (The scopolamine patch is the kind that is often given to limit seasickness.) Unfortunately, her husband did not hear these instructions.

Two days later, the woman began to have hallucinations, she began talking to herself, and she lost her short-term memory. Until one doctor reviewed her emergency room records and realized that she had been given a scopolamine patch, her physicians believed that she was suffering a mental breakdown.

By the time she developed symptoms from the scopolamine patch, she was unable to remember about the patch or to tell anyone else about it.

When the doctors removed the patch, the woman's problems soon disappeared, and she was back to normal.

If you use any medicine that might have side effects, someone else around you should know to be on the lookout for potentially serious problems.

Medical Source ───────────────
The Journal of Family Practice (34,6:676)

When iron supplements are unhealthy

Iron supplements interfere with a common drug?

Many people who've had some form of thyroid disease have to take the drug thyroxine, which is a man-made substitute for the hormone the thyroid gland normally produces.

Taking thyroxine helps these people avoid a condition known as hypothyroidism, in which there is not enough thyroid hormone in the body.

However, some people who take the drug thyroxine might still develop hypothyroidism — if they are taking iron supplements with the thyroxine, that is.

Scientists have known for quite some time that iron supplement pills sometimes interfere with the absorption of other substances from the digestive tract, and they suspected that iron supplements could also interfere with the absorption of thyroxine.

So they recruited 14 volunteers to participate in a study to test the effects of iron supplements on thyroxine absorption. Each of the 14 volunteers suffered from a condition known as Hashimoto thyroiditis or from damage from radioiodine treatment of hyperthyroidism.

These disorders damage the thyroid gland and make it necessary for people to take thyroxine to make up for the thyroid hormone the gland can no longer produce.

All of the volunteers were being treated with thyroxine doses ranging from 0.075 to 0.15 milligrams per day.

At the beginning of the study, the volunteers received a seven-week supply of their thyroid medication as well as a seven-week supply of 300-milligram ferrous sulfate tablets (iron supplement pills).

They were all instructed to take their daily thyroid pill and one iron tablet simultaneously each morning 30 to 60 minutes before eating breakfast.

The volunteers checked into the laboratory every few weeks for monitoring. During the check-up visits, the volunteers completed questionnaires about how well they were following instructions, any unusual symptoms or problems, and other questions regarding the thyroid hormone.

The researchers also took blood samples from each volunteer to check thyroid hormone levels.

At the six-week check-in, the volunteers received a five-week supply of thyroxine and iron supplement pills and were instructed to complete the next five weeks just as they had the first seven-week period of the study.

Again, the volunteers came in every few weeks to allow the scientists to monitor their thyroid hormone levels.

At the end of the 12-week study, the scientists analyzed the questionnaire results and the blood test results and discovered some important news.

According to the test results, 11 of the 14 volunteers suffered from lower levels of thyroid hormone in the blood at the end of 12 weeks compared to the beginning of the study before they began taking the iron supplement pills.

The scientists suspect that the iron molecule chemically binds to the thyroxine molecule in the digestive tract and makes it difficult to absorb the thyroxine into the bloodstream.

In other words, the volunteers were taking the thyroxine medicine, but the thyroxine never made it out of the intestines into the bloodstream.

This is an important discovery, because thyroxine and iron supplement pills are both commonly prescribed medications that people often take together.

The researchers suggest that people who must take thyroxine and iron supplement pills should take the two medications several hours apart to avoid problems with absorption.

Iron supplement pills also interfere with the absorption of medications such as methyl-dopa, penicillamine, tetracycline and quinolone drugs. People taking these medications should avoid taking them with iron supplements. Instead, take the iron at a different time — several hours later.

Talk to your pharmacist or doctor about the drugs you are taking if you use iron supplement pills. They will know if iron interferes with the absorption of the drugs you are taking and can advise you about the best way to take your medications.

Medical Source ————————————————————
Annals of Internal Medicine (117,12:1010)

The wrong way to take birth control pills

Women, beware of taking your birth control pills without water.

A few doctors have reported cases of women who developed ulcers on the esophagus after taking their oral contraceptive pills at night right before going to bed — without washing them down with water.

Apparently, the pills didn't make it to the stomach due to the lack of water and due to the lack of gravitational pull (they went to bed too quickly).

The pills got "stuck" in the esophagus and seemed to irritate the sensitive lining of the esophagus. This resulted in painful esophageal ulcers.

If you take your medications at night (birth control or anything else), make sure you take them with plenty of liquid to wash them out of the esophagus into the stomach and avoid the complications of pills getting stuck in the esophagus.

Medical Source ————————————————
British Medical Journal (303,6813:1344)

INDEX